Ward Rounds in
DERMATOLOGY

Ward Rounds in DERMATOLOGY

SECOND EDITION

Bela J Shah MD
Professor
Department of Dermatology,
Sexually Transmitted Infection (STI) and Leprosy
GCS and RC Medical College
Ahmedabad, Gujarat, India

Santosh Rathod MD(Skin and VD) DNB
Professor
Department of Dermatology
NHL Municipal Medical College
and Smt Shardaben Hospital
Ahmedabad, Gujarat, India
Honorary Secretary of Indian Association of Leprologists (IAL)

Foreword

Sudhir Pujara

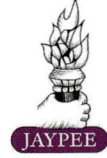

JAYPEE BROTHERS MEDICAL PUBLISHERS
The Health Sciences Publisher
New Delhi | London

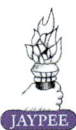 **Jaypee Brothers Medical Publishers (P) Ltd**

Headquarters
EMCA House, 23/23-B
Ansari Road, Daryaganj
New Delhi 110 002, India
Landline: +91-11-23272143, +91-11-23272703
+91-11-23282021, +91-11-23245672
e-mail: jaypee@jaypeebrothers.com

Corporate Office
4838/24, Ansari Road, Daryaganj
New Delhi 110 002, India
Phone: +91-11-43574357
Fax: +91-11-43574314
e-mail: jaypee@jaypeebrothers.com

Overseas Office
JP Medical Ltd.
83, Victoria Street, London
SW1H 0HW (UK)
Phone: +44-20 3170 8910
e-mail: info@jpmedpub.com

EU GPSR Authorised Representative
Logos Europe, 9 rue Nicolas Poussin
17000, La Rochelle, France
Phone: +33 (0) 6 67 93 73 78
e-mail: contact@logoseurope.eu

Website: www.jaypeebrothers.com
Website: www.jaypeedigital.com

© 2026, Jaypee Brothers Medical Publishers

The views and opinions expressed in this book are solely those of the original contributor(s)/author(s) and do not necessarily represent those of editor(s) or publisher of the book.

All rights reserved. No part of this publication may be reproduced, stored or transmitted in any form or by any means, electronic, mechanical, photocopying, recording or otherwise, without the prior permission in writing of the publishers.

All brand names and product names used in this book are trade names, service marks, trademarks or registered trademarks of their respective owners. The publisher is not associated with any product or vendor mentioned in this book.

Medical knowledge and practice change constantly. This book is designed to provide accurate, authoritative information about the subject matter in question. However, readers are advised to check the most current information available on procedures included and check information from the manufacturer of each product to be administered, to verify the recommended dose, formula, method and duration of administration, adverse effects and contraindications. It is the responsibility of the practitioner to take all appropriate safety precautions. Neither the publisher nor the author(s)/editor(s) assume any liability for any injury and/or damage to persons or property arising from or related to use of material in this book.

This book is sold on the understanding that the publisher is not engaged in providing professional medical services. If such advice or services are required, the services of a competent medical professional should be sought.

Every effort has been made where necessary to contact holders of copyright to obtain permission to reproduce copyright material. If any have been inadvertently overlooked, the publisher will be pleased to make the necessary arrangements at the first opportunity.

Inquiries for bulk sales may be solicited at: jaypee@jaypeebrothers.com

Ward Rounds in Dermatology / *Bela J Shah, Santosh Rathod*

First Edition: 2017

Second Edition: **2026**

ISBN: 978-93-6616-772-5

Printed at: Samrat Offset Pvt. Ltd.

DEDICATED TO

My Beloved Parents and Brother Dr Manoj J Shah

—**Bela J Shah**

Three lovely ladies of my life:
My mother, Manjula; my wife, Archana; and
my daughter, Kanvi

—**Santosh Rathod**

Foreword

The Second Edition of *"Ward Rounds in Dermatology"* by Dr Bela J Shah and Dr Santosh Rathod provides an update on the very successful first edition with inclusion of recent advances, newer molecules and updated guidelines about the usage of the drugs in indoor care of the dermatology patients.

The book contains practically everything one would want to know about common, and some not-so-common clinical situations sans the elaborate the theoretical discussions (which one would have anyway read elsewhere to build up the conceptual framework) and provides enough practical details.

This work by two accomplished dermatologists would serve as a quick-reference source to recapitulate what one has already learned earlier; but, it is not just a compilation of facts, it is much more.

Dr Santosh has been known to me as a well-read doctor. I had a pleasure of being Dr Bela's postgraduate examiner for MD degree. She had already demonstrated her potential then. We have also worked together on some projects. I have always appreciated her dedication while we worked together.

I wish them all the success in their future endeavors!

Sudhir Pujara MD DVD DDV
Formerly, Professor and Head
Department of Dermatology
Smt Nathiba Hargovandas Lakhmichand (NHL)
Municipal Medical College
Ahmedabad, Gujarat, India

Preface to the Second Edition

It gives us immense pleasure and joy in the appreciation and response received over the past 8 years for the first edition of *"Ward Rounds in Leprosy"*. In the last 8 years, dermatology has undergone sea-change and our knowledge and armamentarium to treat various diseases, especially with newer drugs like biologics, Janus kinase inhibitors (JAKis) have expanded manifold.

Simultaneously, based on the feedback received to improve certain sections and chapters of this book, we are coming up with this second edition of the book. While maintaining the format we followed in the first edition, we have included new clinical case scenarios, detailed information, and management.

This book is a culmination of knowledge gathered from standard textbooks/journals and authors' own clinical experience of more than 40 years. The information has been produced in a very simplified format to guide the junior residents how to efficiently write detailed history and perform clinical examination as well. This book is a ready-recknor for postgraduates preparing for their MD, the National Board of Examinations (NBE), etc., examinations. The chapter on the drugs is a concise synopsis for a quick revision. At the end, a chapter on frequently asked questions (FAQs) in examinations is included to cover the viva-voce section of practical examination. *"Ward Rounds in Dermatology"* is essentially designed and aimed to help the "Postgraduates in Dermatology". Other specialities such as general practitioners, physicians, and pediatricians can also benefit from this comprehensive textbook.

We hope that you all will appreciate our hard work, and the book makes learning and reading enjoyable.

Happy reading!

Bela J Shah
Santosh Rathod

Preface to the First Edition

Dermatology is a branch of medicine which caters mainly to outdoor patients. Compared to outdoor patients, dermatologists have less workload as far as indoor patients are concerned. The management of indoor patients takes a backseat many a times.

Patients with skin failure need to be monitored round the clock. We have been using dexamethasone cyclophosphamide pulse (DCP) therapy and biologics. This requires admission of the patients in the ward.

Every morning for every admitted patient, we have to have our own checklist which will help us to manage the indoor patients effectively.

We have included all the aspects of history-taking in dermatology in the book.

This book is a culmination of knowledge gathered from standard textbooks/journals and authors' own experience. The information has been produced in the form of questions and answers to guide the residents in their postgraduate examinations. The chapter on the drugs is a concise synopsis for a quick revision. At the end, a chapter on frequently asked questions (FAQs) in examinations is included in the complete question-answer format.

Ward Rounds in Dermatology is essentially designed and aimed to help the beginners and the practitioners alike.

We hope that you all will appreciate our hard work, and the book makes reading enjoyable.

Bela J Shah
Santosh Rathod

Acknowledgments

The book is fruitful amalgamation of the experience gained over the last 40 years in clinical practice (Dr Bela J Shah), with huge number (on an average 800) of op attendees and number of indoor cases as well.

We are grateful to a number of people who have helped us during preparation of the script, without whom this journey would have been impossible.

First and foremost, I (Bela J Shah) thank my revered teacher late Dr Bharat H Shah, who has been a great guide, philosopher, and teacher par excellence. With his blessings only, I am able to pen down this book.

We would like to acknowledge the efforts of our postgraduates who were involved at every stage. We thank our residents, Drs Uzzaif Mansuri, Ankan Gupta, Sonal Patel, Suyog Dhamale, Darshan Karia, and Sonal Tibrewal for their untiring efforts. We would also like to acknowledge the efforts made by the residents of LG Hospital, Ahmedabad, Gujarat, India, especially Dr Shikha Shivhare.

For the second edition of this book, our PGs Dr Deval Mistry, Dr Shikha Shah, Dr Yashika Doshi, Dr Tejasvi, Dr Rutvi, Dr Puja Shah, and many more have put in immense efforts to make the content of the text relatable as well as easily readable.

We are grateful to M/s Jaypee Brothers Medical Publishers (P) Ltd, New Delhi, India, for their continued support in publishing this book.

Lastly, we are thankful to the Almighty who helped us at every step.

Bela J Shah
Santosh Rathod

Contents

SECTION 1: INPATIENT MANAGEMENT OF MAJOR CASES IN DERMATOLOGY

CHAPTER 1:	Autoimmune Vesiculobullous Disorders	3
CHAPTER 2:	Drug Reactions	22
CHAPTER 3:	Systemic Lupus Erythematosus	42
CHAPTER 4:	Systemic Sclerosis, Dermatomyositis, and Other Connective Tissue Diseases	65
CHAPTER 5:	Erythroderma	102
CHAPTER 6:	Lepra Reactions	112
CHAPTER 7:	Cutaneous T-cell Lymphoma	121
CHAPTER 8:	Short Cases: Infantile Hemangioma and Bullous Pyoderma Gangrenosum	135

SECTION 2: THERAPEUTICS

CHAPTER 9:	Immunosuppressants in Dermatology	157
CHAPTER 10:	FAQs on Biologics and JAKis	187
CHAPTER 11:	Antihistamines	205
CHAPTER 12:	Antibiotics in Dermatology	210

SECTION 3: MISCELLANEOUS

CHAPTER 13:	Bedside Tests in Dermatology	221
CHAPTER 14:	Signs in Dermatology	254
CHAPTER 15:	Frequently Asked Questions in Dermatology	257

Index   269

SECTION 1

Inpatient Management of Major Cases in Dermatology

1. Autoimmune Vesiculobullous Disorders
2. Drug Reactions
3. Systemic Lupus Erythematosus
4. Systemic Sclerosis, Dermatomyositis, and Other Connective Tissue Diseases
5. Erythroderma
6. Lepra Reactions
7. Cutaneous T-cell Lymphoma
8. Short Cases: Infantile Hemangioma and Bullous Pyoderma Gangrenosum

CHAPTER 1

Autoimmune Vesiculobullous Disorders

BACKGROUND

Throughout this book, we will follow the format as presented in this chapter, wherein clinical history of a patient admitted to the dermatology ward is followed by frequently asked questions and answers in viva voce during practical examination. We have also tried to update current management guidelines of the given case in the uniform format in all the chapters of the book as well. Autoimmune vesiculobullous disorders especially Pemphigus is one of the most common disease for which admission in dermatology wards is frequently required.

CLINICAL HISTORY OF A PEMPHIGUS VULGARIS[1] CASE

A 32-year-old, female graduate Hindu patient named XYZ, unmarried, from a middle socioeconomic background was admitted in government hospital with chief complaints of: Painful oral erosions limiting oral intake for 9 months and crusted areas over scalp, neck, and back for 3 months.

Origin, Duration, and Progress

Patient was apparently all right before 9 months. Then she developed multiple, painful oral erosions, lip erosions along with throat pain, limiting oral intake—she could only take semisolid food, that even with difficulty. Oral erosions were difficult to heal and persisted even after multiple over-the-counter therapies. After 1 month of the above complaints, she developed multiple fluid-filled lesions over the neck, chest, upper back, and both axillae. The lesions were not tense, appeared on normal-looking skin. The lesions were filled with clear fluid initially. Soon, they ruptured on their own to form raw areas associated with burning sensation, with little tendency to heal, and the raw areas extended at the edges with pressure and soon were covered with crusts as well as oozing serious fluid. Patient also developed fluid-filled lesions around few nails and, within 30 days, involved nails were shading away. There was history of erosions over genitals and perianal region, redness in both eyes, erosions around the lower eyelid, and stickiness of both eyes while waking up in the morning.

No history of tense, large fluid fluid-filled blisters, blistering over palms and soles, photosensitivity and joint pain, drugs, peeling away of skin at the sites of trauma.

Treatment history: Following the above complaints patient was hospitalized in a government hospital for 7 days. She was given daily IV fluids and some tablets in the morning to be taken with milk. Treatment led to improvement in cutaneous lesions, but oral lesions persisted. She discontinued all treatment before 3 months and presented to this hospital with this current flare of the disease.

Past History
No history of diabetes, hypertension, tuberculosis, blood transfusion, or any major medical or surgical illness.

Personal History
- Patient has BA degree and is unemployed.
- *Diet*: Vegetarian
- *Appetite*: Reduced
- *Sleep*: Reduced
- *Habits*: Bowel/bladder—unaltered
- *Addiction*: None

Family History
Patient is unmarried. There was no history of similar complaints in the family.

Menstrual History
The patient has regularly spaced, moderate amounts of bleeding and experiences moderately painful symptoms.

Physical Examination
Examination was done under proper light, adequate exposure and with informed consent in the presence of a female attendant. Patient is moderately nourished and well oriented to time, place, and person.
- *Temperature*: 98.1 F
- *Pulse*: 86 beats/min over right radial artery with adequate volume, amplitude, and rhythm with no radiofemoral delay
- *Blood pressure (BP)*: 126/82 mm Hg in right brachial artery in supine position by auscultatory method
- *Respiratory rate (RR):* 16 breaths/min
- *Tongue*: Moist
- *Thyroid*: Not palpable
- *Nail*: Onychomedesis in few fingernails
- *Conjunctiva*: Clear
- There was no evidence of pallor, icterus, cyanosis, pedal edema, raised jugular venous pressure, or lymphadenopathy.
- *Cardiovascular system*: S1 and S2 heard. No murmurs auscultated.
- *Respiratory system*: Bilateral air entry present. No adventitious sounds were heard.
- *Central nervous system*: Patient is well oriented to time, place, and person.
- *Per abdomen*: Soft, nontender, and no evidence of organomegaly.

Cutaneous Examination

There are multiple, flaccid blisters with multiple erosions and crusting present all over the body.

Clear flaccid bullae, smallest being 1 × 1 cm, largest 3 × 4 cm, present on forehead, axillae, arms, forearms, palms, and thighs. Multiple erosions covered with adherent crusts with foul odor, over scalp, face, trunk, and extremities involving palms and soles were present. 70% of the body surface was involved **(Figs. 1A and B)**.

Patient was emiting "mousy" odor.

Mucosal Examination

Multiple erosions over bilateral buccal mucosa.

Oral cavity examination: Mainly tongue and buccal mucosa were affected. Multiple erosions measuring 0.5 cm covered with whitish slough were present **(Figs. 2A and B)**.

Bedside Tests

Marginal and direct Nikolsky signs: Positive.

Asboe Hansen sign and bulla spread sign: Positive.
Tzanck smear is showing multiple acantholytic cells **(Fig. 3)**.
- *Most probable diagnosis*: Pemphigus vulgaris.

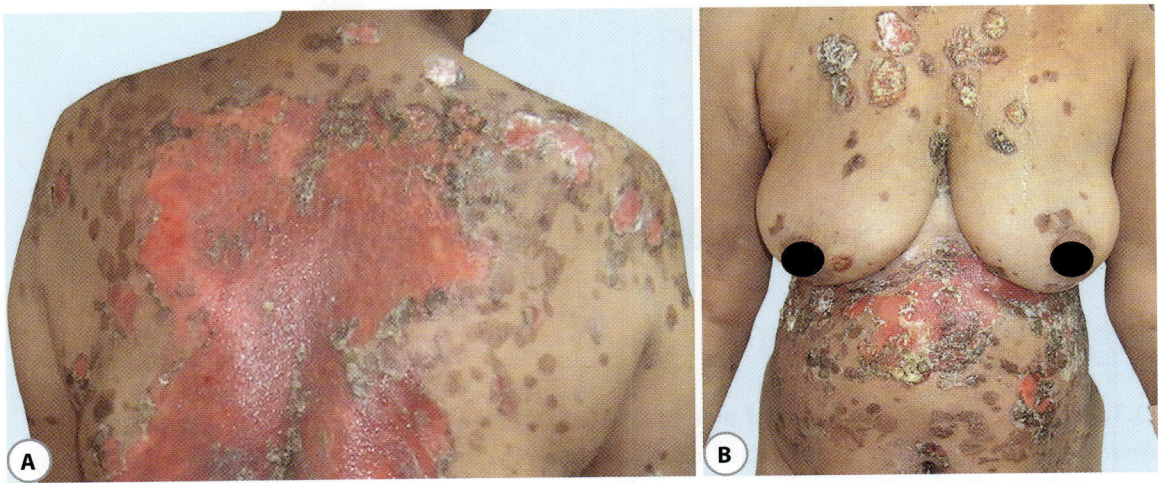

FIGS. 1A AND B: Multiple erosions with erythematous base. Few lesions are discrete, many are coalescing in varying sizes and shapes, with overlying crusts over back and trunk. Postinflammatory hyperpigmentation at few sites over back and trunk.

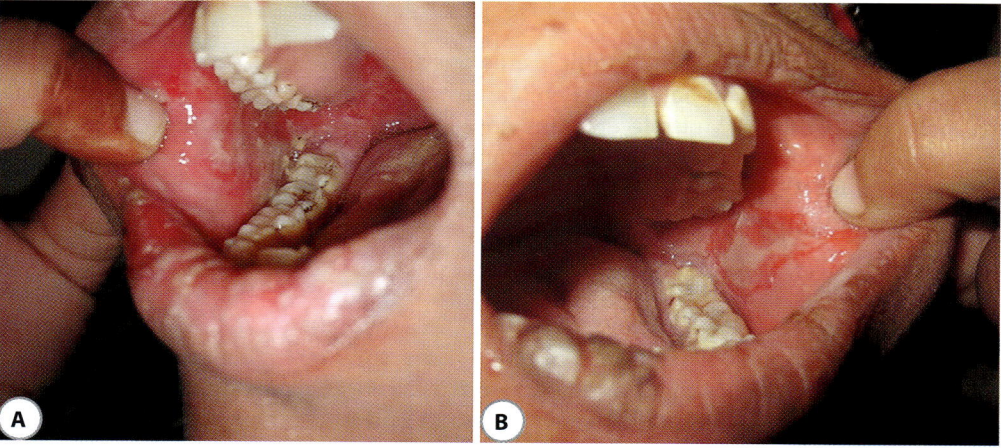

FIGS. 2A AND B: Multiple erosions with erythematous base and overlying white slough present over bilateral buccal mucosa.

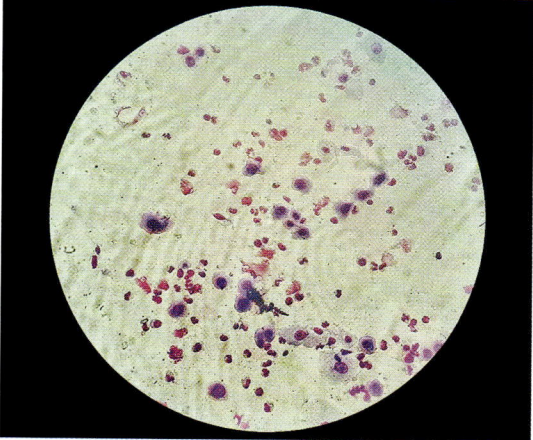

FIG. 3: Acantholytic cells.

Questions and Answers

Q.1. What is the significance of age in context of AI-VBD?
Ans. Pemphigus group of disorders are more common in young patients, while bullous pemphigoid is more common in old age seen after the age of 60 years.

Q.2. What is the importance of residence?
Ans. While PV is more common than pemphigus foliaceus in most parts of the world, there is a localized variant of pemphigus foliaceus which is endemic in certain parts of Brazil, Tunisia, and other

South American countries called Fogo selvagem (meaning "wildfire" in Portuguese), where pemphigus foliaceus is far more common than PV.

Location is also important in deciding the duration of the interval between subsequent follow-ups.

Q.3. What are the sites of predilection in different autoimmune blistering diseases?
Ans. PV commonly starts from the oral mucosa and then spreads to the skin. It commonly affects the scalp and face. Involvement of mucosa to start with carries a poor prognosis in cases of PV. Pemphigus foliaceus usually presents with very superficial blisters which rupture instantly to form crust, especially involving seborrheic sites, such as face, chest, and scalp. Paraneoplastic pemphigus (PNP) involves mucosae severely, including ocular and oral mucosae. Intractable stomatitis is one of the hallmarks of PNP. Bullous pemphigoid usually affects extremities first. Dermatitis herpetiformis localizes to the elbows, knees, and buttocks more often. Patients suffering from epidermolysis bullosa acquisita may have blisters at trauma-prone areas.

Q.4. In cases of PV, what are the differential diagnoses for oral lesions?
Ans. Aphthous ulcers, erythema multiforme, primary herpetic gingivo-stomatitis, and erosive lichen planus.

Q.5. What is the importance of associated symptoms (burning/itching)?
Ans. Intense burning is associated with a particular form of PV known as Fogo selvagem. While, intractable pruritus preceding the development of urticarial wheals and bullae is suggestive of bullous pemphigoid.

Q.6. What is the significance of weight loss?
Ans. Due to underlying malignancy, patients with PNP usually have a history of significant weight loss. Also, weight loss can also be due to severe oral involvement, which restricts oral intake in patients with PV and PNP. In a country like India, if a patient gives giving history of weight loss, we have to suspect tuberculosis. Patients gain weight due to GCS therapy.

Q.7. Why do we ask about burning micturition/difficulty in swallowing/difficulty in vision/pain in the throat?
Ans. Burning micturition can be due to involvement of the urethral mucosa. Similarly, difficulty in swallowing occurs if there is esophageal involvement, stickiness of the eye due to conjunctival mucosa involvement and pain in the throat due to laryngeal or pharyngeal mucosae involvement. Ocular involvement in mucous membrane pemphigoid can lead to loss of vision over a period of time. Hoarseness of voice in MMP cases.

Q.8. In which type of pemphigus can photosensitivity occur?
Ans. One variant of pemphigus foliaceus, "pemphigus erythematosus", in which there are symptoms of both the diseases, pemphigus foliaceus and lupus erythematosus. It is also called "Senear–Usher syndrome." Patients usually present with crusted scaly erythematous plaques over the malar area, which are associated with photosensitivity.

Q.9. Why do we ask about treatment history?

Ans. It is the most important aspect of history, determining how to go about further management of the patient. To understand which treatment has worked for the given patient, whether the patient has been compliant with the previous therapy, and if there are any adverse effects related to prior therapy. Addition of adjuvant immunosuppression can also be decided after the same.

Q.10. What are the drugs causing bullous pemphigoid?

Ans.
- *Topical drugs*: Anthralin, 5-FU, and benzyl benzoate.
- Penicillamine, penicillin, and psoralen + ultraviolet A (PUVA)
- *Nonsteroidal anti-inflammatory drugs (NSAIDs)*: Diclofenac
- *Diuretics*: Furosemide
- Antidiabetics

Q.11. Which are the commonly associated malignancies in PNP?

Ans. Castleman's disease, Waldenstrom macroglobulinemia, non-Hodgkin's lymphoma, chronic lymphocytic leukemia, and thymoma.

Q.12. What dietary advice will you give to patients of pemphigus?

Ans. Apart from the high protein diet, which is necessary to compensate for the loss of proteins via skin, we should also be aware of substances such as thiols, thiocyanates, phenols, and tannins, which can precipitate pemphigus in genetically predisposed individuals. So, we have to have thorough knowledge about food items containing such substances. Some of the food items which should be avoided in pemphigus are garlic, tea, mango, tomatoes, banana, cashew nuts, ice cream, etc.

Q.13. Why should we ask about family history?

Ans. Hailey–Hailey disease is a hereditary condition generally having a positive family history. We can think about adding steroid-sparing agents, such as cyclophosphamide, if the patient's family is complete, as cyclophosphamide has known gonadal toxicity.

Q.14. What is the significance of respiratory system examination in a patient of PNP?

Ans. In patients with PNP, autoantibodies against certain keratinocyte adhesion molecules contribute to acute inflammation of the respiratory epithelium. Therefore, when treating PNP, it is important to consider the potential of developing a life-threatening complication, in the form of bronchiolitis obliterans.

Q.15. What is the significance of central nervous system (CNS) examination in context of AI-VBDs?

Ans. The neurological conditions most commonly linked to BP are amyotrophic lateral sclerosis, Parkinson's disease, multiple sclerosis, epilepsy, dementia, stroke, and Shy–Drager syndrome. The pathophysiological mechanisms behind this association are not yet fully understood; however, it is believed that BPA1 and BPA2 antigens may act as autoreactive antigens in both the skin and brain.

Q.16. How will you differentiate different autoimmune vesiculobullous diseases based on clinical features?
Ans.

TABLE 1: Differentiating features of various autoimmune vesiculobullous diseases.

Site	PV	PF	PNP	IgA pemphigus	BP	Dermatitis herpetiformis
Skin	Flaccid blisters, erosions, crusting	"Cornflake" scaling mainly over seborrheic area. Intact blisters are rare (Fig. 4)	Polymorphous skin lesions with features of both erythema multiforme and pemphigus vulgaris	Flaccid vesicles or pustules on erythematous or normal-looking skin. Pustules tend to form an annular pattern.	Tense blisters over erythematous skin or urticarial plaques. Blisters not seen in very early stage (Fig. 5)	Papulovesicles mainly over elbows, knees, and buttocks
Mucosa	Involved in most cases	Very rare	Severe mucosal involvement	Rare	In around 30% of patients	Very rare

(BP: bullous pemphigoid; IgA: Immunoglobulin A; IgG: immunoglobulin G; PF: pemphigus foliaceus; PNP: paraneoplastic pemphigus; PV: pemphigus vulgaris)

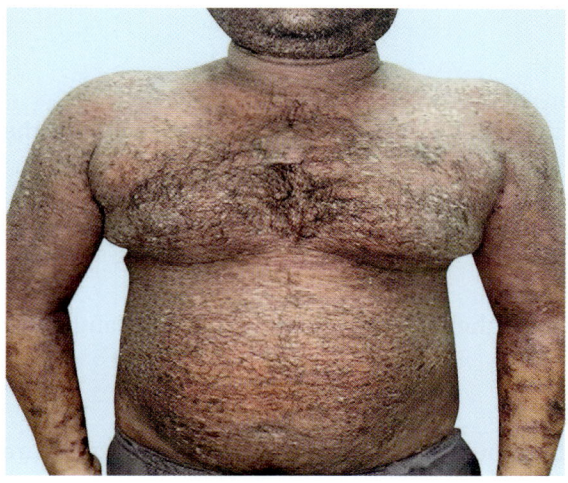

FIG. 4: Diffuse erythema with overlying brown crusting and fine white scaling over trunk in case of pemphigus foliaceus.

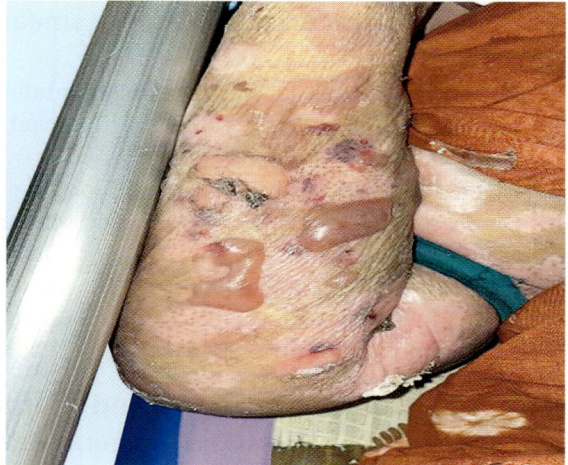

FIG. 5: Bullous pemphigoid—tense blisters on erythematous skin.

Q.17. What are the types of Nikolsky's sign?
Ans.
- *Nikolsky's sign*: The sign is elicited by applying lateral pressure with the thumb on the skin over a bony prominence. (1) Direct—is over normal appearing skin at a distant site. (2) Marginal—is close to an existing lesion. Nikolsky's sign is positive in pemphigus (active disease).
- *Modified Nikolsky's sign*: When pressure is applied to the blister's surface, it extends peripherally. This is helpful for patients who do not have any new blisters to biopsy.

- *Bulla spread sign/Leutz sign*: On applying unidirectional pressure from one side of the lesion using a finger, the bulla extends beyond the marked margin in a rounded manner in the case of bullous pemphigoid and in angulated form in the case of PV.
- *Asboe Hansen sign*: It is a modified version of the bulla spread sign, wherein pressure is applied in the center of the lesion. It is positive in all varieties of pemphigus and subepidermal blisters, such as BP, DH, epidermolysis bullosa acquisita (EBA), mucous membrane pemphigoid (MMP), dystrophic epidermolysis bullosa (DEB), SJS, and toxic epidermal necrolysis (TEN).
- *Pseudo-Nikolsky's sign or epidermal peeling sign*: This is Nikolsky's sign elicited on erythematous skin. It is positive in SJS, TEN, burns, and bullous ichthyosiform erythroderma. It is due to necrosis of epidermal skin and not due to acantholysis.
- *Nikolsky phenomenon,* i.e., instead of immediately forming an erosion as in Nikolsky's sign, the superficial layer of the epidermis is thought to move over the deeper layer.
- Pear sign—is pooling of the fluid at the base of the lesion due to gravity.
- *Sheklakov sign/ false Nikolsky's sign*: It involves pulling of the remnant of the roof of the blister. It is positive in subepidermal blisters such as BP, MMP, Herpes gestationis, linear IgA dermatosis, EBA, junctional and dystrophic EB, porphyrias, and bullous SLE.
- *Microscopic Nikolsky's sign*: It is rubbing the surrounding normal appearing skin with an eraser to cause a microscopic split. This is useful for taking a biopsy.

Q.18. How do you prepare a Tzanck smear?

Ans.
- A fresh vesicle without signs of trauma or infection should be selected.
- The roof of the blister should be removed with a 15-number knife and folded back on the nearby skin.
- Excess fluid may be absorbed by sterile gauze pieces.
- Gently remove the blister contents and scrape the floor and edges of the vesicle with a no. 10 or 15 scalpel blade or curette.
- Make a thin smear with a knife on a glass slide.
- Air dry and stain with Giemsa stain to be visualized in the microscope to check if any acantholytic cells are present or not.

Q.19. What are Sertoli rosettes and streptocytes?

Ans. A "Sertoli rosette" consists of a ring of leucocytes surrounding an epithelial cell. "Streptocytes" are adherent chains of leucocytes formed by filamentous substance.

Q.20. Classify pemphigus.

Ans.
- *Pemphigus vulgaris*:
  - Pemphigus vegetans
- *Pemphigus foliaceus*:
  - *Pemphigus erythematosus*: Localized
  - *Fogo selvagem*: Endemic
- Pemphigus herpetiformis
- Drug-induced pemphigus
- PNP
- *Immunoglobulin A (IgA) pemphigus*:
  - Subcorneal pustular dermatosis type and IgA intraepidermal neutrophilic type.

Q.21. Enlist variants of bullous pemphigoid.
Ans.
- Classical bullous pemphigoid
- *Localized bullous pemphigoid*:
  - Pretibial
  - Vulvar
  - Peristomal
  - Umbilical
  - Distal end of amputated limb (stump pemphigoid)
  - Paralyzed limb
  - Sites of radiotherapy
  - Brunsting–Perry form
- *Dyshidrosiform pemphigoid*: It presents as palmoplantar vesicles and bullae.
- *Pemphigoid vegetans, like BP*: *It presents* with intertriginous vegetating plaques.
- *Pemphigoid nodularis*: Prurigo nodularis-like lesions.
- Large erosive TEN-like lesions.
- Vesicular pemphigoid-dermatitis herpetiformis-like presentation with small-grouped vesicles.
- Eczematous pemphigoid
- Erythrodermic pemphigoid
- Lichen planus pemphigoides

Q.22. What are the recently described variants of pemphigoid?
Ans.
- *Antiepiligrin cicatricial pemphigoid or anti-laminin 5 pemphigoid*: It is considered a separate variant because of its unique immunologic feature-circulating antibodies directed against laminin 5 (epiligrin).
- *B-4 pemphigoid-pemphigoid*: Seen or associated with ocular cicatricial pemphigoid due to mutation of a634 integrin of lamina lucida.
- *Anti-p200 pemphigoid*: With antibodies against a 200 kDa protein of dermoepidermal junction.

Q.23. Which investigations are performed in case of autoimmune blistering disease?
Ans.
- Baseline weight and height of the patient (to assess the dose).
- Abdominal girth (if the patient is being started on steroids).
- Complete blood count to rule out leukocytosis/leucopenia, being a relative contraindication to use immunosuppressants.
- Urine analysis-to look for proteinuria and presence of urine sugar.
- Random blood sugar, fasting, and postprandial blood sugar.
- Liver function tests include serum bilirubin estimation, liver enzymes, namely serum glutamate oxaloacetate transaminase (SGOT), serum glutamate pyruvate transaminase (SGPT), and serum alkaline phosphatase estimation.
- *Renal function tests*: Serum creatinine and blood urea estimation.
- *Serum electrolytes estimation*: Serum Na, serum K, and serum Cl estimation.
- *Chest X-ray*: To screen for tuberculosis.
- Electrocardiogram (ECG)
- Dsg1 and Dsg3
- Histopathology, direct immunofluorescence (DIF), indirect immunofluorescence (IIF), salt-split study, and enzyme-linked immunoassay (ELISA).

Q.24. What are the histopathological, DIF, and IIF findings in autoimmune vesiculobullous diseases?

Ans.

TABLE 2: Histopathology, DIF, and IIF findings in autoimmune vesiculobullous diseases.

Investigation	PV	PF	PNP	BP	IgA pemphigus	Dermatitis herpetiformis
Histopathology	Suprabasal split with "raw of tombstones" appearance. Acantholytic cells can be seen **(Fig. 6)**	Subcorneal split with neutrophils in the cavity. Eosinophilic spongiosis in the early lesions. Acantholytic cells can be seen	Suprabasal acantholysis with individual keratinocyte necrosis. Lymphocytes within the epidermis. Features of interface dermatitis can be seen	Subepidermal blister accompanied by eosinophils and mononuclear cells **(Fig. 7)**	Intraepidermal pustule or vesicle, which predominantly contains neutrophils. Acantholysis is usually not seen.	Small areas of subepidermal detachment with concentrated groups of neutrophils and occasional eosinophils at the papillary tips, leading to the formation of microabscesses
DIF	Intercellular IgG and C3 in entire epidermis "Fish-net pattern" **(Fig. 8)**	Intercellular IgG and C3 at superficial epidermis	Intercellular IgG and C3, linear IgG and C3 at basement membrane zone	Linear IgG and C3 at basement membrane zone	Intercellular IgA and C3	Granular IgA deposits at dermal papilla **(Fig. 9)**
IIF	Intercellular IgG (monkey esophagus)	Intercellular IgG (monkey esophagus or guinea pig esophagus)	Intercellular IgG (rat bladder)	Epidermal IgG (salt split skin)	Intercellular IgA (monkey esophagus)	IgA against endomysium of smooth muscle cells (monkey esophagus)

(BP: bullous pemphigoid; IgA: Immunoglobulin A; IgG: immunoglobulin G; PF: pemphigus foliaceus; PNP: paraneoplastic pemphigus; PV: pemphigus vulgaris)

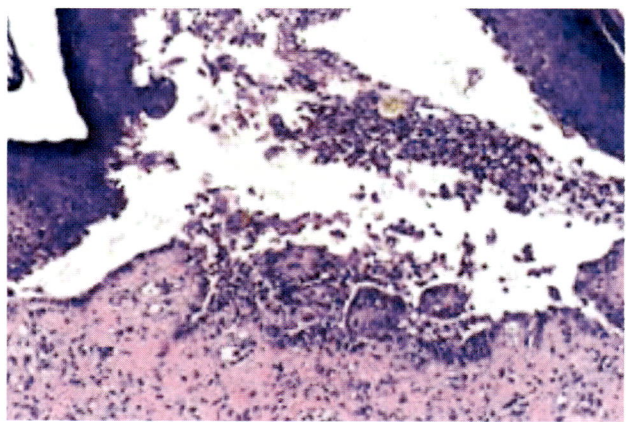

FIG. 6: Pemphigus vulgaris—suprabasal cleft.

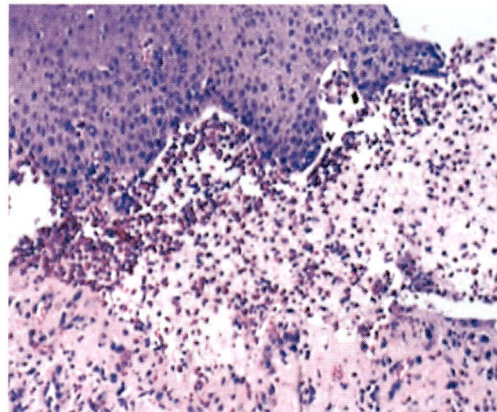

FIG. 7: Bullous pemphigoid—subepidermal cleft.

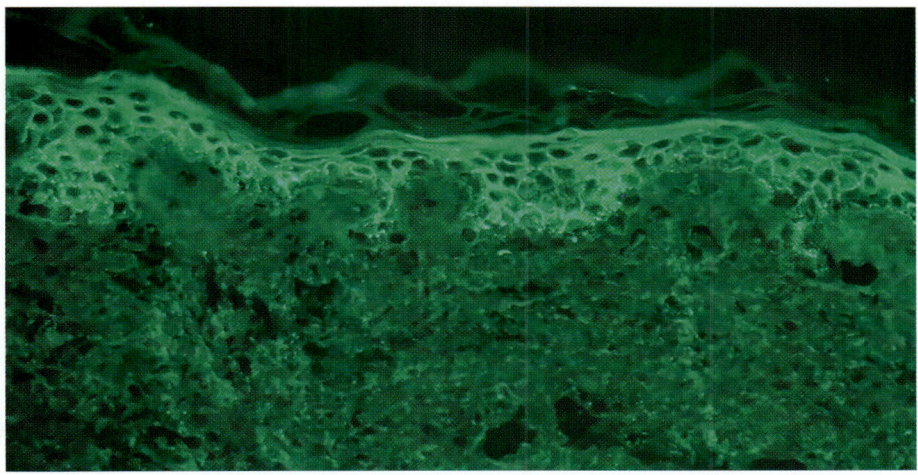

FIG. 8: Immunoglobulin G (IgG) deposition in intercellular area (fish-net pattern)—pemphigus vulgaris.

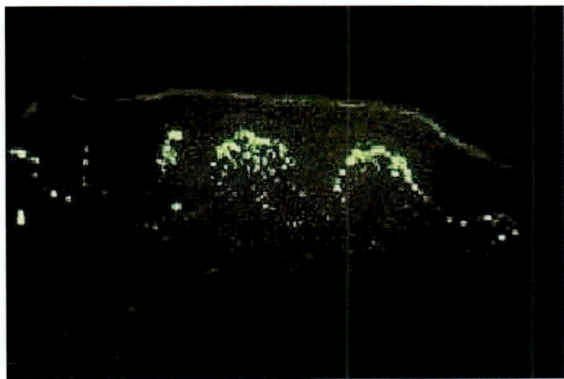

FIG. 9: Granular deposits of immunoglobulin G (IgA) at the tips of dermal papillae—dermatitis herpetiformis.

Q.25. Where do we get false-positive DIF and IIF? Enumerate.

Ans.
- *False-positive DIF*: It is nonspecific staining due to the presence of serum in the intercellular substance in spongiotic dermatitis, psoriasis, bullous impetigo, epidermis adjacent to ulcers secondary to disease varicosities. It is stained with IgA, fibrinogen, and fibrin.
- *False-positive IIF*: After burns, toxic epidermal necrolysis, bullous pemphigoid and cicatricial pemphigoid, systemic lupus erythematosus, lichen planus, neoplasia, and penicillin reactions.

Q.26. What are the target antigens in autoimmune vesiculobullous diseases?
Ans.

TABLE 3: Target antigens in autoimmune vesiculobullous diseases.	
Disease	Target antigens
Pemphigus vulgaris	Desmoglein 1 and 3 (3>1)
Pemphigus foliaceus	Desmoglein 1
Paraneoplastic pemphigus	Desmoglein 1 and 3, periplakin, envoplakin, plactin, desmoplakin, and BPAG-1
IgA pemphigus	Desmocollin-1, desmoglein 1, and 3
Bullous pemphigoid	BPAG-1 and BPAG-2
Dermatitis herpetiformis	Epidermal transglutaminase

Q.27. What are the recent developments in understanding the pathogenesis of PV?
Ans.
- The desmoglein compensation hypothesis suggests that the profiles of anti-Dsg1 and 3 antibodies in pemphigus sera, along with the normal epidermal distribution of Dsg1 and 3, influence the locations of blister formation. It proposes that either Dsg1 or Dsg3 alone is adequate to sustain keratinocyte adhesion.
- Desmoglein sloughing hypothesis. Dsg antibodies "witness" rather than trigger PV, thereby production of these autoantibodies is the result rather than the cause of epidermal blistering in pemphigus.
- *"Multiple hit" hypothesis*: Anti-ACHR antibodies induce acantholysis by disrupting the cohesion of adjacent keratinocytes, which is caused by the inhibition of the normal regulation of their polygonal shape and intercellular adhesion.
- The various alternative hypotheses regarding Dsg3 alterations, proposed by different authors, share a common theme. They all assume that the outside-in signals triggered by the binding of PV IgG to keratinocytes originate solely from Dsg3.
- Apoptolysis

Q.28. What is apoptosis?
Ans. Hypothetical model of keratinocyte apoptosis in PV:
- *Step 1*: Pathogenic antibodies bind to keratinocytes through a receptor-ligand interaction, triggering a range of agonist- and antagonist-like signals.
- *Step 2*: Activation of Src, EGFRK, p38 MAPK, mTOR, and other signaling molecules downstream of ligated PV antigens, along with an increase in intracellular Ca^{2+}, collectively initiate enzymatic cell death cascades.
- *Step 3*: Suprabasal acantholysis begins as basal cells shrink due to reorganization of cortical actin filaments, collapse and retraction of tonofilaments (TFs) cleaved by executioner caspases, and dissociation and internalization of intercellular adhesion complexes, caused by phosphorylation of adhesion molecules and their cleavage by caspases.
- *Step 4*: Acantholysis progresses with the continued breakdown and extensive collapse of structural proteins by the same cell death enzymes, causing the separation of pre-existing desmosomes from the cell membrane through shear forces, thereby separating the collapsing cells and stimulating the production of secondary (scavenging) antibodies.
- *Step 5*: Acantholytic cells in the lower epidermal compartment round up and die as a result of irreversible damage to mitochondrial and nuclear proteins.

Q.29. How do you categorize the disease severity in the case of pemphigus vulgaris?
Ans.

TABLE 4: Severity grading of pemphigus vulgaris based on clinical parameters.[2]

Grade	Oral mucosa (Agarwal and Saraswat)	Skin area involvement (Bellani)	Number of new lesions/day (Agarwal)	Nikolsky sign (Agarwal)	Peripheral extension of blister (Agarwal)
No disease	No	0	0	Negative	Nil
Mild disease	1 site	<10%	1–5	Perilesional	Mild
Moderate disease	2 sites	10–25%	6–10	Distant	Moderate
Severe disease	>2 sites	>25%	>10	Distant	Extensive

Q.30. What are the therapeutic options available to us for the treatment of autoimmune vesiculobullous diseases?
Ans.

TABLE 5: Various available treatment modalities for autoimmune vesiculobullous diseases.

Route	Drugs

Systemic	• *Oral corticosteroids*: Immunosuppressants, i.e., azathioprine, cyclophosphamide, and mycophenolate mofetil
	    ○ Cyclosporine
	    ○ Rituximab
	    ○ Plasmapheresis, intravenous immunoglobulin (IVIg), and extracorporeal photopheresis
	• *Miscellaneous*: Dapsone, tetracyclines, and nicotinamide

Topical	• Corticosteroids • *Immunomodulators*: Tacrolimus
Intralesional	Corticosteroids and rituximab

Q.31. What are the end points of therapy regarding the treatment of pemphigus?
Ans.

TABLE 6: Summary of end points of therapy in case of pemphigus.[3]

End points	Definition
Baseline	The day when treatment starts by the physician
Control of disease activity	It is the period from baseline until new lesions stop forming, and existing lesions start to heal, signaling the onset of the consolidation phase
End of consolidation phase	This is characterized by a period where no new lesions appear for at least 2 weeks, and about 80% of the existing lesions have healed. At this stage, clinicians begin to reduce corticosteroid dosage
Complete remission on therapy	It is defined as the absence of both new and existing lesions for a minimum of 2 months while the patient is on minimal treatment
Minimal therapy	It is defined as the use of ≤10 mg/day of prednisolone (or its equivalent) and/or minimal adjunctive therapy for a duration of at least 2 months
Minimal adjuvant therapy	It is defined as half the dose needed to classify the condition as treatment failure

Continued

Continued

End points	Definition
Complete remission off therapy	It is defined as the absence of both new and existing lesions for at least 2 months, with the patient having discontinued all systemic therapy for the same duration
Relapse/Flare	It refers to the development of three or more new lesions per month that do not heal on their own within one week, or the extension of existing lesions, in a patient who has previously achieved disease control

Q.32. What is the management of a blister?
Ans.
- Cleanse the blister gently with an antimicrobial solution, taking care to avoid rupturing it.
- Use a sterile needle to pierce the base of the blister, with the bevel facing upwards. Choose a site where the fluid can drain by gravity, preventing refilling.
- Apply gentle pressure with sterile gauze swabs to promote drainage and absorption of the fluid.
- Avoid deroofing the blister.
- Once the fluid has drained, clean the area again with an antimicrobial solution.
- A nonadherent dressing may be necessary.
- For larger blisters, a bigger hole may be required for adequate drainage—use a larger needle, and multiple piercings may be needed.
- Many patients experience pain or a burning sensation during blister treatment; consider offering analgesia before beginning the procedure.
- Record the number and location of new blisters on the blister chart.

Q.33. How do you administer corticosteroids in a patient of PV?
Ans. Initiate treatment with prednisolone 1–2 mg/kg/day or equivalent. Milder cases may be treated with 0.5–1 mg/kg. If there is no response within 5–7 days, the dose should be increased in 50–100% increments until the disease control is achieved.

When to taper the steroids: After almost 2 weeks (when there are no new lesions and healing of most of preexisting lesions).

Tapering schedule: Decrease the initial dose to 80 mg, then by 20 mg (up to 40 mg), by 10 mg (up to 20 mg), by 5 mg (up to 10 mg), and then by 2.5 mg. Tapering is to be done weekly.

Alternate day therapy: Consider once the dose of prednisolone reaches 30 mg. Increase the dose on day by 5 mg, while decreasing it on the off day by 5 mg. Continue each dosing level for at least two cycles.

Maintenance dose: 5–7.5 mg of prednisolone may be required in patients who relapse when a dose below 10 mg is reached.

Breakthrough lesions: Double the dose at which breakthrough lesions occur; taper slowly once the critical dose is reached.

Q.34. What is pulse therapy?
Ans. Pulse therapy involves the administration of high (suprapharmacologic) doses of medications at intervals, aiming to maximize therapeutic benefits while minimizing side effects.

Methylprednisolone pulse therapy: Methylprednisolone is a potent, intermediate-acting anti-inflammatory corticosteroid with a lower propensity for sodium and water retention compared to hydrocortisone. Its biological half-life ranges from 12 to 36 hours, and its potency is 1.25 times greater than that of prednisolone.
- *Dosage*: The typical dose for methylprednisolone pulse therapy is 20–30 mg/kg (500–1,000 mg/m²) per pulse, with a maximum dose of 1 g.

Dexamethasone pulse therapy: Dexamethasone is a fluorinated long-acting glucocorticoid, with a half-life of 36–72 hours. It is 6.7 times more potent than prednisolone and has minimal mineralocorticoid effects, with negligible sodium retention and a small equivalent volume.
- *Dosage*: Dexamethasone is typically administered at a dose of 4–5 mg/kg (100–200 mg)/pulse.

Administration of pulse therapy: In the past, pulse therapy[4] infusions were administered over 10–20 minutes. However, rapid infusions are known to increase the risk of hemodynamic abnormalities. So currently, corticosteroids are dissolved in 150–200 mL of 5% dextrose and infused intravenously slowly over a period of 2–3 hours.

Advantages of corticosteroids as pulse therapy:
- It produces an immediate and significant anti-inflammatory effect with fewer toxicities compared to traditional high-dose oral therapy. Faster resolution of symptoms than oral therapy, and clinical improvement lasts about 3 weeks after a single pulse.
- It does not result in prolonged suppression of the hypothalamic–pituitary axis.

Laboratory monitoring: Before starting the therapy, it is essential to admit all patients who are scheduled to undergo pulse therapy. Initial laboratory tests to be performed during the first visit include a hemogram, serum electrolytes, renal and liver function tests, blood glucose (including hemoglobin A1c), urine microscopic examination, chest X-ray, electrocardiogram, and pregnancy test. Additionally, blood glucose levels, serum electrolytes, urine examination, body weight, and BP should be monitored both at baseline and during each follow-up visit.

During and following therapy, heart rate, RR, and BP should be monitored and recorded every 15–30 minutes. Immediately stop the infusion if an arrhythmia is suspected. An electrocardiogram should be performed, and blood levels of sodium, potassium, calcium, and magnesium should be measured and corrected as necessary. Continuous screening for the onset or worsening of infections is crucial. Blood glucose and electrolyte levels should be assessed every alternate day.

Contraindications:
- Invasive fungal infections, systemic fungal or other infections, uncontrolled hypertension, and steroid preparation hypersensitivity.
- Absolutely contraindicated in pregnant, lactating, and unmarried patients.

Adverse effects: Serious adverse effects in children include:
- Elevated BP during or after the infusion.
- Seizures, especially in children with systemic lupus erythematosus, are potentially linked to rapid flux of electrolytes.
- Anaphylactic shock, which may occur even after a previous infusion, is often related to the succinate ester form of methylprednisolone.

Common side effects include:
- Behavioral changes such as mood swings, hyperactivity, psychosis, disorientation, and sleep disturbances are some acute adverse events observed in approximately 10% of patients.

- Hyperglycemia, hypokalemia, and an increased risk of infection. The likelihood of infections is higher with cumulative doses of methylprednisolone exceeding 5 g.

Side effects peculiar to pulse therapy:
- Hiccups
- Facial flushing
- Weakness
- Generalized swelling and weight gain
- Joint and muscle pains
- Arrhythmias and shock

Types of steroid pulse therapy:
- *Minipulse corticosteroid therapy*: Administering oral betamethasone at a dose of 10 mg once a week, divided into two equal doses, taken on two consecutive days each week. This treatment has been used with varying success for skin conditions, such as Alopecia areata, vitiligo, and lichen planus.
- *Topical corticosteroid pulse therapy*: It involves intermittent application of superpotent corticosteroids, which is beneficial to maintain remissions, reduce total cost of therapy and side effects associated with prolonged continuous treatment, like telangiectasias, cutaneous atrophy, hypothalamic–pituitary–adrenal (HPA) axis suppression, and tachyphylaxis.
- Clobetasol propionate (0.05%), weekly topical treatment with three consecutive applications at 12-hour intervals, is used mainly in psoriasis.

Dexamethasone-cyclophosphamide pulse (DCP) therapy is divided into four phases (Pasricha regimen).
- *First phase*: Slow IV infusion of dexamethasone 100 mg in 5% dextrose is administered over 2 hours for 3 consecutive days. Cyclophosphamide 500 mg is also infused on one of those days. DCPs are repeated every 28 days until no new lesions appear between pulses. On the remaining days, oral cyclophosphamide 50 mg/day is given. During this phase, the patient may experience recurrences in between DCPs, and in such cases, conventional oral corticosteroid doses can be used to achieve a faster response.
- *Second phase*: Remission phase while on treatment. DCPs are given for a period of 9 months.
- *Third phase*: Monthly pulses are discontinued, and oral cyclophosphamide is continued for another 9 months.
- *Fourth phase*: Treatment is halted, and patients are monitored through follow-up for the next 10 years.

Dexamethasone azathioprine pulse therapy: For unmarried patients or those who have not yet completed their family, cyclophosphamide is substituted with 50 mg of azathioprine daily during the first three phases of treatment.

Dexamethasone methotrexate pulse therapy: During the first three phases of pulse therapy, cyclophosphamide is replaced with 7.5 mg of methotrexate, administered once a week, orally.

Q.35. How is DCP therapy given in diabetics?

Ans. Diabetic patients need to be given 10 units of soluble insulin for every 500 mL bottle of 5% dextrose dissolved in the same drip. In addition, the patient's regular treatment for diabetes mellitus is continued.

Adjuvant therapy: Patient should be started on prophylactic therapy for osteoporosis from day 1 with adequate calcium and vitamin D supplementation.

Chapter 1: Autoimmune Vesiculobullous Disorders

Additional key points in management: If complete blood count (CBC) is showing leukocytosis, erosions are secondarily infected, local pus swabs and blood culture and sensitivity should be performed, and the patient put on appropriate antibiotic therapy.

Q.36. What is the dosage of weekly cyclophosphamide pulse in pemphigus?

Ans. Intravenous cyclophosphamide is given weekly in a dosage of 500 mg to those pemphigus patients who fail to respond to corticosteroids (oral prednisone 1–2 mg/kg/day) alone.

Patients with pemphigus receiving weekly cyclophosphamide therapy in addition to corticosteroids improve quickly, without many side effects. Usually, 4–6 cycles are adequate.

Q.37. Describe about the steroid-sparing drugs used in autoimmune vesiculobullous diseases.

Ans.

TABLE 7: Summary of various steroid-sparing agents along with their mechanism of action, dose, monitoring guidelines, and side effects used in the treatment of autoimmune vesiculobullous disease.

Drug	Mechanism of action	Dose	Monitoring	Side effects
Azathioprine	Purine analogue that inhibits DNA replication	2–4 mg/kg/day (usually 100–300 mg/day)	CBC, LFT biweekly for the first 2 months, every 2–3 months thereafter	Gastrointestinal toxicity, hepatotoxicity, alopecia, pancreatitis, lymphoproliferative diseases, and increased infection rate
Cyclophosphamide	An alkylating agent that binds DNA during the cell cycle	1–3 mg/kg/day (usually 50–200 mg/day)	CBC, urine analysis weekly for 2–3 months, then biweekly after 2–3 months. LFT monthly and then after 3–6 months	Acute myelosuppression, mucosal ulcers, alopecia, nephrotoxicity, cardiotoxicity, hepatotoxicity, interstitial lung fibrosis, and azoospermia
Mycophenolate mofetil	Inhibits purine synthesis during DNA replication	2–3 g/day	CBC, RFT, LFT every 2-4 weeks following dose escalation, every 2–3 months once dose is stable	Gastrointestinal distress, anemia, leukopenia, thrombocytopenia, an increased rate of infection
Cyclosporine	Suppresses T-cell proliferation by forming a complex with cyclophilin, which blocks calcineurin activation	3–5 mg/kg/day	CBC, RFT, LFT, lipid profile every 2 weeks for the first 1–2 months, then monthly	Electrolyte abnormalities, renal toxicity, tremors, hirsutism, hyperlipidemia, hypertension, and gingival hyperplasia
Methotrexate	Inhibits dihydrofolate reductase required for DNA synthesis	7.5–20 mg/week	• CBC, LFT every 1–2 weeks for 3–4 weeks • RFT once or twice yearly	Hepatotoxicity, bone marrow suppression, ulcers, alopecia, interstitial pneumonitis and fibrosis, nephrotoxicity
Dapsone	Sulphone antibiotic that inhibits neutrophil toxicity and chemotaxis	25–100 mg/day	CBC every week for 4 weeks, then every 2 weeks until week 12, then every 3–4 months. Reticulocyte count as needed. LFT, RFT every 3–4 months	Hemolytic anemia, methemoglobinemia, idiosyncratic, peripheral motor neuropathy, psychosis, agranulocytosis, and dapsone hypersensitivity syndrome

(DNA: deoxyribonucleic acid; CBC: complete blood count; LFT: liver function test; RFT: renal function test)

Q.38. What is the role of IVIg in pemphigus?

Ans. A randomized, placebo-controlled, double-blind study showed that pemphigus patients who received a single cycle of high-dose IVIg (400 mg/kg/day over 5 consecutive days) experienced prolonged remission.

The side effects are generally mild and self-limiting, including headaches, back pain, chills, flushing, fever, hypertension, myalgia, nausea, and vomiting. These symptoms may improve by reducing the infusion rate or using NSAIDs, antihistamines, or low-dose corticosteroids.

Mild skin reactions such as erythema, pain, and phlebitis can occur at the infusion site. More severe side effects may include anaphylaxis (especially in IgA-deficient individuals), renal failure, aseptic meningitis, and infections.

The typical dosing regimen consists of 2 g/kg, divided into two or three equal doses, administered over 3 consecutive days and repeated every 4 weeks.

Q.39. What is the role of rituximab in PV?

Ans. Rituximab is now a first-line drug approved by the United States Food and Drug Administration (US FDA) in the treatment of moderate to severe forms of PV.

- The anti-CD20 mAb rituximab, first approved for use in B-cell malignancies, is increasingly used to treat a variety of autoimmune disorders.
- Rituximab induces not only depletion of all B cells and a decline of antidesmoglein autoantibodies but also decreases desmoglein-specific T cells. Furthermore, B-cell populations recovered after treatment are modified.
- Rituximab is recommended for pemphigus patients who do not respond or experience relapse after treatment with conventional medications, in those for whom systemic corticosteroids and/or other immunosuppressive drugs are contraindicated or cause severe side effects that necessitate discontinuation.
- Baseline investigations prior to rituximab:
  - Complete hemogram
  - Liver function tests
  - Renal function tests
  - Chest X-ray and Mantoux test
  - Screening for viral infection, including Hepatitis B surface antigen (HBsAg), antibody against the Hepatitis B core antigen (anti-HBc), antibody against the Hepatitis C virus (anti-HCV), and human immunodeficiency virus types 1 and 2 (HIV-1 and HIV-2).
  - ECG and echocardiography.

Q.40. Which are the newer anti-CD20 antibodies?

Ans. Ocrelizumab, obinutuzumab, and veltuzumab.

Q.41. What is efgartigimod?

Ans. Efgartigimod is a first-in-class antibody fragment to target the neonatal Fc receptor (FcRn). It is currently being evaluated for the treatment of patients with severe autoimmune diseases,[2] including PV.[4]

Q.42. What is the management of pemphigus during pregnancy?

Ans.
- Commonly used treatments are *oral corticosteroids*. The treatment depends on which trimester the patient is in. In the first trimester, usage of corticosteroids in dosages higher than 20 mg can lead to

teratogenic effects; hence, they should be used carefully and according to risk—benefit ratio. After the first trimester, the use of prednisolone has not been associated with a significant increase in the risk of stillbirth, preterm delivery, or congenital malformations.
- Systemic immunosuppressive medications like cyclophosphamide, mycophenolate mofetil, and methotrexate should be avoided due to their established risks to fetal development.
- Azathioprine, in conjunction with corticosteroids, has been effectively employed in the treatment of pemphigus during pregnancy.
- Rituximab, when used in later months of pregnancy, can be associated with immunosuppression in the child.
- IVIg is safe in pregnancy.

Q.43. How do you daily assess the patient with pemphigus in the ward?
Ans.
- Look for appearance of new lesions and daily lesion count
- Perform direct and marginal Nikolsky's sign.
- Monitoring of fluid intake and urine output
- Check vitals, such as pulse, BP, and RR.

Q.44. What are the prognostic factors in pemphigus?
Ans.
- Age at the time of disease onset.
- Extent of disease.
- Disease progression before initiating therapy.
- A dose of steroid is required to control the disease.

Q.45. What are the causes of death in PV?
Ans. The leading cause of death is septicemia. The extent of cutaneous involvement is the single most important factor leading to death in pemphigus patients secondary to sepsis due to entry of bacteria, especially *Staphylococcus aureus*. Other causes include bronchopneumonia, electrolyte imbalance, and pulmonary thromboembolism. Hypoalbuminemia, along with electrolyte and fluid losses, leads to decreased intravascular volumes. If hypovolemia is left uncorrected, it may lead to hemodynamic alterations, renal failure, and increase the risk of aseptic shock.

Corticosteroid use is associated with several morbidities, including osteoporosis, avascular necrosis of the bone, peptic ulcer disease, cataract formation, and the potential onset or uncovering of diabetes mellitus.

REFERENCES

1. De D, Mehta H, Shah S, Ajithkumar K, Barua S, Chandrashekar L, et al. Consensus Based Indian Guidelines for the Management of Pemphigus Vulgaris and Pemphigus Foliaceous. Indian Dermatol Online J. 2025;16(1):3-24.
2. Grover S. Scoring systems in pemphigus. Indian J Dermatol. 2011;56(2):145-9.
3. Rao PN, Lakshmi TS. Pulse therapy and its modifications in pemphigus: A six year study. Indian J Dermatol Venereol Leprol 2003;69:329-33.
4. Pasricha JS. Pulse therapy as a cure for autoimmune diseases. Indian J Dermatol Venereol Leprol. 2003;69:323-8.

CHAPTER 2

Drug Reactions

INTRODUCTION

Severe cutaneous drug reactions are one of the most common conditions for hospital admission in dermatology. Severe cutaneous adverse reactions (SCARs) refer to those drug reactions that usually require hospitalization, often in intensive care for close monitoring of the vital signs and bodily function.

According to the World Health Organization (WHO) definition, a drug reaction is termed as serious, "if it results in death, requires hospitalization or prolongation of existing hospital stay, results in persistent or significant disability/incapacity, or is life-threatening".

Severe cutaneous adverse reactions include the following **(Box 1)**:
- Anaphylaxis
- Acute generalized exanthematous pustulosis (AGEP)
- Drug rash with eosinophilia and systemic symptoms (DRESS)/drug-induced hypersensitivity syndrome (DIHS), drug hypersensitivity syndrome (DHS), and drug-induced delayed multiorgan hypersensitivity syndrome (DIDMOHS)
- Generalized bullous fixed drug eruption
- Stevens–Johnson syndrome and toxic epidermal necrolysis
- Anticoagulant-induced skin necrosis

CASE HISTORY

A 36-year-old male came to skin department with chief complaints of eye, oral, and genital lesions for past 6 days associated with peeling of skin over face, upper limbs, and trunk since 3 days. According to patient's wife, he developed redness and watering from eyes and burning sensation in mouth as well as body. There was history of painful urination 6 days back, after which he developed reddish slightly raised lesions first over the chest then on face, whole trunk, and upper limbs. The lesions spontaneously led to peeling of skin **(Figs. 1A and B)**.

BOX 1	Risk factors for development of severe cutaneous adverse reactions (SCARs).

- Female gender
- Immunosuppression (individuals with HIV are at a 10–50 times higher risk of experiencing an exanthematous eruption from sulfamethoxazole)
- Dermatomyositis (particularly for hydroxychloroquine use)
- Specific HLA alleles

(HIV: human immunodeficiency virus; HLA: human leukocyte antigen)

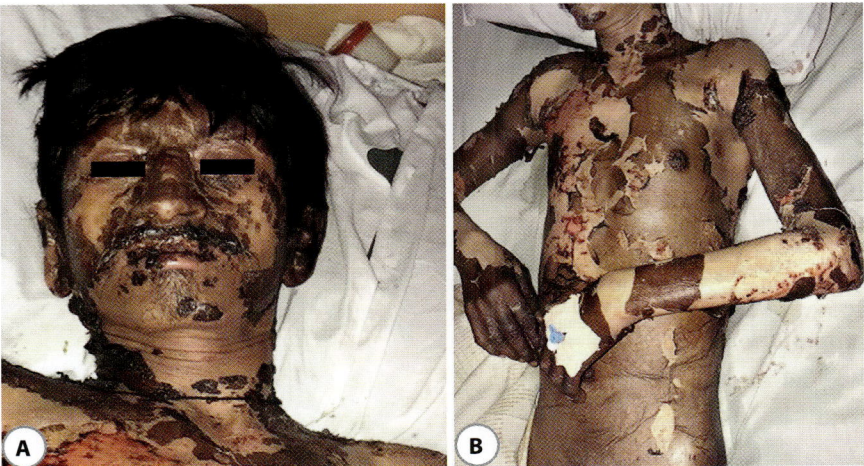

FIGS. 1A AND B: Toxic epidermal necrolysis.

Essential points in the history taking of suspected drug reaction patient are given here.

The patient history is crucial in diagnosing a drug reaction. Any exanthem in a hospitalized adult should raise suspicion for a drug-induced reaction. It is important to ask specific and focused questions regarding the potential offending drugs, which includes:
- Obtain a complete list of all drugs; prescription medicines, eye/ear drops, nasal sprays, injections, and immunizations. Enquire regarding use of over-the-counter medications (herbal medications, laxatives, sleeping pills, etc.).
- History of any prior drug reactions and assess whether the patient has taken the current medications before.
- *Length of treatment:* The timing of the reaction, including both onset and resolution, is important. When a patient is exposed to a medication for the first time, an allergic reaction typically cannot occur within the first 4–8 days. However, reactions due to re-exposure, cross-reactions, or pseudoallergic responses can occur more quickly, sometimes even immediately, as seen in cases such as anaphylaxis.
- Inquire about any other symptoms like fever, chills, diarrhea, or joint pain.
- If the patient is known to have contact allergy to paracompounds, this could account for reactions to sulfonamides, oral hypoglycemic agents, thiazide diuretics, or ester -caine type local anesthetics. Likewise, sensitivity to ethylenediamine may explain reactions to theophylline and similar substances.
- History of drug reactions in any family members should be taken.
- Route of drug administration is important as risk of sensitization is highest with topical agents followed by oral > intramuscular > intravenous (IV), in that order.

Physical Examination

A thorough physical examination should be carried out from head to toe including all mucosae.

General examination:
- Temperature
- Pulse

- Blood pressure
- Respiratory rate
- Nail
- Conjunctiva
- Tongue

Local examination:
- *Cutaneous examination*:
    - Sites involved
    - Type of lesion
    - % Body surface area (BSA)
- *Mucosal examination*:
    - Conjunctival
    - Oral
    - Genital
    - Nasal
    - Perianal
- Hair
- Nails

Clinical Outline of Severe Cutaneous Drug Reactions

Toxic epidermal necrolysis (TEN) and Stevens–Johnson syndrome (SJS) are uncommon, severe, and potentially fatal muco-cutaneous conditions that are almost invariably caused by drugs.

Classification of SJS–TEN[1]
- *SJS:* <10% BSA detachment + widespread purpuric macules or flat atypical target lesions + involvement of two or more mucosae
- *Overlap SJS/TEN:* 10–30% of the BSA detachment + widespread purpuric macules or flat atypical target lesions + involvement of two or more mucosae
- *TEN with spots:* Detachment of >30% of the BSA + widespread purpuric macules or flat atypical target lesions + involvement of two or more mucosae
- *TEN without spots*: Detachment of >30% of the BSA + with large epidermal sheets without purpuric macules or target lesions.
   Risk factors for development of SJS and TEN are given in **Box 2**.

Pathogenesis

Drug-induced SJS/TEN are serious hypersensitivity reactions involving MHC I-restricted drug presentation and the expansion of cytotoxic T lymphocytes (CD8+), which ultimately cause widespread keratinocyte death. Several mechanistic models have been proposed to explain the immunogenic response triggered by these drugs, including **(Figs. 2 and 3)**:
- Hapten/prohapten model
- p–i model
- Altered repertoire model

| BOX 2 | Risk factors for development of Stevens–Johnson syndrome (SJS) and toxic epidermal necrolysis (TEN). |

- Old age
- *Pharmacokinetics:* Slow acetylators phenotype
- *Immunosuppression:* Conditions such as lymphoma and human immunodeficiency virus (HIV) infection
- Concurrent use of radiotherapy and anticonvulsants (particularly in patients with brain tumors)
- *Genetics:* Individuals from specific ethnic groups with certain human leukocyte antigen (HLA) subtypes have a higher risk of developing SJS/TEN when exposed to particular drugs.
  - HLA-A*3101— in Europeans exposed to carbamazepine
  - HLA-B*5701 and HLA B*5801—confers increased risk of abacavir and allopurinol-induced hypersensitivity reaction, respectively.
  - HLA-A*0206—in Japanese and Korean exposed to NSAIDs
  - HLA-B*4403—in Indians and Caucasians exposed to NSAIDs
  - Interferon (IFN) gamma gene polymorphism—linked to SJS in the Mexican population
  - HLA-B*1502—Carbamazepine-induced SJS/TEN in Asian population

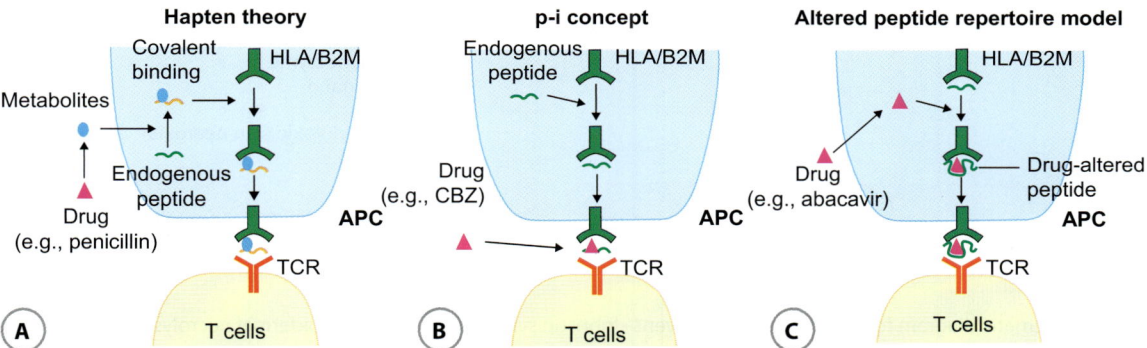

FIGS. 2A TO C: Models to explain pathogenesis of drug-induced Stevens–Johnson syndrome (SJS)–toxic epidermal necrolysis (TEN).
(APC: antigen-presenting cells; CBZ: carbamazepine; HLA: human leukocyte antigen; TCR: T-cell receptor)

STEVENS–JOHNSON SYNDROME

Stevens–Johnson syndrome is an immune-complex-hypersensitivity disease that typically involves the skin and the mucous membranes.

Prodromal symptoms range from thick productive cough, to headache, malaise, and arthralgia. Rash may start from face with burning sensation and progress to involve trunk. Rash begins as macules that develop into papules, vesicles, bullae, urticarial plaques, or confluent erythema.

Lesions usually start as nonpruritic urticarial lesions. Lesions may be bullous, which rupture to leave behind denuded skin. Mucosa may be erythematous, edematous, sloughed, ulcerated or covered with hemorrhagic crust or can be necrosed **(Fig. 4)**.

Toxic epidermal necrolysis **(Fig. 5)** is a severe, life-threatening condition marked by widespread erythema, necrosis, and bullous separation of the epidermis and mucous membranes, with erosions affecting >30% of the BSA. It results in exfoliation and possible sepsis and/or death. Mucous membrane

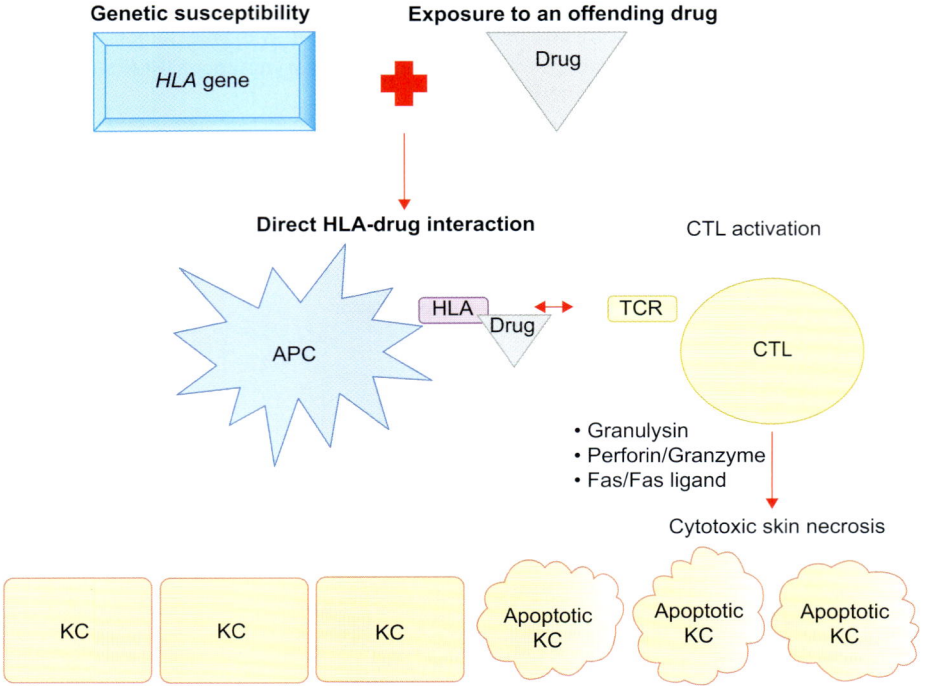

FIG. 3: Schematic diagram for pathogenesis of Stevens–Johnson syndrome (SJS)–toxic epidermal necrolysis (TEN).
(APC: antigen-presenting cells; CTL: cytotoxic T lymphocytes; HLA: human leukocyte antigen; KC: keratinocyte)

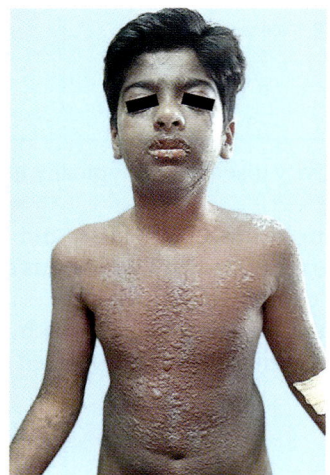

FIG. 4: Stevens–Johnson syndrome.

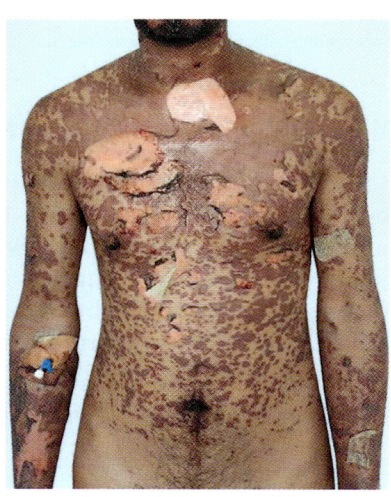

FIG. 5: Toxic epidermal necrolysis.

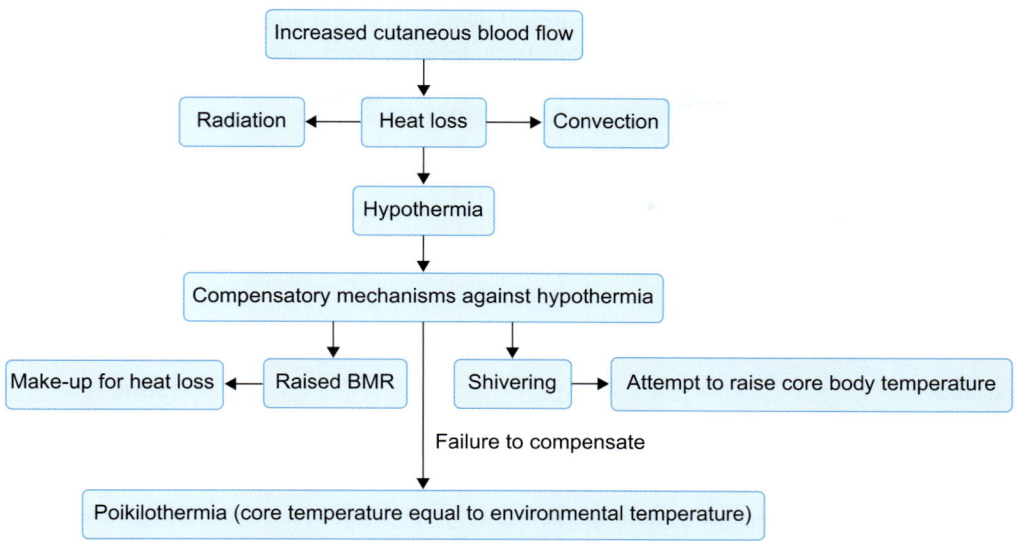

FLOWCHART 1: Pathogenesis of altered temperature regulation in acute skin failure.
(BMR: basal metabolic rate)

involvement can be severe involving gastrointestinal hemorrhage, respiratory failure, ocular abnormalities, and genitourinary complications. SJS-TEN is one of the common causes of acute skin failure.

Acute skin failure: "It is loss of normal temperature control with inability to maintain the core body temperature and failure to prevent percutaneous loss of fluid, electrolytes and protein, with resulting imbalance and failure of the mechanical barrier to prevent penetration of foreign materials" **(Flowchart 1)**.

DRUG REACTION WITH EOSINOPHILIA AND SYSTEMIC SYMPTOMS OR DRUG HYPERSENSITIVITY SYNDROME OR DRUG-INDUCED HYPERSENSITIVITY SYNDROME

Synonyms: DIHS, DIDMOHS, anticonvulsant hypersensitivity syndrome, or drug induced pseudolymphoma

The exact pathogenesis of DRESS remains unclear, although several potential mechanisms have been suggested, including:
- Specific changes in the metabolism of certain drugs
- Certain HLA alleles have been linked to a markedly higher risk of developing drug-specific DRESS **(Table 1)**
- IL-5 is involved in the development of eosinophilia and the activation of drug-specific T cells in the skin and internal organs.

Reactivation of human herpes viruses (HHV), particularly HHV-6, HHV-7, *Cytomegalovirus* (CMV), and Epstein–Barr virus (EBV), has been observed. Clinically, this hypersensitivity syndrome typically emerges 2–6 weeks after starting the offending drug, making it a later onset compared to many other immunologically mediated skin reactions. The most common symptoms include fever and a morbilliform rash. Rash becomes edematous in few days. Typical areas affected include face, upper trunk, and extremities. Facial edema is a key characteristic. Both cutaneous and visceral symptoms may persist for weeks, even after the drug has been discontinued. DRESS can present as erythroderma as well. Systemic involvement is common in DRESS **(Figs. 6A and B)**.

Histologically, several inflammatory patterns may be observed, such as eczematous, interface dermatitis, AGEP-like, and erythema multiforme-like reactions. A notable feature is peripheral blood eosinophilia, which is highly characteristic. This is often associated with mononucleosis-like atypical lymphocytosis.

TABLE 1: Criteria for drug rash with eosinophilia and systemic symptoms (DRESS).	
Clinical feature	**Score**
Extent of rash >50% body surface area	1 point
Rash suggestive of DRESS	1 point
Systemic involvement: Lymphadenopathy[a], eosinophilia, atypical lymphocytosis[b], and organ involvement[c]	Maximum 6 points
Relevant negative serological tests[d]	1 point

[a] ≥2 sites, ≥1 cm. A maximum 1 point gained from lymphadenopathy.
[b] *Eosinophilia:* 10–19% of total white cell count = 1 point; ≥20% = 2 points (if total leucocytes <4 × 10^9/L and an eosinophil count 0.7–1.5 × 10^9 = 1 point, an eosinophil count of ≥ 1.5 × 10^9/L = 2 points); atypical lymphocytes = 1 point
[c] *Liver:* Transaminases > 2 × upper limit of normal (ULN) on two successive dates or bilirubin × 2 ULN on 2 successive days or aspartate aminotransferase (AST), γ-glutamyltransferase (GGT), and alkaline phosphatase >2 × ULN on one occasion. *Renal:* Creatinine 1.5 × patient's baseline. *Cardiac:* Echocardiographic evidence of pericarditis. Maximum of *2 points* for internal organ involvement.
[d] *≥3 of the following performed and negative:* Hepatitis A, B, and C; *Mycoplasma/Chlamydia*; antinuclear antibody; blood culture (performed ≤3 days after hospitalization). A maximum of 1 point gained for relevant negative serological tests.

Note: 5 points—Definite case.

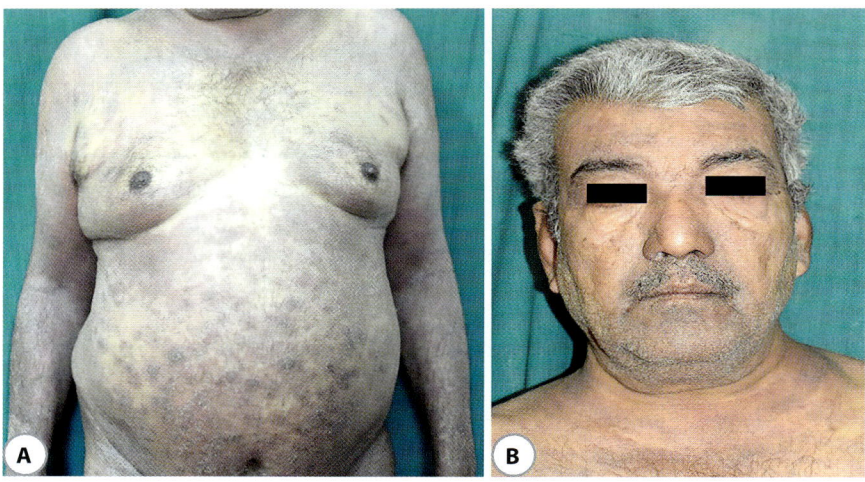

FIGS. 6A AND B: Imatinib-induced drug reaction with eosinophilia and systemic symptoms [drug rash with eosinophilia and systemic symptoms (DRESS)].

ACUTE GENERALIZED EXANTHEMATOUS PUSTULOSIS

Acute generalized exanthematous pustulosis is also known as exanthemic pustular psoriasis, toxic pustuloderma or pustular drug rash.

It is characterized by fever exceeding 38°C and a cutaneous eruption characterized by nonfollicular sterile pustules on an edematous, erythematous base. The time between drug administration and the onset of the eruption can range from 24 hours to 3 weeks. A longer interval typically suggests primary sensitization, while a shorter interval may indicate unintentional re-exposure. The eruption begins on the face or intertriginous area and disseminates within few hours. Subcorneal aseptic pustules are characteristic and easily recognized. But targetoid skin lesions, purpura, and vesicles may occur too. Usually it is a self-limiting condition, which resolves on its own within two weeks **(Fig. 7)**.

Bullous Fixed Drug Eruption

Bullous fixed drug eruption is characterized by fluid-filled lesions occurring at the same site after taking a drug, mostly involving lips, genitals, and hands and feet. The lesions occur around 1–2 weeks after the intake of culprit drug, as a hyperpigmented/dusky macule, which develops a central fluid-filled lesion. The most common causes include antibiotics, especially tetracyclines, though sulfonamides, nonsteroidal anti-inflammatory drugs (NSAIDs), and antifungals are not uncommon. The pathogenesis involves memory CD8+ T cells and the diagnosis can be confirmed by an in-vivo patch test at the site of the lesion (and absence at the other sites) after a refractory period. This provocation test is only prudent in diagnosis of *fixed drug eruption* and not in other forms of drug reactions.

ERYTHEMA MULTIFORME MAJOR

Erythema multiforme (EM) is an acute, self-limiting skin condition marked by the sudden appearance of symmetrical, fixed red papules, some of which may develop into typical or occasionally, "atypical" target lesions. The eruption is commonly triggered by an infection, most notably herpes simplex virus (HSV). EM is classified into two forms: (1) EM minor and (2) EM major **(Table 2)**. Though EM has

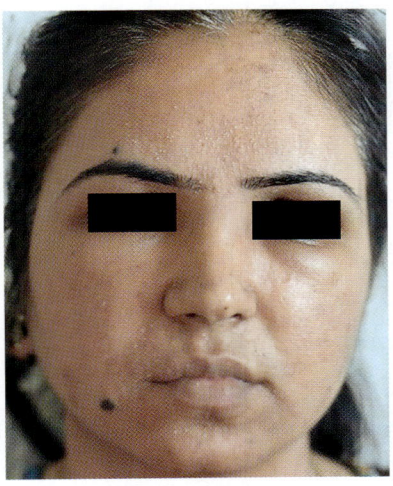

FIG. 7: Acute generalized exanthematous pustulosis.

TABLE 2: Difference between erythema multiforme (EM) minor, EM major, and Stevens–Johnson syndrome (SJS).

	Type of skin lesions	Distribution	Mucosal involvement	Systemic symptoms	Progression to TEN	Precipitating factors
EM minor	Typical targets ± Papular atypical targets	Extremities (especially elbows, knees, wrists, and hands), face	Absent or mild	Absent	No	*Herpes simplex virus:* Other infectious agent
EM major	• Typical targets ± Papular atypical targets • Occasionally bullous lesions	Extremities and face	Severe	*Usually present:* • Fever • Arthralgias	No	*Herpes simplex virus:* • *Mycoplasma pneumoniae* • Other infectious agents • Rarely, drugs
SJS	• Dusky and/or dusky-erythematous macules with epidermal detachment and erosions • Macular atypical targets • Bullous lesions • Isolated lesions confluence (+)	Trunk and face	Severe	*Usually present:* • Fever • Lymphadenopathy • Hepatitis • Cytopenia	Possible	• Drugs • Occasionally, *ycoplasma pneumoniae* • Rarely, immunizations

wide range of etiological factors, drugs constitute a major part of causative factors. The common drugs implicated in causation of EM are:
- *Antibiotics*:
    - Cephalosporins
    - Erythromycin
    - Penicillins and ampicillin
    - Quinolones
    - Sulfonamides
    - Tetracyclines
- *Antifungals*:
    - Griseofulvin
    - Nystatin
    - Terbinafine
- *Antiretroviral drugs*:
    - Abacavir
    - Nevirapine
- *NSAIDs*:
    - Ibuprofen
    - Paracetamol (acetaminophen)
- *Anticonvulsants*:
    - Barbiturates
    - Carbamazepine
    - Hydantoin derivatives
    - Lamotrigine

A typical target lesion is defined as a lesion with central area of dusky erythema or purpura, middle paler zone of edema, and outer ring of erythema with a well-defined edge **(Table 3)**.

TABLE 3: Difference between typical and atypical target lesion.	
Typical target/iris lesion/bull's eye lesion	**Targetoid/atypical target lesion**
Dusky center present	Present
Zone of pale edema present	Absent
Peripheral zone of erythema with well-defined edges	Present but with poorly defined edges

Questions and Answers

Q.1. What is "Herpes iris of Bateman"?
Ans. Herpes iris of Bateman is a distinct skin lesion seen in patients of vesiculobullous form of EM having an erythematous macule/plaque often with central bulla and a marginal ring of vesicles **(Table 4)**.

TABLE 4: Difference between urticaria and erythema multiforme.

Urticaria	Erythema multiforme
Transient duskiness or normal skin in the central zone	The central area consists of damaged skin, which may appear dusky, bullous, or crusted
Individual lesions are evanescent, lasting <24 hours	Individual lesions are fixed for a minimum of 7 days
Appearance of daily new lesions	All lesions develop within the first 72 hours
May be accompanied by facial swelling, edema of hands and/or feet, and angioedema	Not associated with edema

Mechanisms of cutaneous drug reactions:
- *Immunological mechanisms*:
    - *IgE-mediated type-I reactions*: These include *urticaria* and *anaphylaxis*
        - *Common drugs:* Penicillins—
            - Cephalosporins
            - Aminoglycosides
            - Tetracyclines
            - Sulfonamides
            - Blood products
            - Insulin
            - Vaccines containing egg protein
    - *Antibody mediated type II reactions:* These include—
        - *Thrombocytopenic purpura*: Quinidine
        - Hemolytic anemia:
            - Penicillin
            - Quinine
            - Sulfonamides
            - Methyl dopa
    - *Delayed T-cell-mediated type IV reactions*: These include—
        - SJS; TEN; DRESS; fixed drug eruption (FDE); EM
            - Anticonvulsants
            - NSAID
            - Beta-lactam antibiotics
            - Antimalarials
            - Quinolones
            - Dapsone
    - *Immune-complex mediated type III reactions*:
        - *Vasculitis:* Common drugs include—
            - Allopurinol
            - Amiodarone
            - Diuretics
            - Ampicillin
            - Aspirin and other NSAIDs

- Arsenic
- Captopril
- Phenytoin
- Sulfonamides
- *Serum sickness:* Common drugs include—
  - Heterologous serum
  - Aspirin
  - Penicillins and cephalosporins
  - Ciprofloxacin
  - Cotrimoxazole
  - Sulfonamides
  - Sulfasalazine
  - IV streptokinase
- *Nonimmunologic mechanisms (sometimes predictable)*:
  - Overdose
  - Pharmacologic side effects
  - Cumulative toxicity
  - Delayed toxicity
  - Drug–drug interactions
  - Changes in metabolism
  - Aggravation of disease
- *Idiosyncratic with a possible immunologic mechanism (unpredictable)*:
  - DRESS
  - SJS/TEN
  - Drug reactions in the setting of HIV infection
  - Drug-induced lupus erythematosus

Diagnostic Workup
Diagnostic workup includes the following:
- *Blood workup:* A comprehensive blood workup is essential for assessing the extent of internal organ involvement in patients with DRESS, DHS, SJS, and TEN. Key tests include:
  - *CBC with differential:* This may reveal atypical lymphocytosis, leukopenia, leukocytosis, and eosinophilia.
  - Liver function tests, serum creatinine, urinalysis, and TSI.
  - Abnormal blood test results should be retested during recovery, and TSI should be re-evaluated after three months.
- Cultures (skin and blood), erythrocyte sedimentation rate (ESR), ANA, and other tests may be ordered to rule out or confirm alternative conditions.
- If palpable purpuric lesions are present, a thorough laboratory examination is necessary to exclude vascular diseases, vasculitis, and other causes like infections or collagen vascular diseases.
- *Skin biopsy* should be considered to confirm the diagnosis.
- Although there are no reliable tests to determine whether a drug is the cause of an adverse reaction apart from rechallenge test, it is no longer done for ethical reasons aside.

Q.2. What is ALDEN?

Ans. It stands for algorithm for drug causality for epidermal necrolysis (ALDEN). It is a set of questionnaires that gives an objective assessment of the chances a drug has to cause the adverse drug reaction. Other similar questionnaire is Naranjo scale to establish drug causality.

Q.3. What is EMPACT?

Ans. Patients taking phenytoin for the prevention of seizures brought on by brain metastases may develop a particular type of EM minor in the radiation field, i.e., EM associated with phenytoin and cranial radiation therapy (EMPACT).

Q.4. What is SCORTEN?

Ans. The severity-of-illness score for TEN (SCORTEN) score is used to predict the mortality risk in patients with SJS and TEN. One point is assigned for each of the seven criteria that are present at the time of admission **(Box 3)**.

> **BOX 3** The risk of dying from SJS/TEN depends on the score.
>
> SCORTEN and predicted mortality rates:
> - SCORTEN 0–1 > 3.2%
> - SCORTEN 2 > 12.1%
> - SCORTEN 3 > 35.3%
> - SCORTEN 4 > 58.3%
> - SCORTEN 5 or more > 90%

The SCORTEN criteria are:
- Age > 40 years
- Presence of a malignancy (cancer)
- *Heart rate*: >120 beats/min
- *Percentage of epidermal detachment:* If initially >10%
- Serum urea level of >10 mmol/L
- Serum glucose level of >14 mmol/L
- Serum bicarbonate level of <20 mmol/L

Q.5. What are the diagnostic criteria for drug hypersensitivity syndrome?

Ans. The diagnostic criteria for DIHS, as established by a Japanese consensus group, include:
- Development of a maculopapular rash >3 weeks after the initial administration of a limited number of drugs.
- Persistence of clinical symptoms for >2 weeks after discontinuing the suspected drug.
- Fever (>38°C).
- Liver abnormalities, such as alanine aminotransferase levels exceeding 100 IU/L.
    - Leukocyte abnormalities, with at least one of the following:
        - Leukocytosis (>11 × 10^9/L)
        - Atypical lymphocytosis (>5%)
        - Eosinophilia (> 1.5 × 10^9/L)
- Lymphadenopathy
- Reactivation of HHV-6

Typical DIHS or DRESS is characterized by the presence of all seven criteria, while atypical DIHS is identified when five criteria (1–5) are present. Other organ abnormalities, such as those affecting the kidneys, liver, heart, and skeletal muscles may also occur **(Figs. 6A and B)**.

Q.6. What are the causes of acute skin failure?

Ans. They are as outlined as follows:
- *Erythroderma*:
    - Primary (idiopathic)
    - Dermatitis (atopic, seborrheic, and contact dermatitis)
    - Psoriasis and pityriasis rubra pilaris
    - Exfoliative drug rash
    - Disorders of keratinization
    - Cutaneous T-cell lymphoma
    - Graft-versus-host disease
- Severe cutaneous[2] drug reactions including SJS and TEN
- Acute generalized pustular psoriasis
- Immunobullous disorders, such as extensive pemphigus vulgaris and pemphigus foliaceus, involving large areas of the body.
- Staphylococcal scalded skin syndrome

Q.7. What are the consequences of acute skin failure?

Ans. They are as follows:
- Altered hemodynamics
- Altered thermoregulation
- Metabolic abnormalities
- Fluid and electrolyte imbalance
- Loss of nutrients
- Pulmonary complications
- Altered immune function
- Peripheral edema
- Infections

Q.8. What are the long-term complications of acute skin failure?

Ans. The common long-term complications of acute skin failure are **(Table 5)**.

TABLE 5: Long-term complications of acute skin failure.	
Organ involved	**Complications**
Eye	Ectropion, entropion, corneal scarring, symblepharon, and secondary sicca syndrome
Mucosal involvement	• *Esophagus:* Dysphagia resulting from stricture *Urethra:* Stricture and phimosis • *Vagina:* Synechiae
Skin	Pigmentary changes (hypo- and hyperpigmentation), hypohidrosis, and contracture
Hair	Scarring alopecia
Nail	Beau's lines, splinter hemorrhage, distal onycholysis, dystrophy, and total shedding of nails

Q.9. What are the histopathological findings of lesional skin in SJS-TEN?
Ans.
- In the early stages of SJS and TEN, apoptotic keratinocytes are observed scattered in the basal and immediate suprabasal layers of the epidermis. This corresponds with the dusky to grey coloration, which clinicians experienced with SJS/TEN recognize as a warning sign of impending extensive epidermal necrosis and detachment.
- In the later stages, biopsy samples from lesions reveal a subepidermal blister with widespread necrosis of the entire epidermis. A sparse perivascular infiltrate, mainly composed of lymphocytes, is also present.

Q.10. What is dapsone hypersensitivity syndrome?
Ans. Dapsone-induced idiosyncratic drug rash was first identified as an infectious mononucleosis-like eruption in patients treated for lepromatous leprosy. Symptoms typically appear 3–12 weeks after starting therapy and include fever, a widespread skin eruption, and internal organ involvement. The skin manifestations can range from a maculopapular rash to toxic epidermal necrolysis. Hepatitis in these patients typically presents with a mixed pattern, showing both hepatocellular and cholestatic features. Patients often exhibit signs of severe hypersensitivity such as peripheral eosinophilia, and fatalities have been reported. Although initially observed in leprosy patients, dapsone hypersensitivity syndrome has also been noted in those using dapsone for other skin disorders. Corticosteroids are the preferred treatment.

Q.11. What is the role of genetics in pathogenesis of DRESS?
Ans. Multiple specific HLA alleles have been linked to a notably higher risk of developing drug-specific DRESS. The different associated HLA alleles are as follows:
- *HLA B 5701:* Abacavir
- *HLA B 5801:* Allopurinol
- *HLA A 3101:* Carbamazepine
- *HLA DRB1*01*01:* Nevirapine

Q.12. What are the most common drugs implicated in DRESS?
Ans.
- *Anticonvulsants:* Carbamazepine, lamotrigine*, phenobarbital, phenytoin, oxcarbazepine, zonisamide > valproic acid
- *Antimicrobials:* Ampicillin, cefotaxime, dapsone, ethambutol, isoniazid, linezolid, metronidazole, minocycline, pyrazinamide, quinine, rifampin, sulfasalazine, streptomycin, trimethoprim–sulfamethoxazole, teicoplanin, and vancomycin
- *Antiretrovirals:* Abacavir, nevirapine, and zalcitabine
- *Antidepressants:* Bupropion and fluoxetine
- *Antihypertensives:* Amlodipine and captopril
- *NSAIDs:* Celecoxib and ibuprofen
- *Miscellaneous:* Allopurinol, azathioprine, imatinib, mexiletine, ranitidine, and ziprasidone

Q.13. What are the clinical features of AGEP?
Ans. The key features of AGEP include **(Fig. 7)**:
- *Skin rash:* Small nonfollicular pustules on an erythematous background, typically appearing in skin folds such as the neck, axilla, and groin, as well as on the trunk and upper extremities.

Patients may also experience a burning sensation and generalized edema, particularly on the face.
- *Fever:* A temperature exceeding 38°C, which appears on the same day as the rash
- Increased neutrophil count
- *Histopathology:* Subcorneal pustules, papillary dermal edema, and a perivascular polymorphic infiltrate
- *Spontaneous resolution:* Typically occurs within 15 days

Q.14. What are the common drugs causing AGEP?

Ans. The most common drugs implicated in AGEP are as follows:
- Acetaminophen
- *Antibiotics:* Penicillins, aminopenicillins, cephalosporins, clindamycin, pristinamycin, sulfonamides, metronidazole, carbapenems, quinolones, and macrolides.
- Calcium channel blockers, especially diltiazem
- Carbamazepine
- Cetirizine
- Herbal medicines
- Antimalarials, especially hydroxychloroquine
- NSAIDs, including oxicam derivatives and COX-2 inhibitors
- Proton pump inhibitors
- Terbinafine

Q.15. What are the differential diagnoses of AGEP?

Ans. The differential diagnoses of AGEP are:
- Pustular psoriasis
- Subcorneal pustular dermatosis
- DRESS
- Candidial infection

Q.16. How to manage a patient of SCAR in an emergency room?

Ans.
Critical care management:
- Stop all the medications
- Perform an initial ABC assessment of the patient
- Measures to assist skin healing include maintaining a warm environment for the patient and warming peripheral areas of the skin to prevent a core-peripheral temperature gradient of >2°C. As patients with TEN often require prolonged ICU care, arterial and central venous access should be obtained through unaffected areas of skin. Noninvasive cardiac output monitoring is typically used to guide fluid management and determine the need for inotropic or vasopressor medications.
- Avoidance of vasopressors unless severe hypotension occurs

Fluid management:
- Unless resuscitation has already started, the patient should be presumed to be hypovolemic.
- Initial fluid needs can be estimated using a modified version of the Baxter–Parkland formula, which is calculated as: Skin area affected × body weight × 3 mL.

This amount represents approximately two-thirds of the total resuscitation fluid required and should be administered over the first 24 hours.
- Fluid management beyond the initial 24-hour period should be adjusted based on the patient's clinical condition.

Skin care in TEN:
- Routine de-roofing of blisters is not advised, as the blistered skin serves as a natural biological dressing that promotes re-epithelialization.
- There is no conclusive evidence supporting the use of one dressing type over another. However, current recommendations suggest the use of nanocrystalline silver dressings due to their enhanced antimicrobial properties and reduced need for frequent dressing changes.

Pain management: There are two types of pain—
1. *Procedural pain:* During procedures, more intensive and short-lived
2. *Background pain:* Present at rest, of low intensity
   - It is individualized as follows:
     - *For procedural pain:* Oral, transmucosal short-acting, medium potency opioids
     - *For rest pain:* Anxiolytics such as low dose benzodiazepines.

Ophthalmology assessment:
- Ophthalmic involvement in TEN can result in blindness and the formation of adhesions. The corneal team should be alerted upon admission and should evaluate the patient within 2 hours.
- *Current recommendations include*:
  - Application of topical eye lubricants every 1–2 hours
  - Use of preservative-free topical antibiotics
  - Amniotic membrane application to the cornea, under the guidance of the corneal team, to prevent symblepharon formation.

Therapeutics: Prophylactic antibiotic administration is not indicated.
- *Systemic corticosteroids*: Their usage remains controversial
  - Corticosteroids may be most effective as an anti-inflammatory treatment when started early.
  - However, current evidence does not support the routine use of corticosteroids, especially once significant skin loss has occurred. High-dose corticosteroids may be considered for patients presenting with early-stage TEN during the erythrodermic phase, before skin loss begins. Even then, their use should be restricted to the first 48 hours to minimize the risk of severe complications.
- *Cyclosporine*:
  - It has a potent immunosuppressive effect by inhibiting T-cell activation and tumor necrosis factor-alpha (TNF-α), leading to an antiapoptotic response. Disease progression typically halts within 24–36 hours, and complete re-epithelialization occurs more rapidly.
  - The recommended dosage is 3–5 mg/kg daily, either intravenously or orally, for 8–24 days (until re-epithelialization is achieved), followed by a gradual reduction in dose over the next 2 weeks.
- *Intravenous immunoglobulin (IVIg)*:
  - The use of IVIg remains controversial, with limited evidence supporting its benefit and some concerns about potential harm. As there is no consensus on its effectiveness, the decision to use IVIg is left to the discretion of the dermatology team.

- IVIg works by blocking Fas–Fas Ligand interactions between effector cells and keratinocytes, thereby preventing keratinocyte apoptosis. Recently, the use of whole blood has been recommended as an alternative to IVIg, offering better cost-effectiveness and pharmacological advantages.

Management of DRESS:
- *For patients with non-life-threatening and non-organ-threatening disease:*
  - Discontinue the offending anticonvulsant and replace with a safer one, e.g., topiramate or levetiracetam.
  - Supportive therapy (anti-histamines, topical corticosteroids, and emollients) are used. Investigate for the organ involvement and assessment of the severity of organ involvement
  - Skin biopsy performed, if blistering or pustular eruption is present.
  - The patient is advised about the possibility of cross-reactivity.
- *For patient with life-threatening or organ-threatening disease*:
  - Earlier mentioned measures +
  - Use of oral prednisolone or pulse methyl prednisolone
  - IVIg and cyclosporine can be used as alternatives or adjuvants

Management of AGEP:
- On discontinuation of offending drug AGEP usually resolves spontaneously
- Topical steroids, antipyretics, and emollients are commonly used to support the healing process.

METHOTREXATE TOXICITY

A 56-year-old male patient, a known case of psoriasis since 18 years came with burning sensation over body, pedal edema, generalized weakness, increased body lesions, and oral ulceration. He was being treated with tablet methotrexate in various doses since 4 years on a weekly basis but owing to the flare of the disease, he consumed methotrexate daily for 14 days and presented to us in the present condition **(Figs. 8 and 9)**

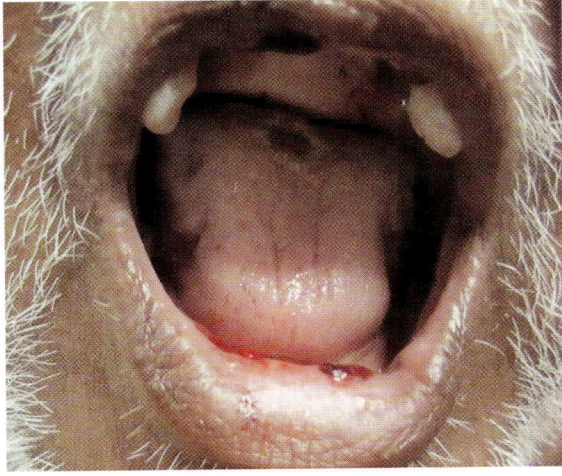

FIG. 8: Ulceration with hemorrhagic crusting over lip and tongue.

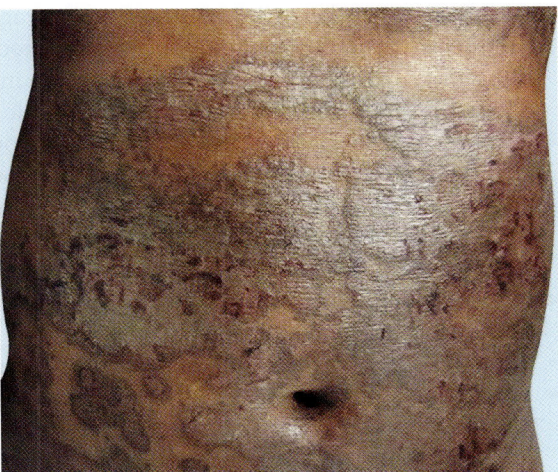

FIG. 9: Erythematous to brown colored scaly plaques with overlying erosions over the trunk.

Approach

Investigations:
- *CBC:* Pancytopenia
- *Liver enzymes (especially transaminases):* Raised
- *Renal function test:* Deranged
- *Serum methotrexate level:* >1 µmol/L

Q.17. How will you manage the case?

Ans. Patient was treated with injection leucovorin 20 mg IV 6 hourly for 4 days. Hemogram profile show consistent decrease in white blood count (WBC) count. Patient was then given injection. Filgrastim subcutaneous (SC) once a day for 5 days after this WBC count increased above 10,000.

Q.18. How does methotrexate toxicity occur?

Ans.
- Methotrexate is a potentially toxic, antimetabolite, anticancer drug, which in low dose is effective and safe therapy for psoriasis, if careful monitoring is done according to the recommended guidelines.
- Failure to adhere to the guidelines can lead to methotrexate toxicity. Well-known signs of toxicity include bone marrow suppression and oral and gastrointestinal ulcerations.
- Methotrexate toxicity can present in various forms, including hepatotoxicity, pulmonary toxicity, acute kidney failure, pancytopenia, stomatitis, and ulcerations or erosions of gastrointestinal tract.
- In rare cases, it can also cause skin-related side effects such as a burning sensation, skin peeling at pressure points, severe mucositis, SJS and, ulceration or pain of psoriatic plaques.

TREATMENT OF TOXICITY

Treatment of toxicity involves the following:
- Folinic acid (leucovorin) acts as a counteragent to methotrexate by bypassing the dihydrofolate reductase (DHFR) enzyme pathway required for deoxyribonucleic acid (DNA) synthesis. In the absence of DHFR, folinic acid is converted in the body to tetrahydrofolate, offering an alternative source of precursors for DNA and ribonucleic acid (RNA) synthesis.
- Folinic acid should be given within 24–36 hours following the last dose of methotrexate, with the required dose determined by the serum methotrexate level. Since folinic acid has minimal toxicity, an oral dose of 10 mg/m² can be administered promptly at the first sign of toxicity, even before waiting for serum levels to be tested. In cases where a serum assay is not available, 15–25 mg of folinic acid can be taken orally every 6 hours for a duration of 6–10 doses.
- Filgrastim (G-CSF) administration is done at a dose of 5 µg/kg/day SC until absolute neutrophil count reaches 10,000/µL.
- Supportive therapy in the form of systemic antibiotics and antifungals.
- Proper hydration is crucial to optimize renal excretion. If renal function is compromised, urine alkalinization using sodium bicarbonate may be necessary to prevent methotrexate from precipitating in the renal tubules.

REFERENCES

1. Bastuji-Garin S, Rzany B, Stern RS, Shear NH, Naldi L, Roujeau JC. Clinical classification of cases of toxic epidermal necrolysis, Stevens-Johnson syndrome, and erythema multiforme. Arch Dermatol. 1993;129(1):92-6.
2. Hung SI, Mockenhaupt M, Blumenthal KG, Abe R, Ueta M, Ingen-Housz-Oro S, et al. Severe cutaneous adverse reactions. Nat Rev Dis Primers. 2024;10(1):30.

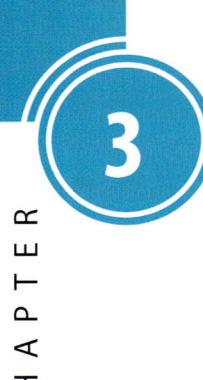

CHAPTER 3

Systemic Lupus Erythematosus

INTRODUCTION

Among autoimmune connective disorders, systemic lupus erythematosus (SLE) remains the leading cause of admission in the ward.

CLINICAL HISTORY

A 22-year-old female, college student, presented with *chief complaints of:*
- Recurrent skin lesions over face and bilateral arms for 4 year
- Low grade fever, joint pains for 4 years
- Hair loss for 1 year
- Aggravation of skin lesions since past 1 month

ORIGIN, DURATION, AND PROGRESS

Patient was relatively asymptomatic 4 years ago when she started to develop reddish skin lesions first over the face followed by bilateral arms, which aggravated on sun exposure. The lesions were initially transient and gradually they turned persistent. She had been suffering from diffuse hair fall since the past 1 year. She was experiencing body ache and fatigue for 4 years.

The patient was apparently well before 1 year, when she noticed reddish lesions over her central face that were associated with burning, tingling sensation, and redness, which increased on exposure to sun. The patient also developed reddish lesions over her forearms and hands since last 6 months that gradually developed a central area of white discoloration. These lesions were associated with burning sensation on sun exposure. Since 10 months, the patient started experiencing more pain over small joints of both hands and knees that is present throughout the day and restricts her daily routine but denied any history of associated joint swelling and any deformity. 4 months back, patient developed shortness of breath on climbing stairs. Now she had such episodes more frequently including her daily chores at times. Patient gave history of low-grade fever, easy fatigability, non-productive cough with chest pain, vague abdominal pain, and diffuse hair loss **(Figs. 1 and 2)**.

NEGATIVE HISTORY

There was no history of seizures, loss of consciousness/concentration, mood changes, difficulty in oral opening/swallowing, chest pain, palpitation, heartburn, postprandial abdominal pain, blood

in urine/frothy urine, decreased urine output, difficulty in getting up from sitting position/climbing stairs/combing hair, tingling or numbness in the extremities associated with color change on exposure to cold, dryness of mouth and eyes, fluid filled lesions, or antecedent drug intake.
- It is important to consider the patient's history of drug use, as drug-induced lupus, which is reversible, accounts for approximately 10% of cases and is more commonly seen in older individuals, particularly males.
- Systemic lupus erythematosus (SLE) have a higher frequency of allergic reactions to sulfa drugs compared to the general population with over 30% of SLE patients reportedly experiencing such reactions, including a potential worsening of their lupus symptoms.
- Burning sensation in mouth associated with difficulty in eating
- Frothy urine or decreased urine output, swelling over face
- Headache, seizures, or altered behavior
- Bluish discoloration of fingers on cold exposure
- Palpitation
- Difficulty in getting up from squatting position or raising arms
- Tightness of skin over both the hands and face
- Dryness in mouth and eyes
- Vesiculo-bullous lesions

PERSONAL HISTORY

The patient experienced decrease in her appetite and sleep. Bowel and bladder movements were unaltered. She had no addictions.

PAST HISTORY

There was no past history of diabetes, hypertension, thyroid disorder, tuberculosis, blood transfusion, and surgical illness.

FAMILY HISTORY

The patient was younger one of two siblings, elder sister being 25 years old. There was no history of similar illness in any family member.

OBSTETRIC/MENSTRUAL HISTORY

The patient had achieved menarche at 15 years of age. Her cycles were painless, regularly spaced at 28–30-day intervals, and were 3–5 days long.

GENERAL EXAMINATION

The patient was moderately built and nourished.
She was vitally stable. There was no evidence of jaundice, pallor, cyanosis, clubbing, edema, or lymphadenopathy.

SYSTEMIC EXAMINATION

Summary of systemic examination is given in **Table 1**.

TABLE 1: Summary of systemic examination in case of systemic lupus erythematosus (SLE).

System	Finding	Inference
Musculoskeletal	Tender, swollen joints (especially, bilateral knees, wrists, PIP, and MCP joints)	Nonerosive, nondeforming, and symmetric arthropathy
	Difficulty in combing hair, climbing stairs or getting up from sitting position with or without elevated muscle enzymes	Proximal muscle inflammation
Gastrointestinal	Oral ulcers (painless)	Flare of disease
	Abdominal pain	Steroid-induced gastritis, pancreatitis, ischemic bowel perforation, or mesenteric vasculitis
	Rebound tenderness, fever, nausea, vomiting, and diarrhea	Lupus panniculitis (due to mesenteric ischemia/bowel perforation)
Cardiovascular	Chest pain that eases when sitting upright and intensifies when leaning backward, with or without the presence of a pleural or pericardial rub	Pericarditis
	Fever, conduction abnormalities, elevated serum creative phosphokinase (CPK), skeletal myositis, and serositis	Myocarditis
	Systolic cardiac murmurs; usually over mitral and aortic areas	Libman–Sachs endocarditis (APLA associated); anemia, hypoxemia, and fever
	Tachycardia	Autonomic dysregulation
	Loud P2 with or without elevated aPTT	Pulmonary hypertension (usually with APLA)
Pulmonary	Pin pricking chest pain worsened by lying in ipsilateral position and on deep breaths	Pleuritis and pleural effusion (usually exudative—protein >3 g)
	Hemoptysis	• Pneumonitis • Pulmonary embolus
	Shrinking lung	Diaphragmatic weakness/paralysis
Central nervous system	Seizures (MC: GTCS)	• Lupus vasculitis • Acute thrombosis • Hypertension due to steroid therapy • Uremia
	Lack of sleep, concentration mood changes, and depression	Disease itself
	Intracranial hemorrhage and chorea	APLA syndrome

(ALPA: antiphospholipid antibody; aPTT: activated partial thromboplastin time; GTCS: generalized tonic–clonic seizure; MC: myoclonic)

CUTANEOUS EXAMINATION

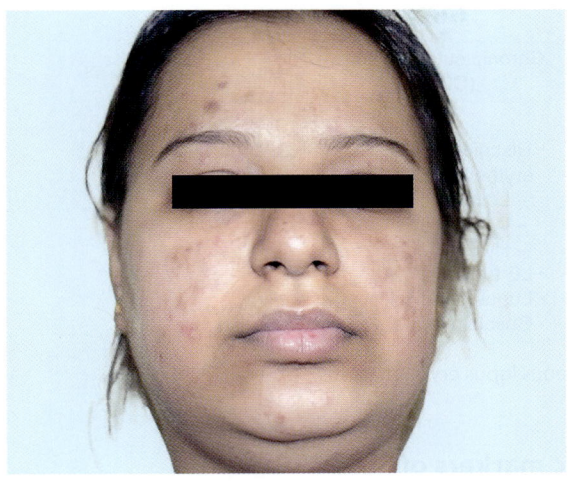

FIG. 1: Multiple discrete erythematous papules and plaques present over bilateral malar area and forehead.

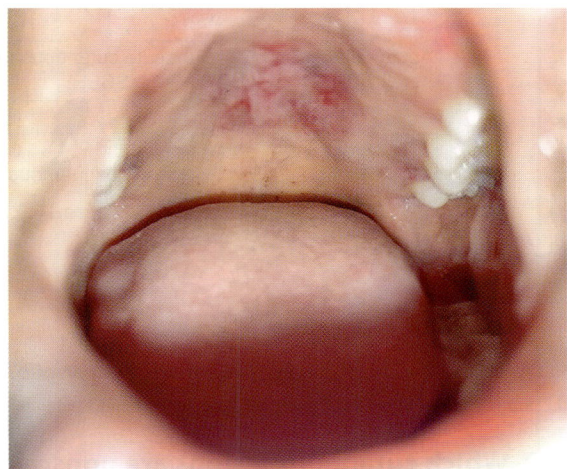

FIG. 2: Oral ulcer over hard palate.

Questions and Answers

Q.1. What are the risk factors for SLE?
Ans.
- *Gender:* Women with SLE outnumber men by 9:1 whereas women with only cutaneous lesions have a predominance of 3:1.
- *Age:* Lupus is uncommon in prepubertal children; most commonly affects women during their child-bearing age.
- *Hormonal susceptibility:* Early menarche, pregnancy, estrogen-containing pills, and hyperprolactinemia
- *Ethnicity:* African American women have a fourfold higher risk
- *Genetics:* HLA-DR, PTPN22, STAT4, IRF5, TREX1, C1Q
- Ultraviolet (UV) radiation (UVB > UVA)
- Cigarette smoking
- Drugs
- *Viruses:* Epstein–Barr virus (EBV)
- Mental/Physical stress

Q.2. Discuss the Gilliam and Sontheimer classification of cutaneous lupus erythematosus.
Ans. Gilliam and Sontheimer classification of cutaneous lupus erythematosus is given in **Flowchart 1**.

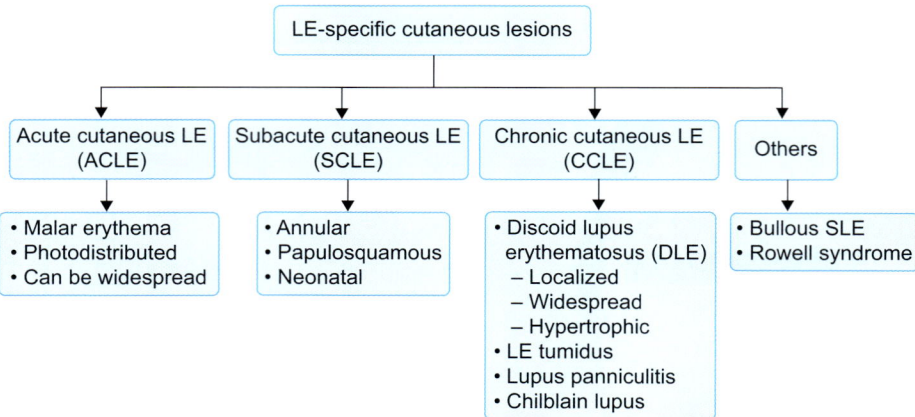

FLOWCHART 1: Gilliam and Sontheimer classification of cutaneous lupus erythematosus.

(LE: lupus erythematosus; SLE: systemic lupus erythematosus)

Q.3. Which cutaneous lesions are nonspecific markers of SLE?

Ans. Nonspecific markers of SLE are listed in **Box 1**.

BOX 1 | **Nonspecific cutaneous lesions of systemic lupus erythematosus (SLE).**

- Diffuse nonscarring alopecia
- Raynaud phenomenon
- Nail fold (periungual) telengiectasias and erythema
- *Vasculitis:*
    - Urticarial vasculitis
    - Small-vessel vasculitis (palpable purpura)
    - Polyarteritis nodosa like lesions
    - Ulcerations
- *Cutaneous signs of antiphospholipid syndrome:*
    - Livedo reticularis
    - Ulcerations
    - Acrocyanosis
    - Atrophie blanche-like lesions
    - Degos-like lesions
    - Livedoid vasculopathy
- Palmar erythema
- Papular and nodular mucinosis
- Sweet syndrome-like neutrophilic dermatoses

Q.4. How would a patient of acute cutaneous lupus erythematosus (ACLE) commonly present?

Ans.
- *Localized ACLE:* A butterfly-shaped rash or distinct maculopapular eruption with fine scaling or edema on the butterfly area of cheeks, typically sparing the nasolabial folds.

- *Generalized lupus erythematosus (LE):* A widespread or papular erythema on the face, upper trunk, and limbs resembling a viral exanthem or drug-induced eruption **(Fig. 3A)**.
- *Toxic epidermal necrolysis (TEN)-like lupus erythematosus (LE) or acute syndrome of apoptotic panepidermolysis (ASAP):* Clinically and histopathologically indistinguishable from drug-induced TEN **(Fig. 3B)**.

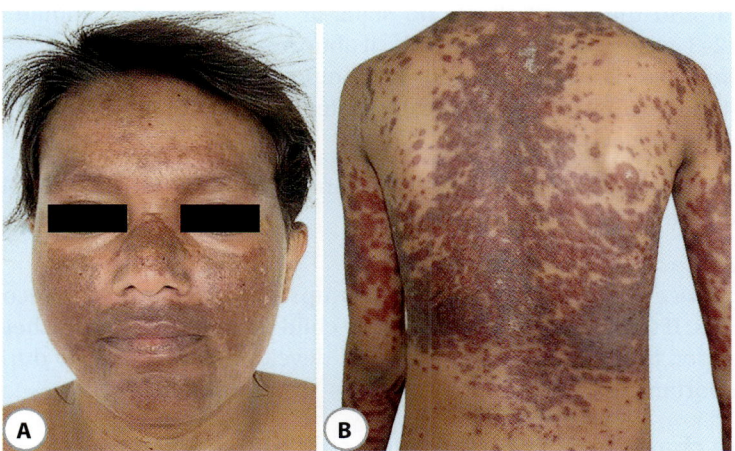

FIGS. 3A AND B: (A) Acute cutaneous LE; (B) Toxic epidermal necrolysis (TEN)-like presentation of lupus erythematosus (LE) over bilateral malar area (in butterfly pattern) in back.

Q.5. How would a patient of subacute cutaneous lupus erythematosus (SCLE) present?

Ans. A patient with SCLE may present with:
- Non-scarring papulo-squamous eruptions in about two-thirds of cases
- Annular polycyclic lesions in approximately one-third of cases
  The borders of the lesions may display vesiculation, crusting, and occasionally bullae. As they heal, they often leave behind grey–white hypopigmentation and telangiectasia. Erythroderma, pityriasiform, and poikilodermatous lesions have also been observed **(Figs. 4A and B)**.

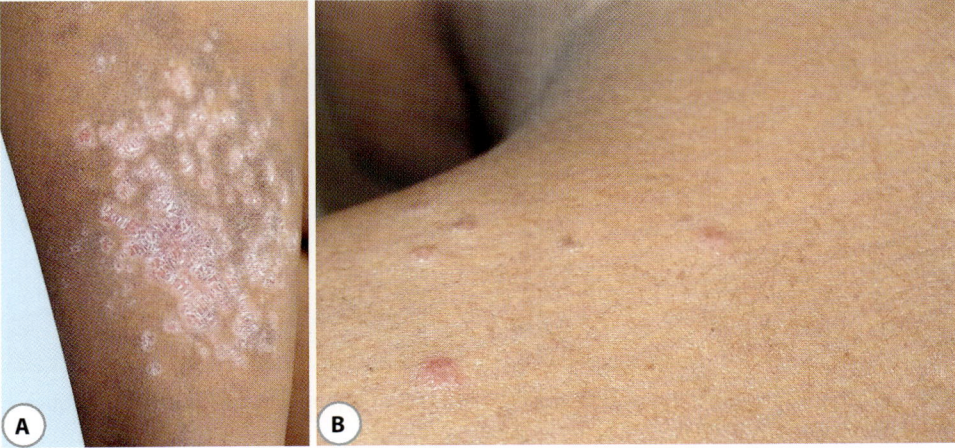

FIGS. 4A AND B: Erythematous scaly annular polycyclic plaques in subacute cutaneous lupus erythematosus (SCLE).

Q.6. How do you evaluate neonatal LE?

Ans. History, review of systems and physical examination, and regular monitoring of growth and head circumference are essential to check for macrocephaly/hydrocephalus.

- *Laboratory studies:* Initial tests may include an electrocardiogram (ECG), echocardiogram, complete blood count (CBC) with differential and platelet count, and liver function tests. If these tests are normal and the infant shows no signs or symptoms, they should be repeated every 2–3 months for 2–3 cycles, or more frequently, if abnormalities are present.
- *Family counseling and care coordination:* It is important to discuss the risk of neonatal lupus erythematosus (NLE) in future pregnancies, the potential for autoimmune connective tissue disease (AI-CTD) in the mother, and possibly the child.

Pre-emptive treatment: For mothers of infants with cardiac NLE, consider prescribing hydroxychloroquine during subsequent pregnancies.

Long-term follow up the child with neonatal LE:
- *History and physical examination:* Periodic follow-ups as per pediatrician's recommendation
- *Laboratory studies:* If tests remain normal and the child remains healthy, further testing may not be necessary. However, monitoring for the potential development of AI-CTD during adolescence or adulthood is important.

Q.7. Describe the characteristic lesion of discoid lupus erythematosus (DLE).

Ans. It appears as single or multiple well demarcated red, scaly patch, or plaque of varying sizes, which eventually heal with atrophy, scarring, and pigmentation.

Presentation:
- *Localized DLE:* It is limited to the head and neck.
- *Disseminated DLE:* It is much more extensive disease, potentially affecting any area of the skin **(Figs. 5 and 6)**.

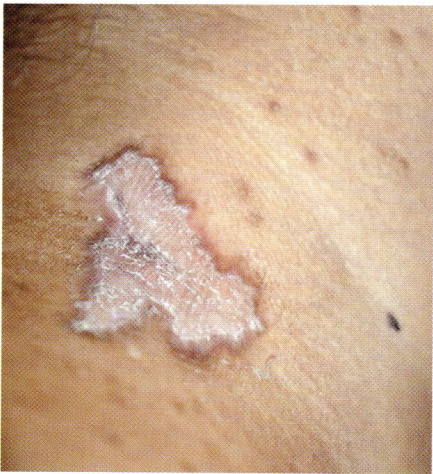

FIG. 5: Erythematous scaly plaque with surrounding hyperpigmentation.

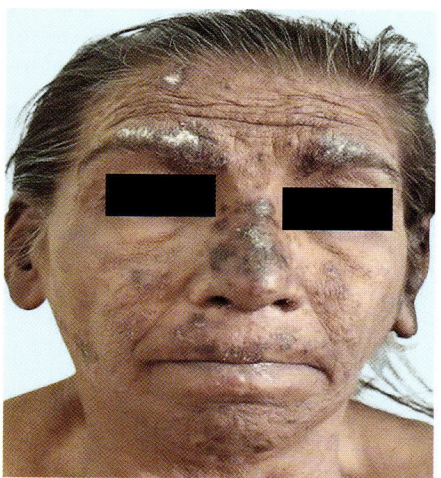

FIG. 6: Hyperpigmented thick scaly plaques.

Q.8. What is the tin-tack/cat tongue sign?
Ans. When the adherent scale is lifted, the surface beneath displays keratinous plugs that have filled the expanded pilosebaceous follicles. It is seen in DLE as well as pemphigus foliaceous.

Q.9. What is Shuster sign?
Ans. In patients with DLE, wide follicular pits are found in the concha or triangular fossa of the ear **(Fig. 7)**.

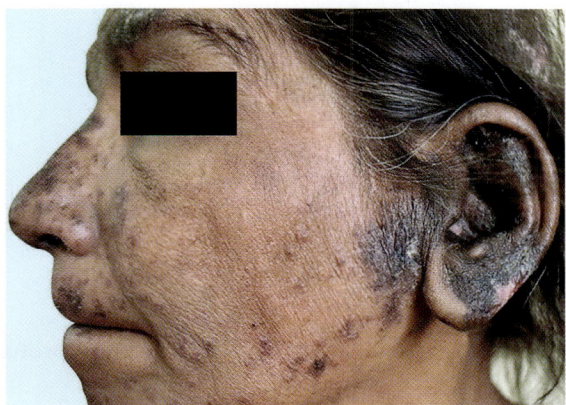

FIG. 7: Shuster sign of discoid lupus erythematosus (DLE) (wide follicular pits in concha).

Q.10. What is the risk of progression from DLE to SLE?
Ans. 5% cases of DLE whereas 20% cases of diffuse discoid lupus erythematosus (DDLE) show progression to SLE.

Q.11. What are dermoscopic findings in the lesion of DLE?
Ans. Branching and linear blood vessels, keratin plugging, perifollicular whitish halo, rosettes, and structureless brown and white areas are the dermoscopic findings in the lesion of DLE.

Q.12. How does tumid LE present?
Ans. Tumid LE presents as firm erythematous, indurated plaque resembling urticarial vasculitis typically lacking scale or follicular plugging on the face and trunk. Surface changes are minimal.

Q.13. When do you suspect lupus panniculitis?
Ans. It appears as indurated erythematous plaques on the face, scalp, upper arms, upper trunk, breasts, buttocks, and thighs, which may progress into disfiguring, depressed areas **(Fig. 8)**.

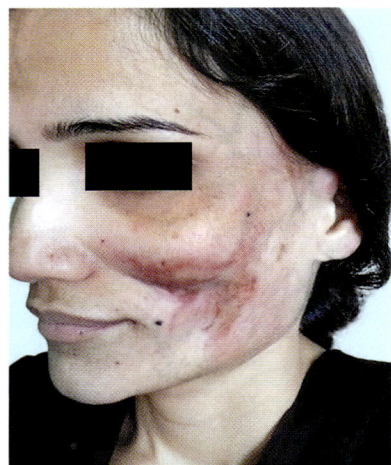

FIG. 8: Lupus panniculitis.

Q.14. What is lupus profundus?

Ans. Discoid lesions overlying the panniculitis are referred to as lupus profundus.

Q.15. What is lupus pernio?

Ans. Chilblains lupus manifests as red or purplish papules and plaques on the toes, fingers, and occasionally on the nose, elbows, knees, and lower legs. These lesions are triggered or worsened by cold, especially cold moist environments.

Q.16. What is Aicardi Groutières syndrome?

Ans. Aicardi Groutières syndrome is a primarily autosomal recessive autoinflammatory disorder characterized by recurrent sterile fevers, progressive developmental delay, and chilblains due to mutations in *TREX1*, *SMAHD1*, *ADAR1*, *IFIH1*, and *RNASEH2A/B/C* genes.

Q.17. What is Rowell syndrome?

Ans. Rowell's syndrome refers to the occurrence of erythema multiforme-like lesions in conjunction with distinctive immunological features, such as a speckled pattern of antinuclear antibodies (ANA), the presence of anti-Ro or anti-La antibodies, and a positive rheumatoid factor in lupus patients. Major criteria include (1) LE—SLE, DLE, and SCLE; (2) erythema multiforme-like lesions (with/without involvement of the mucous membranes); (3) speckled pattern of ANA. Minor criteria were (1) chilblains, (2) anti-Ro antibody or anti-La antibody, and (3) positive RF. All three major criteria and at least one minor criterion is required for a diagnosis of RS **(Figs. 9A and B)**.

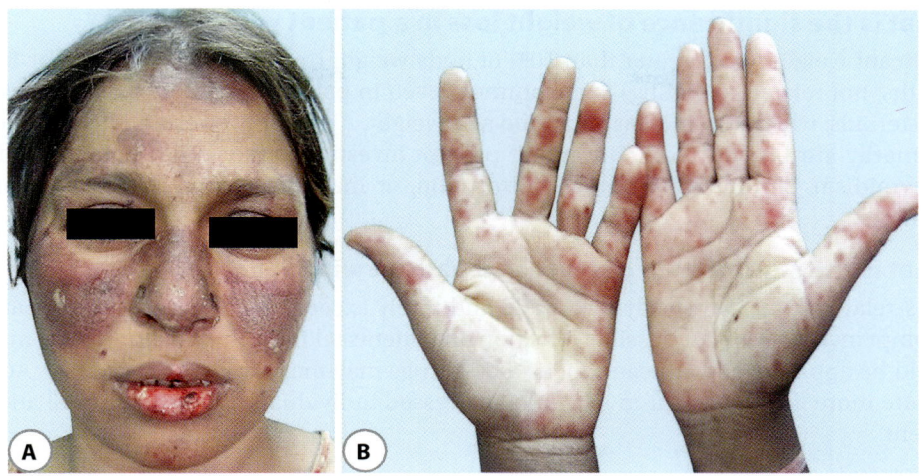

FIGS. 9A AND B: (A) Acute cutaneous lupus erythematosus (ACLE) rash with lesions on palms hemorrhagic cheilitis and (B) erythematous.

Q.18. Discuss Kikuchi–Fujimoto disease.
Ans. Kikuchi–Fujimoto disease is a benign and typically self-limiting condition characterized by histiocytic necrotizing lymphadenitis of unknown etiology. The condition typically presents with tender lymphadenopathy, most often affecting the cervical lymph nodes, with fever, weight loss, and night sweats in more severe cases. Skin manifestations are usually nonspecific and may include erythematous papules, patches, plaques, and less commonly, nodules, bullae, or acneiform eruptions.

Q.19. What is Sneddon syndrome?
Ans. Sneddon syndrome is characterized by widespread livedo racemosa or livedo reticularis, accompanied by cerebrovascular lesions that lead to focal neurological symptoms or signs.

Q.20. How do you assess photosensitivity in the patient?
Ans. The American College of Rheumatology (ACR) defines photosensitivity as an atypical response to sunlight, as noted by the patient's history or the physician's observation. Photosensitivity does not strongly correlate with disease activity and may be linked to lower mortality rates. The severity of a photosensitive rash is assessed based on four factors: (1) The extent of the rash, (2) the degree of erythema, (3) the thickness of the lesions, and (4) the presence of scarring.

Q.21. What is the significance of fatigue in a patient with SLE?
Ans. Fatigue or reduced stamina is almost universally experienced by individuals with active lupus. It can often be the earliest sign of an impending flare and is frequently the first symptom to improve once the flare is managed. Fatigue that limits the ability to perform daily tasks or engage in recreational activities is considered severe fatigue. In SLE, a distinct pattern of fatigue is observed compared to other connective tissue diseases. In SLE, fatigue tends to be milder in the morning and worsens in the evening, whereas in conditions like scleroderma, the reverse is true.

Q.22. What is the significance of weight loss in a patient with SLE?

Ans. Significant weight loss (greater than 10% of body weight over the past 6 months or 5% over the last 3 months, not related to dieting) is uncommon, even in patients with active disease, likely due to the use of steroids, which can increase appetite and weight. As a result, substantial weight loss should not be primarily attributed to SLE, but rather prompt investigation for other potential causes, such as hyperthyroidism, chronic infection, malabsorption, or inadequate food intake, malignancy, etc., should be done.

Q.23. What is the significance of fever in a patient with SLE?

Ans. Lupus-related fever is typically low-grade and rarely exceeds 102°F. A temperature above 102°F should prompt investigation for possible infection. In patients taking immunosuppressive medications, fever should be approached with caution, as these drugs may mask or reduce the fever. Additionally, infections are more likely to occur in immunosuppressed individuals, requiring special attention and management.

Q.24. What is lupus hair?

Ans. Broken and unruly hair along the front hairline, known as lupus hair, is a characteristic feature of nonscarring alopecia in SLE. This pattern of hair loss may be visible upon examination, even if the patient does not report any hair loss.

Q.25. Describe alopecia in SLE.

Ans. Alopecia in SLE may be *scarring* as in DLE or *nonscarring* as in telogen effluvium **(Fig. 10)**.

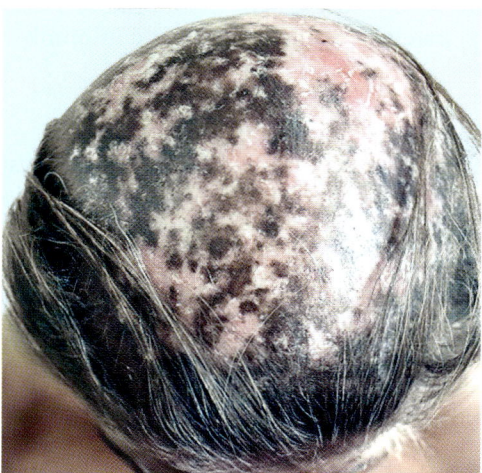

FIG. 10: Scarring alopecia in discoid lupus erythematous (DLE).

Q.26. Discuss mucosal lesions in SLE.

Ans. Painless oral, nasal, or genital ulcers may develop. They indicate a flare of disease activity **(Fig. 11)**.

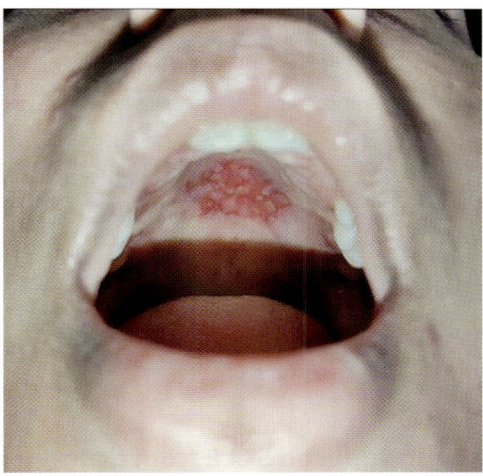

FIG. 11: Mucosal lesions of systemic lupus erythematosus (SLE) (erythematous erosions over hard palate).

Q.27. How does vasculitis present in SLE?

Ans. Vasculitis typically presents as small-vessel leukocytoclastic vasculitis, characterized by palpable petechiae or purpura in dependent areas. When medium **(Figs. 12A and B)** or large vessels are involved, it may appear as retiform or stellate purpura, with or without necrosis and ulceration or as subcutaneous nodules. Additional symptoms may include gangrene, periungual infarcts, splinter hemorrhages, as well as urticarial and bullous lesions **(Table 2)**.

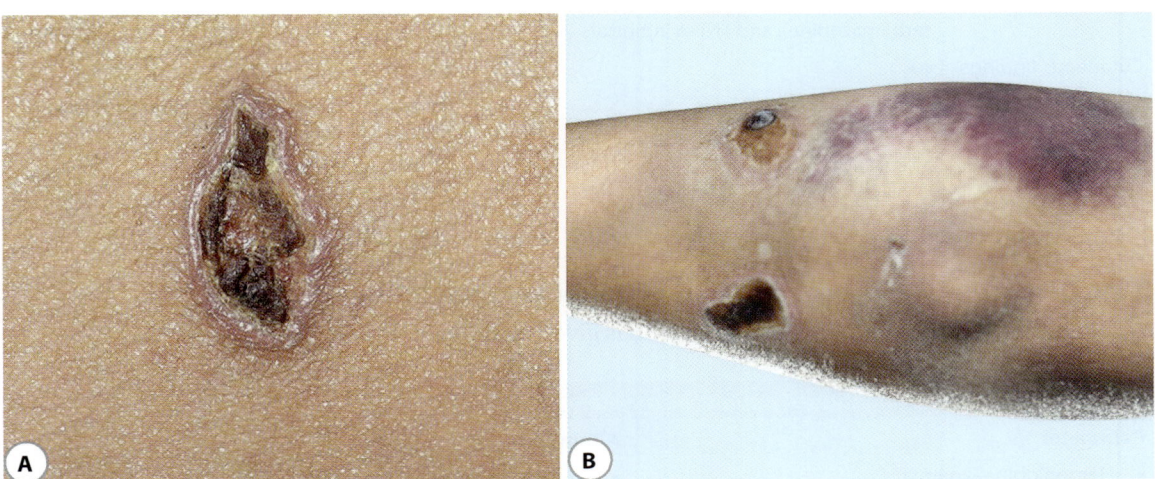

FIGS. 12A AND B: Medium vessel vasculitis: Irregularly shaped punched out ulcers with necrotic base and ecchymosis over leg.

TABLE 2: Vascular manifestations of systemic lupus erythematosus (SLE).

Manifestations	Vessel involved and site
Leukocytoclastic angitis (urticaria and palpable purpura)	Postcapillary venules and upper dermis
Atrophie blanche	Small vessels, middle and lower dermis
Subcutaneous nodules	Medium-sized arteries, panniculitis, and lower dermis
Livedo reticularis	Medium-sized arteries, panniculitis and lower dermis
Coronary arteritis	Coronary arteries
Mononeuritis multiplex	Vasa nervorum
Cerebral infarcts	Primary small vessels
Mesenteric infarcts	Small and medium-sized arteries
Retinopathy	Arterioles and venules

Q.28. How to differentiate drug-induced SCLE from drug-induced LE?

Ans. Differences between drug-induced SCLE and drug induced LE are given in **Table 3**.

TABLE 3: Differences between drug-induced (DI) subacute cutaneous lupus erythematosus (SCLE) and drug induced lupus erythematosus (LE).

	DI-SCLE	DI-SLE
Drugs responsible	Terbinafine, griseofulvin, proton pump inhibitors (such as omeprazole, lansoprazole, and pantoprazole), ranitidine, thiazide diuretics (like hydrochlorothiazide), calcium channel blockers (e.g., diltiazem, nifedipine, and verapamil), ACE inhibitors (e.g., enalapril and lisinopril), β-blockers, statins, antiepileptics (e.g., carbamazepine), and TNF-α inhibitors	Hydralazine, procainamide, isoniazid, quinidine, methyldopa, chlorpromazine, minocycline, and TNF-α inhibitors
Cutaneous findings	++	+/-
Systemic findings	Usually absent, athralgias	Serositis (arthralgia, pleuritis, and pericarditis) Fever, weight loss, and myalgia
Associated auto-antibodies	Anti Ro/SSA	• Anti-histone, • Anti-dsDNA (reported with TNF-α inhibitor)

(ACE: angiotensin-converting enzyme; DNA: deoxyribonucleic acid; TNF: tumor necrosis factor)

Q.29. Discuss laboratory evaluation of patient with SLE.

Ans. Laboratory evaluation of patient with SLE is given in **Table 4**.

TABLE 4: Laboratory evaluation of patient with systemic lupus erythematosus.

Parameter	Alteration
• Hemoglobin—anemia • DCT, and ICT	• Anemia of chronic disease • Iron deficiency anemia • Autoimmune hemolytic anemia • Drug-induced myelotoxicity

Continued

Continued

Parameter	Alteration
	• Anemia of chronic renal disease • Pure red cell aplasia • Aplastic anemia • Reactive hemophagocytic syndrome
White blood cells	• Leukopenia • Lymphopenia
Platelets	Thrombocytopenia
ESR and CRP	Raised
• RFT with electrolytes • Urine protein to creatinine ratio • 24-hour urinary protein	>100 mg/24 hours
LFT	Hypoproteinemia
URM (3 or more days prior to or after cessation of menstrual periods)	• Proteinuria, hematuria • Dysmorphic (irregular or fragmented) erythrocytes suggest inflammatory glomerular or tubulointerstitial disease, while monomorphic (normal) erythrocytes point to bleeding in the lower urinary tract, such as from infection, urolithiasis, or tumors. Granular and fatty casts are typically seen in proteinuric conditions, while red blood cells (RBCs), white blood cells (WBCs), and mixed cellular casts are associated with inflammatory (nephritic) states. Broad and waxy casts are indicative of chronic renal failure
Immunoglobulins	Polyclonal gammopathy
C3, C4	Hypocomplementemia
CXR	
ECG, 2D echocardiogram	
Biopsy and direct immunofluorescence	
Fundoscopy, perimetry, and visual acuity assessment	Ophthalmological screening before starting hydroxychloroquine

(CRP: C-reactive protein; CXR: chest X-ray; DCT: direct Coombs test; ECG: electrocardiogram; ESR: erythrocyte sedimentation rate; ICT: indirect Coombs test; LFT: liver function test; RFT: renal function test)

Q.30. Discuss the various stages of lupus nephritis.

Ans. The various stages of lupus nephritis are given in **Table 5**.

TABLE 5: Characteristic features and clinicopathological correlations in lupus nephritis.

	World Health Organization (WHO) class of lupus nephritis					
	I. Minimal	II. Mesangial	III. FPLN	IV. DPLN	V. Membranous	VI. Sclerosing
Normal urine	X					
Hematuria		X	X	X	+	
Cellular casts			X	X		
Broad, waxy casts			+	+	+	X

Continued

Continued

	World Health Organization (WHO) class of lupus nephritis					
	I. Minimal	II. Mesangial	III. FPLN	IV. DPLN	V. Membranous	VI. Sclerosing
Proteinuria		+	X	X	X	+
Nephrotic syndrome				X	X	
Azotemia				X	+	X
Hypertension				X	+	X

(FPLN: focal proliferative lupus nephritis; DPLN: diffuse proliferative lupus nephritis)

- *Normal or minimal glomerular abnormality:* No glomerular changes were observed under light microscopy.
- *Mesangial nephropathy:* It features mesangial expansion, including increased cellularity, matrix, and immune complex deposits.
- *Focal proliferative glomerulonephritis:* It is characterized by segmental hypercellularity and necrosis affecting <50% of glomeruli, leading to compromised capillary loop circulation and mesangial and subendothelial immune complex deposits.
- *Diffuse proliferative glomerulonephritis:* Typically, it exhibits global yet irregular hypercellularity, necrosis, and possible cellular crescents in >50% of glomeruli; may include sclerosis, atrophy, and fibrosis, with mesangial, subendothelial, and sometimes subepithelial immune complex deposits.
- *Membranous nephropathy:* It is marked by diffuse thickening of capillary loops, with immune complex deposits in the mesangium and subepithelial regions.
- *Sclerosing nephropathy:* It predominantly involves hyalinized glomeruli, tubular atrophy, and interstitial fibrosis, with little to no immune complex deposits.

Q.31. What are extractable nuclear antigens (ENAs)?

Ans. Extractable nuclear antigens are soluble cytoplasmic and nuclear components that are antibody targets with over 100 different antigens described.

Extractable nuclear antigen-4 and its importance: The concept of "ANA-negative lupus" originated from older, less sensitive testing methods and cross-sectional studies, where ANA titers can fluctuate over time and may become negative with treatment. Modern assays using human epithelial cells show that nearly all patients with clinical SLE test positive for ENAs, even if their ANA is negative, and most ANA-negative individuals will have had a positive ANA at some point. However, once ANA levels are documented, tracking titers is not useful for monitoring disease activity. Similarly, specific antibodies such as anti-Ro (anti-SSA), anti-La (anti-SSB), anti-SM, anti-RNP, and anticardiolipin (ACL) antibodies can aid in diagnosis but do not provide insight into whether the disease is currently active.

Q.32. What is ANA-negative lupus?

Ans. A positive ANA test is essential for diagnosing SLE. "ANA-negative lupus", previously thought to represent up to 5% of SLE cases, refers to clinical lupus without typical autoantibodies. In the past, sera from SLE patients could test negative on rodent cells, particularly when the predominant antibodies were those associated with anti-Ro/SSA, seen in conditions such as SCLE and Sjögren's syndrome (SIS). However, with the use of human Hep-2 cells for testing, only about 1–2% of SLE patients now show negative ANA results. As a result, "ANA-negative SLE" is largely considered a historical concept.

Q.33. What is relevance of ANA-titer?
Ans. Relevance of ANA-titer is given in **Tables 6 and 7**.

TABLE 6: Antinuclear antibody (ANA) titers and their clinical significance.	
Titer	**Significance**
<1:40–1:80	Insignificant
1:160 or greater	AI-CTD, 5% of normal individuals
Negative	1–2% cases of SLE

(AI-CTD: autoimmune connective tissue disease; SLE: systemic lupus erythematosus)

TABLE 7: Correlation of antinuclear antibody (ANA) titers and pattern with autoimmune connective tissue disease.	
ANA pattern	**Disease**
Peripheral/Rim	SLE
Homogenous	SLE
Nucleolar	PSS
Fine speckled	SLE, PSS, MCTD, Sjögren's
Coarse speckled	CREST

(CREST: calcinosis, Raynaud's phenomenon, esophageal dysmotility, sclerodactyly, and telangiectasia; MCTD: mixed connective tissue disease; PSS: progressive systemic sclerosis; SLE: systemic lupus erythematosus)

Q.34. Discuss relevance of various ANAs.
Ans. The relevance of various ANAs is given in **Table 8**.
- *Anti-deoxyribonucleic acid (DNA) antibodies:*
  - These are the most well-known specific autoantibodies identified in patients with SLE.
  - Antibodies targeting DNA can be classified into two main types: (1) Those that react with denatured (single-stranded) DNA and (2) those that bind to native (double-stranded) DNA.
  - They are relatively specific (97%) for SLE, making them very useful for diagnosis.
  - *Titers rise when disease is active* and usually fall (generally into the normal range) when the flare subsides.
  - High levels of IgG anti-dsDNA titers are known to be associated with active *glomerulonephritis*; there also appear to be highly enriched amounts of anti-dsDNA antibodies in the glomerular deposits of immune complexes found in patients with lupus nephritis.
- *Anti-Smith antibodies:*
  - The Smith antigen, a nuclear nonhistone protein, was identified in 1966 and was the first nuclear protein autoantigen associated with SLE.
  - Complexes formed by nuclear proteins and RNAs are known as small nuclear ribonucleoprotein particles (snRNPs), which play a crucial role in the splicing of precursor messenger RNA, an essential step in RNA processing from DNA.
  - Anti-Sm antibodies are not highly sensitive (18–30%, depending on the assay) but are highly specific for SLE. These antibodies typically remain detectable even when anti-DNA antibody levels return to normal and the clinical activity of SLE diminishes. Therefore, measuring anti-Sm titers can be diagnostically useful, especially when DNA antibodies are no longer detectable.

- *Antihistone antibodies*: Up to 80% of individuals with SLE and as many as 95% of those with drug-induced lupus erythematosus (DIL) exhibit autoantibodies against histone proteins. The presence of antihistone antibodies provides strong, statistically significant evidence that a patient's symptoms are attributable to DIL.
- *Anti-RNP antibodies:*
    - These antibodies target proteins that contain only U1-RNA. The U1-RNP particle plays a key role in splicing heterogeneous nuclear RNA into messenger RNA.
    - While anti-RNP antibodies are not specific to SLE, they are a hallmark of the related condition known as mixed connective tissue disease.
- *Anti-Ro/Anti-SSA antibodies*: These antinuclear antibodies target cellular proteins with molecular weights of approximately 52 and 60 kDa. The 60 kDa protein is associated with the HY1-5 species of small nuclear RNAs.
  They are frequently found in patients with SLE as well as those with Sjögren's syndrome.
- *Antibodies to ribosomal P proteins:*
    - The targets of these antibodies are three phosphoproteins phloem-specific protein (P proteins) located on the 60S subunit of ribosomes.
    - These antibodies are believed to play a role in protein synthesis, particularly in the interaction between EF-1α, EF-2, and ribosomes.
    - *Ribosomal P protein antibodies and lupus cerebritis:* The presence of ribosomal P protein antibodies has been strongly linked to lupus cases involving psychosis and/or depression.
    - *Antibodies to ribosomal P protein and non-CNS lupus–renal disease:* Some studies have found an association between anti-ribosomal P antibodies and lupus nephritis, including fluctuations in antibody levels corresponding to changes in renal disease activity. However, other studies have not observed such a connection.
    - An association between anti-ribosomal P protein antibodies and antibodies to cardiolipin has been reported, though it remains unclear whether the co-occurrence of these antibodies increases the risk of neuropsychiatric symptoms.
- *Antiphospholipid*: Antiphospholipid antibodies, such as lupus anticoagulants (LAS), ACL antibodies, and $β_2$ glycoprotein I antibodies are known causes of thromboembolic phenomenon, thrombocytopenia, and several adverse obstetrical outcomes.

TABLE 8: Antinuclear antibody (ANA) in various autoimmune connective tissue disease.

Antibodies to	SLE	Sjögren's	SS	DM-PM	MCTD
Ds DNA	+	–	–	–	–
U1RNP	+	–	+	+	+
Sm	+	–	–	–	–
SS-A/Ro	+	+	–	–	–
SS-B/La	+	+	–	–	–
Scl-70	–	–	+	–	–
Centromere	–	–	+	–	–
DM/PM antigens (Jo-1, Mi2, and PI-7)	–	–	–	+	–

(SLE: systemic lupus erythematosus; SS: systemic sclerosis; DM: dermatomyositis; PM: polymyositis; MCTD: mixed connective tissue disease)

Q.35. What are "LE cells"?

Ans.
- LE cells are polymorphonuclear leukocytes that have engulfed nuclear material from disintegrating white blood cells in the presence of antibodies against deoxyribonucleoprotein. This is also referred to as the "LE phenomenon".
- LE cells are found in SLE, chronic DLE, systemic sclerosis, rheumatoid arthritis, DIL.

Q.36. What is lupus band test?

Ans. Deposition of immunoglobulin generally IgM and IgG and/or complement at the dermoepidermal junction in patient with LE is known as lupus band test **(Table 9)**.
- *IgG, IgM, IgA, and C3:* Most common
- *85%:* Multiple immune deposits
- *45%:* IgG and lg M+/-C3
- *Patterns:* Linear, granular, and shaggy
- The intensity of fluorescence is directly related to the levels of dsDNA antibodies and thus reflects the activity of the disease.

TABLE 9: Lupus band test in various subtypes of lupus.

Subtype	Lesional	Nonlesional sun exposed	Nonlesional nonsun exposed
SLE	++	++	++
SCLE	+	+/−	−
DLE	+	−	−

(DLE: discoid lupus erythematosus; SCLE: subacute cutaneous lupus erythematosus; SLE: systemic lupus erythematosus)

Q.37. What are the 2019 EULAR criteria for the diagnosis of SLE?

Ans.
Entry criterion: ANA of ≥ 1;80 on Hep-2 cells or an equivalent positive test
- *If absent:* Do not classify as SLE.
- *If present:* Apply additive criteria.

Additive criteria:
- Occurrence of a criterion at any one occasion is sufficient.
- Criteria need not occur simultaneously.
- SLE classification requires at least one clinical criterion and a score of >10.
  Classify as SLE if the entry criterion is fulfilled and there is a score of 10 or more **(Tables 10 and 11)**.

TABLE 10: Criteria and weighting system for clinical domains in systemic lupus erythematosus (SLE) diagnosis.

Clinical domain	Criteria	Weight
Constitutional	Fever	2
Hematological	• Leukopenia • Thrombocytopenia • Autoimmune hemolysis	3 4 4
Neuropsychiatric	• Delirium • Psychosis • Seizures	2 3 5

Continued

Continued

Clinical domain	Criteria	Weight
Mucocutaneous	• Nonscarring alopecia	2
	• Oral ulcers	2
	• SCLE/DLE	4
	• ACLE	6
Serositis	• Pleural/Pericardial effusion	5
	• Acute pericarditis	6
Musculo-skeletal	Joint involvement	6
Renal	• >0.5 g/24 hours proteinuria	4
	• Renal biopsy class II or V nephritis	8
	• Renal biopsy class III or IV nephritis	10

(ACLE: acute cutaneous lupus erythematosus; DLE: discoid lupus erythematosus; SCLE: subacute cutaneous lupus erythematosus)

TABLE 11: 2019 EULAR criteria for the diagnosis of systemic lupus erythematosus (SLE).[1]

Immunological domain	Criteria	Weight
Antiphospholipid antibodies	• Anticardiolipin	2
	• Anti-beta-2 glycoprotein-1	
	• Lupus anticoagulant	
Complement proteins	• Low C3 or low C4	3
	• Low C3 and low C4	4
SLE-specific antibodies	• Anti-ds-DNA antibody or	6
	• Anti-Smith antibody	

(DNA: deoxyribonucleic acid; EULAR: The European Alliance of Associations for Rheumatology)

Q.38. What are clinical and immunologic criteria used in the Systemic Lupus International Collaborating Clinics (SLICC) classification system?

Ans.

Clinical criteria:
- *ACLE, including*:
  - Lupus malar rash (do not count if malar discoid)
  - Bullous lupus
  - Toxic epidermal necrolysis variant of SLE
  - Maculopapular lupus rash
  - Photosensitive lupus rash in the absence of dermatomyositis
- SCLE (nonindurated psoriasiform and/or annular polycyclic lesions that resolve without scarring, although occasionally with postinflammatory dyspigmentation or telangiectasias)
- *Chronic cutaneous lupus, including*:
  - Classic discoid rash
  - Localized (above the neck)
  - Generalized (above and below the neck)
  - Hypertrophic (verrucous) lupus
  - Lupus panniculitis (profundus)
  - Mucosal lupus
  - Lupus erythematosus tumidus

- Chilblains lupus
- Discoid lupus/lichen planus overlap
- *Oral ulcers*:
  - Palate
  - Buccal
  - Tongue
  - Nasal ulcers in the absence of other causes, such as vasculitis, Behçet's disease, infection (herpes virus, inflammatory bowel disease, reactive arthritis, and acidic foods
- Non-scarring alopecia (diffuse thinning or hair fragility with visible broken hairs) in the absence of other causes such as alopecia areata, drugs, iron deficiency, and androgenic alopecia
- Synovitis involving two or more joints, characterized by swelling or effusion or tenderness in two or more joints and at least 30 minutes of morning stiffness
- *Serositis*:
  - Typical pleurisy for >1 day; or pleural effusions; or pleural rub
  - Typical pericardial pain (pain with recumbency improved by sitting forward) for more than 1 day pericardial effusion; or pericardial rub; or pericarditis by electrocardiography in the absence of other causes, such as infection, uremia, and Dressler's pericarditis
- *Renal:*
  - Urine protein-to-creatinine ratio (or 24-hour urine protein) representing 500 mg protein/24 hours
  - Red blood cell casts
- *Neurologic:*
  - Seizures
  - Psychosis
  - Mononeuritis multiplex (In the absence of other known causes such as primary vasculitis)
  - Myelitis
  - Peripheral or cranial neuropathy the absence of other known causes such as primary vasculitis, infection, and diabetes mellitus
  - Acute confusional state
  - In the absence of other causes, including toxic/metabolic, uremia, and drugs
- Hemolytic anemia
- Leukopenia (–4,000/mm^3 at least once) in the absence of other known causes such as Felty's syndrome, drugs, and portal hypertension
- Lymphopenia (–1,000/mm^3 at least once) in the absence of other known causes such as corticosteroids, drugs, and infection.
- Thrombocytopenia (–100,000/mm^3) at least once in the absence of other known causes such as drugs, portal hypertension, and thrombotic thrombocytopenic purpura.

Immunologic criteria:
- ANA level above laboratory reference range
- Anti-dsDNA antibody level above laboratory reference range or 2-fold the reference range if tested by enzyme-linked immunosorbent assay (ELISA)
- *Anti-Sm:* Presence of antibody to Sm nuclear antigen
- *Antiphospholipid antibody positivity as determined by any of the following*:
  - Positive test result for lupus anticoagulant
  - False-positive test result for rapid plasma regain
  - Medium- or high-titer ACL antibody level (IgA and IgG) or IgM
  - Positive test result for anti-beta-2 glycoprotein I (IgA, IgG, or IgM)

- *Low complement*:
  - Low C3
  - Low C4
  - Low CH50
- Direct Coombs test positive in the absence of hemolytic anemia

Note: The patient must satisfy *at least 4 criteria*, including at least one clinical criterion and one immunologic criterion or the patient must have biopsy-proven lupus nephritis in the presence of ANA or anti-dsDNA antibodies.[2]

Q.39. What are the differences between pediatric and adult SLE?

Ans. The clinical presentation, progression, and treatment are similar to those in adults; however, children generally experience a more acute and severe form of the disease.

Onset of pediatric SLE is described even in children younger than 2 years of age.
- The F/M ratio with pediatric SLE ranges from 4:3 with disease onset during the first decade of life to 4:1, during the second decade, to 9:1 in adult SLE, and decreases to 5:1 in SLE commencing after the age of 50 years.
- At disease onset, fever, malar rash, vasculitis, and arthralgia are found more common in childhood LE.
- Lupus nephritis, hematological disorders, photosensitivity, butterfly rash, and mucosal ulceration are more common in pediatric LE.
- Childhood SLE is more frequently associated with neurological symptoms, renal involvement is more severe, and also enlargement of the liver, spleen, and lymph nodes is frequent.
- Cardiovascular mortality is more prevalent in adult SLE, and in children, mortality is more due to renal cause.
- Anti-SSA, anti-SSB, and antiphospholipid antibodies are found at notably higher levels in adults with SLE compared to pediatric patients.
- Children are more frequently treated with high-dose intravenous immunoglobulin and mycophenolate mofetil than adults.
- These differences highlight that pediatric and adult-onset lupus exhibit distinct characteristics, underscoring the need to recognize these variations to ensure the best treatment and prognosis for each group.

Q.40. What are the causes of death in systemic lupus erythematosus?

Ans. Deaths related to SLE often occur within the first 5–10 years after the onset of symptoms.
- During the early stages of the disease, mortality is typically due to severe SLE manifestations, such as central nervous system (CNS), renal, or cardiovascular involvement, or complications from infections caused by immunosuppressive treatments.
- In contrast, later deaths, typically after age 35 years, are usually linked to myocardial infarction or stroke, which are a result of accelerated atherosclerosis. The presence of lupus nephritis may further elevate these risks.

Q.41. What are the predictors of systemic disease in patients with DLE?

Ans.
- Generalized DLE lesions, i.e., DDLE
- Palmoplantar DLE
- DLE in setting of genetic complement deficiencies

- DLE associated with constitutional symptoms
- DLE associated with acute phase reactants or complement activation
- DLE with an ANA at significant titers (fine speckled >1:320)
- DLE with a specific ANA (anti-Sm and Ro)
- DLE in male patients

Q.42. How to differentiate CNS lupus flare from corticosteroid-induced psychiatric reactions?

Ans. Differences between CNS lupus flare and corticosteroid-induced psychiatric reactions are given in **Table 12**.

TABLE 12: Difference between central nervous system (CNS) lupus flare and corticosteroid-induced psychiatric reaction		
	CNS lupus flare	**Corticosteroid-induced psychiatric reactions**
Onset	After decrease in steroid-dose or ongoing low-dose treatment	Generally, 2 weeks after corticosteroid dosage
Corticosteroid dosage (mg/kg of prednisolone)	Variable	• Common if ≥ 60 mg/day • Rare if <40 mg/day
Psychiatric manifestations	Psychosis, delirium, mood disorders, and cognitive impairment (new onset)	Mania, mixed states, depression (often with mood disorders and psychotic features), psychosis, and delirium
Systemic SLE symptoms	Often present, coincide with onset of psychiatric symptoms	Often present, but precede onset of psychiatric symptoms
Laboratory evaluation	Indices of inflammation	No specific lab findings
Quantitative brain MRI	White matter changes, micro-infarcts, and cortical atrophy	No specific findings
Response to corticosteroid trial	Improvement	Exacerbation or persistence of symptoms

Q.43. Explain lupus foot.

Ans. Lupus foot is a deforming arthropathy of the feet in SLE.
- It includes hallux valgus, subluxation of the metatarsophalangeal joints, and widening of the forefoot.

Q.44. How will you evaluate pregnant women with autoimmune disorders?

Ans. Initial screening is done by ELISA in first trimester **(Flowchart 2)**.

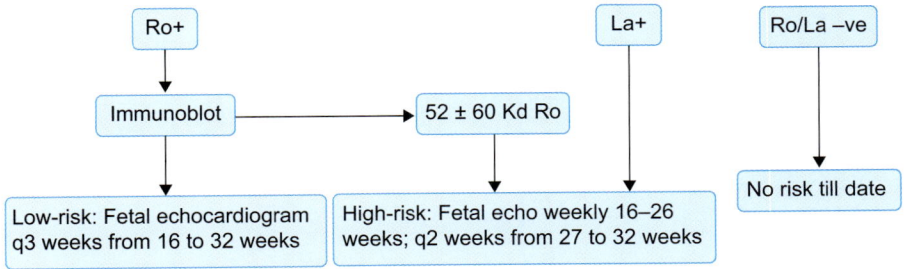

FLOWCHART 2: Evaluation of pregnant women with autoimmune disorders.

REFERENCES

1. Fanouriakis A, Kostopoulou M, Andersen J, Aringer M, Arnaud L, Bae SC, et al. EULAR recommendations for the management of systemic lupus erythematosus: 2023 update. Ann Rheum Dis. 2024;83:15-29.
2. Petri M, Orbai AM, Alarcón GS, Gordon C, Merrill JT, Fortin PR, et al. Derivation and validation of the Systemic Lupus International Collaborating Clinics classification criteria for systemic lupus erythematosus. Arthritis Rheum. 2012;64(8):2677-86.

CHAPTER 4

Systemic Sclerosis, Dermatomyositis, and Other Connective Tissue Diseases

INTRODUCTION

This chapter discusses the 2 cases. One is systemic sclerosis (SSc) and other is dermatomyositis (DM) patient who may require admission in the ward.

It includes salient aspects of history taking and examination, and lab evaluation to arrive at diagnosis and management of the patient. It is followed by frequently asked questions during viva voce for this long case.

CASE 1: SYSTEMIC SCLEROSIS

A 38-year-old, female presented with:

Chief Complaints
- Painful bluish discoloration of fingers on exposure to cold × 15 years.
- Tightness of skin over hands, feet, and face × 10 years.
- Breathlessness on exertion and pain, and stiffness of the knee joint, the elbow joint, and the back × 5 years.
- Difficulty in swallowing solid food × 4 years.
- Ulceration over fingertips and blackening of toes × 1 year.

History of Present Illness

The patient was relatively asymptomatic 15 years ago. Then, she started to experience painful discoloration of fingers and toes. They turned blue on exposure to cold that lasted for approximately 10 minutes and reverted to normal color on rewarming. After 5 years, she noticed a gradual tightening of her skin first over her hands, followed by her feet, than her face, which then spread to involve the most of her body over 1 year. Since the past 5 years, the patient started developing breathlessness on exertion and daily activities associated with a nonproductive cough. She also developed stiffness and pain first in the knee joint, followed by the elbow joint, and back, chiefly in the morning, lasting for <30 minutes. There was aggravation of symptoms on doing physical exertion. For the past 4 years, there has been difficulty in opening her mouth and difficulty in swallowing, especially for solid food and increased hair fall since 2 years. She had developed ulcers over finger tips since the past 1 year. She experienced increased fatigability and malaise since 1 month.

There was no history of headache, seizures, visual disturbances, oral lesions, chest pain, post prandial abdominal pain, palpitations, vomiting, heart burn, constipation, diarrhea, increased flatulence, bloating, decreased urine output, pedal edema, swelling around eyelids, cloudy urine, blood in urine, recurrent abortions, fever, or weight loss.

Treatment History

The patient had been given tablet. Prednisolone in various doses and azathioprine 50 mg twice, tablet. Nifedipine (10 mg) twice, Tadalafil (20 mg) ½ once. She had been given injection cyclophosphamide pulse (4) by a rheumatologist.

Past History

No history of Diabetes, hypertension, thyroid disorder, tuberculosis, jaundice, or any major medical or surgical illness.

Personal History

The patient is illiterate and unemployed.
- *Diet*: Mixed
- *Appetite*: Reduced
- *Sleep*: Reduced
- *Bowel*: Unaltered
- *Bladder*: Unaltered
- *Addiction*: None

Family History

There is no history of similar complaints in the family. The patient is unmarried and the eldest of four siblings.

Menstrual History

The patient has regularly spaced, moderately long, and painless cycles.

Physical Examination

Examination is done under proper light, adequate exposure, and with a female attendant. Patient is malnourished and well oriented to time, place, and person.
- *Temperature*: 98.4°F
- *Pulse*: Felt with difficulty, 88 beats/min, right radial artery with adequate volume, amplitude, and rhythm with no radioradial or radiofemoral delay
- *Blood pressure*: 110/88 mm Hg in the right brachial artery in the supine position by auscultatory method.
- *Respiratory rate*: 18 breaths/min, abdomino-thoracic.
- Pallor is present. No jaundice, cyanosis, clubbing, or lymphadenopathy. Jugular venous pressure (JVP) is not raised.

SYSTEMIC INVOLVEMENT IN SYSTEMIC SCLEROSIS

CARDIOVASCULAR SYSTEM

Cardiac involvement is very common in SS. It is major cause of mortality in SS. The various manifestations are myocarditis pericardial effusion tamponade, myocardial fibrosis with resultant diastolic dysfunction, cardiac arrhythmia, and pulmonary hypertension. Heart failure is not because of coronary artery disease, but due to adverse myocardial remodeling and fibrosis, leading to increased stiffness and diminished compliance of the heart chambers. Clinically, this manifests as left ventricular (LV) diastolic dysfunction, which is highly prevalent in SS and is associated with increased mortality.

A careful cardiac examination, including physical examination, ECG, and echocardiogram, should be part of the comprehensive evaluation of potential cardiac symptoms. ECG shows a bifid P-wave and T-wave changes indicating atrial and ventricular myocardial involvement.

Warning Signs: Abnormalities on the echocardiogram, including right ventricular systolic pressure of 40 mm Hg, suggest the presence of pulmonary disease and warrant intervention like right heart catheterization. Unexplained new-onset fatigue, dyspnea, or palpitations with a normal echo should prompt consideration for right heart catheterization.

RESPIRATORY SYSTEM

Check for respiratory rate, chest expansion during maximal inspiration, and auscultate for bilateral symmetry for air entry and/or any abnormal sounds. Chest expansion is measured at the level of T4. In a normal person, chest expansion is 6 cm, while <3 cm at maximum inspiration is suggestive of reduced chest expansion. Interstitial lung disease (ILD)[1,2] and pulmonary artery hypertension (PAH) are two of the most common and two of the most dreaded complications of SS. ILD is now the leading cause of death for patients with SS followed by PAH, and both result in cardiopulmonary failure **(Table 1)**.

TABLE 1: Patterns of lung involvement.	
Interstitial lung disease (ILD)	**Pulmonary artery hypertension (PAH)**
Seen in 70% of patients at autopsy	Seen in 5% of patients at autopsy
More common in diffuse systemic sclerosis	More common in limited systemic sclerosis
Clinical feature: Dyspnea on exertion and then at rest, persistent dry cough	*Clinical feature*: Chest pain, dyspnea at rest, out of proportion
Starts as microvascular injury and alveolitis	• On examination: Accentuated P2 • Right ventricular heave (due to right ventricular hypertrophy) • Systolic pulmonary artery pressure >35 mm Hg represents pulmonary artery hypertension
Cyanosis, clubbing, and cor pulmonale can develop	

GASTROINTESTINAL SYSTEM

Any part of the gastrointestinal (GI) tract can be affected, from the mouth to the anus, with any site of involvement capable of contributing to the severe impairment of quality of life with pervasive manifestations, such as pain, nausea, malnutrition, food intolerance, diarrhea, colonic inertia, and fecal incontinence.

- *Esophagus*: Involved in 75–90% case, weakness and incoordination in esophageal smooth muscle cause lower esophageal sphincter incompetence and decreased peristalsis in lower two-thirds of esophagus leads to dysmotility and gastroesophageal reflux (twice more common than dysphagia) leading to chronic esophagitis, causing ulceration, bleeding, Barret's metaplasia, distal dysphagia due to decreased peristalsis and decreased propulsive activity.
- *Stomach*: Because of atrophy of smooth muscle and fibrotic changes, feeling of bloating due to decreased peristalsis. Dilatation and delayed gastric emptying lead to telangiectasia of gastric antral vessels, which further leads to bleeding, resulting in anemia and hematemesis.
- *Duodenum*: Fibrotic changes in the second and third parts of the duodenum cause hypomotility, leading to dilatation and aperistalsis, which also causes postprandial abdominal pain, bloating, regurgitation, and vomiting.
- *Small and large intestine*: Fibrosis leads to hypomotility, which gives rise to pseudo-obstruction, abdominal distention, colicky abdominal pain, and volvulus of the small intestine. Malabsorption leads to bacterial overgrowth, which causes diarrhea and weight loss. Wide-mouthed colonic diverticula can be found on the inferior surface of the transverse colon, which can promote bacterial growth, diarrhea, chronic obstruction, megacolon, or even perforation, thereby causing peritonitis. Loss of muscle in the rectal muscle can result in anal sphincter incontinence and rectal prolapse. Death may occur due to paralytic ileus.

Pancreatic function is abnormal in 15% of patients.

MUSCULOSKELETAL SYSTEM

Bone Involvement

- Generalized arthralgia and morning stiffness (often preceding skin changes), severe mortar deformity of the distal interphalangeal joints resembling flexion contractures.
- Acro-osteolysis (resorption of the distal end of the phalanx) due to long-standing digital ischemia. It also shows the pestle and mortar deformity of the distal interphalangeal joint, resembling psoriatic arthropathy. Differential diagnosis is gout and psoriatic arthropathy. Other sites of osteolysis are the distal radius, mandibular condyles, cervical spine, and superior portion of posterior ribs.
- Bulbous terminal phalanges.
- Juxta-articular osteoporosis, osteopoikilosis (multiple small islands of dense bone occurring at epiphysis and metaphysis).
- A vascular necrosis of the femoral head due to vasculitis.
- Carpal tunnel syndrome

Tendon Involvement

Fibrosis occurs, which leads to leathery, audible, palpable friction rubs on moving tendons actively or passively. It is seen in 25% of patients and is a characteristic feature of SSc and may precede joint involvement.

Muscle Involvement

Systemic sclerosis can cause myopathy:
- *Site*: Forearm, hand, and proximal muscles
- *Myopathy in SSc can be of two types*:

1. *Noninflammatory*: In 60–80% cases of myopathy in SSc. It presents with mild weakness and a minimally elevated creatine phosphokinase level.
2. *Inflammatory myositis*: Accounts for 6–12% of myositis in SSc. Raised creatine levels.
- EMG is abnormal in 50% of SSc patients in the early stage and in 93% in late disease.

CUTANEOUS EXAMINATION

Of the various affected sites, the hand, face, and lips show typical cutaneous changes.
- *Skin thickening*: It typically occurs after the onset of Raynaud's phenomenon (RP) and is often linked to internal organ involvement, highlighting the importance of initiating rheumatologic care before the skin changes worsen. Initially, the skin may exhibit swelling or a doughy texture starting at the distal parts of the limbs. In cases of diffuse cutaneous systemic sclerosis (dcSSc), the thickening then spreads proximally, extending beyond the elbows and/or knees. As the condition progresses, the skin may become tightly bound, leading to a rigid, hide-bound appearance. This can result in joint contractures due to the involvement of the skin, fascia, and muscles.
- Taut, shiny skin with a firm and thickened feel, tightly bound to underlying subcutaneous tissue.
- Decreased ability to make a skin fold; fading away of skin creases.
- Fading of dorsal veins.
- Hair loss
- Decreased sweating.
- Sclerosis starts acrally and progresses proximally symmetrically, though not always in a continuous pattern.
- *First sign to appear in SSc*:[1] Bulbous swelling of the fingers, also called the round finger pad sign.
- Facial features in a patient of SSc **(Figs. 1A and B)**.
  - Face is involved in both limited and diffuse SSc. Forehead is smooth, shiny with hide-bound skin, lines of facial expression are smoothened, and the patient has mask-like facies.
  - Parrot beak-like nose, i.e., pinched nose.
  - Radial furrows around the mouth giving a purse-string appearance **(Figs. 1A and B)**.
  - Thinning of the upper lip

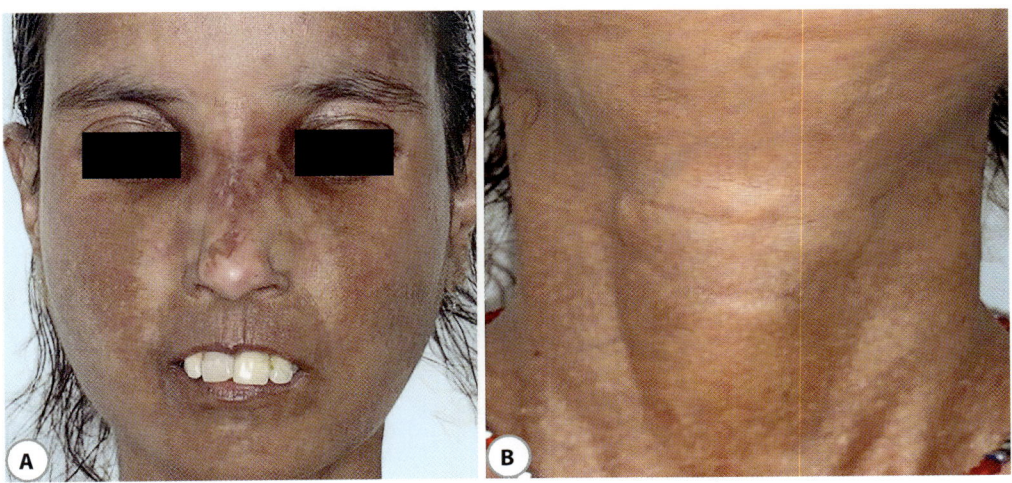

FIGS. 1A AND B: Diffuse pigmentation on face and neck (mottled depigmentation is visible), mask like facies.

Differential diagnosis of mask-like face: An expressionless physiognomy or complete lack of facial effect is called a mask, such as facies, seen in SS.[1]
- Parkinsonism
- Moebius syndrome
- Hereditary congenital facial paresis
- Myotonic dystrophy
- Infantile botulism
- Prader–Willi disease
- Wilson syndrome
- Facioscapulohumeral-type muscular dystrophy.

Reduced oral aperture leading to microstomia due to perioral skin involvement.

When to label decreased oral opening in SS as microstomia?: It is objectively measured by the use of a vernier calliper. Central incisor teeth distance is measured by vernier callipers: In males, <4.5 cm, and in females, <3.9 cm is considered microstomia.

Lip retraction leading to prominent central incisors and an impossible normal mouth closure.

Frenulum sclerosis causing restricted movement of the tongue.

The lower eyelid cannot be depressed easily (Ingram's sign).

Sclerodactyly: The term sclerodactyly is derived from Greek word "skleros", meaning hard, and "dakrylos", meaning a finger or toe, i.e., hard finger or toes. Thus, sclerodactyly is a localized thickening and tightness of the skin of fingers or toes **(Fig. 2)**. It is found in:
- Scleroderma
- Mixed connective tissue disease
- CREST syndrome
- Graft-versus-host disease (GVHD)
- Pseudoscleroderma
- Diabetic sclerodactyly

Flexion contracture: Fingers held in semiflexion and even the elbow in advanced cases due to taut skin.

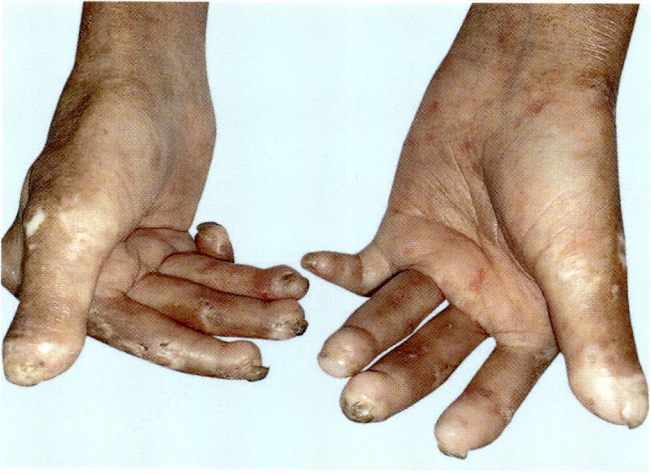

FIG. 2: Sclerodactyly with stellate scars on finger tips.

Ulcers/pits on fingertips, bony prominences: Elbow, malleoli, and dorsal aspect of proximal interphalangeal joint (PIP).

Other findings may include: Reabsorption of terminal phalanges
- *Leg ulcers (40% of cases)*: Nonhealing
- Erythema over the thenar and hypothenar eminence
- Livedo reticularis and small areas of atrophie blanche around ankles, even without ulceration.
- Hyperkeratotic plaque over phalanges (3–20 mm in diameter): Due to amyloid material deposition in the dermal papillae.

Cobblestone appearance: As the sclerosing process leads to blockage of lymphatic channels, causing multiple small papules of lymphangiectasias, giving a cobblestone appearance.

Pigmentary changes: In 50% of patients, a salt and pepper appearance due to hyperpigmentation alternating with hypopigmentation. Tanned appearance-mostly face, followed by leg, thigh, lower abdomen, axillary folds (dense warty pigmentation like acanthosis), and dorsum of hands.

Telangiectasia: A more prominent skin manifestation of localized cutaneous systemic sclerosis (IcSS) are rhomboid-shaped (mat-like), 2–20 mm in diameter, dilated capillary clusters that are typically found on the face, oral mucosa, lips, fingers, and palms. Telangiectasias are often a prognostic feature of SS that is associated with vasculopathy and predictive for the presence of occult or potential development of PAH and heart involvement.

Calcinosis cutis: It refers to the deposition of calcium in the skin. It presents as multiple, firm, whitish dermal papules, plaque, nodules, or subcutaneous nodules in vicinity of joints **(Fig. 2)**. It is seen on:
- Fingers, palmar aspect of terminal phalanges. It is 10 times more common in females.
- Soft tissue around the iliac crest, alongside the spine between vertebrae
- Around elbows, where olecranon bursa may be involved.
- Dorsa of feet
- Around knees

Calcification can occur in internal organs, and while the deposits tend to be large in size, they are generally less widespread compared to the calcification observed in the muscles of healed DM.[3] Calcium deposits may break down with spontaneous ulceration, extruding a chalky white material.

Questions and Answers

Q.1. How to investigate a patient with SS?

Ans. A patient with SS needs to be investigated with the following parameters to find out: Confirmation of diagnosis, to determine the extent of systemic involvement and also understand the likely prognosis, and to exclude if any contraindications exist in the patient before starting systemic immunosuppressive therapy.
- *Complete blood count with differential count*: It may show—normocytic normochromic anemia—due to chronic inflammation. Microcytic anemia—due to iron deficiency secondary to GI bleeding. Macrocytic anemia—due to resultant folate deficiency and bacterial overgrowth in the intestines. Microangiopathic hemolytic anemia—associated with a positive Coombs' test in around 25% cases.
- *Erythrocyte sedimentation rate (ESR)*: Raised in half of patients; other acute phase reactants are normal.
- *Serum complements levels*: Usually normal. It may be elevated in around 8% cases.
- *Rheumatoid factor*: Around 30% of the patients.

- *Anticardiolipin antibodies*: Around 25% of the patients. Various antibodies, their target antigens, frequency, and clinical associations are depicted **Table 2** and **Figure 3**.

TABLE 2: Characteristics of various antibodies in systemic sclerosis.[2]

Antibody	Target antigen	Frequency	Clinical association
Anti-centromere	An antibody that reacts with the kinetochore of a metaphase chromosome	• LcSS 60% • DcSS 2% • CREST 40–70%	• LcSS • Isolated pulmonary hypertension • Severe cutaneous disease favorable prognosis
Anti scl-70	Antibody to topoisomerase 1-Unique to systemic sclerosis	• DcSS 40% • LsSS 15%	• Diffuse skin sclerosis • Pulmonary fibrosis
RNAP	RNA polymerase 3	• DcSS 25% • LsSS 2%	• Diffuse skin sclerosis, hypertensive renal crisis
Nrnp	Ul RNP	15% of SS	Overlap of SS and SLE
PM-SCl		15% of SS	Myositis SS overlap

(CREST: calcinosis, Raynaud's phenomenon, esophageal dysfunction, sclerodactyly, and telangiectasis; DcSSc: diffuse cutaneous systemic sclerosis; LcSSc: localized cutaneous systemic sclerosis; PM-Scl: polymyositis-systemic sclerosis overlap; RNA: ribonucleic acid; RNAP: ribonucleic acid polymerase; RNP: ribonucleoprotein; SS: synovial sarcoma; SLE: systemic lupus erythematosus)

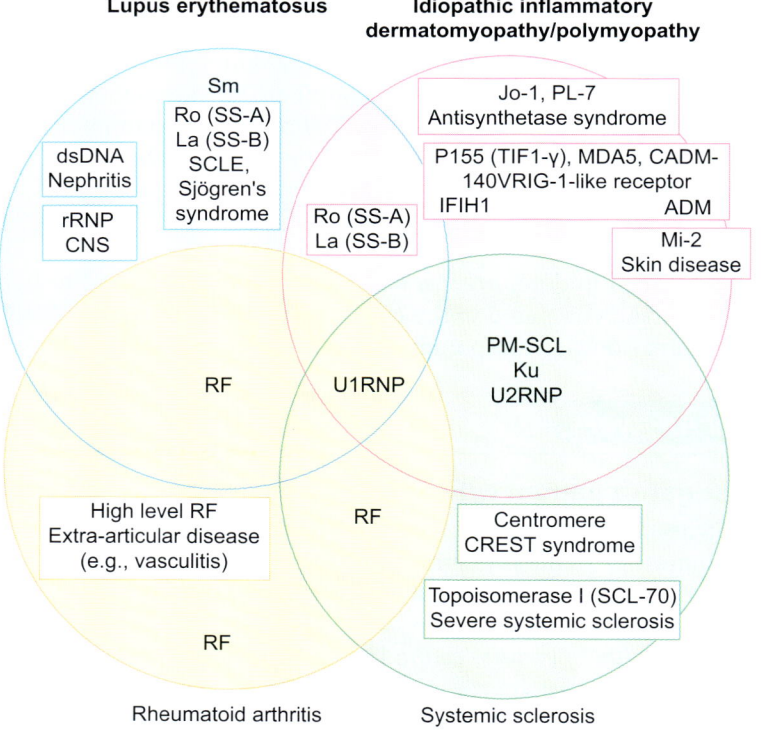

FIG. 3: ANA in various AICTD.

(AICTD: autoimmune connective tissue disease; ANA: antinuclear antibody; CNS: central nervous system; CREST: calcinosis, Raynaud's phenomenon, esophageal dysfunction, sclerodactyly, and telangiectasis; MDAS: malondialdehyde modified epitopes; RF: rheumatoid factor; RNA: ribonucleic acid; rRNP: ribonucleoprotein; SS: synovial sarcoma; SLE: systemic lupus erythematosus)

Urine analysis and renal function test: To monitor and to diagnose scleroderma renal crisis. It had the worst prognosis and highest mortality before the advent of angiotensin-converting enzyme (ACE) inhibitors. Increased risk in patients with diffuse SS and rapidly progressive skin thickening can lead to increased risk for acute renal crisis, which manifests as:
- Headache
- Vision disturbances
- Cramps
- Left ventricular hypertrophy
- Retinopathy
- End-organ damage is present with encephalopathy, with generalized seizures, and pulmonary edema. Renal crisis usually occurs within 4 years of diagnosis in 75% of patients.

Diagnostic criteria:
- Proteinuria <1 g/24 h
- Azotemia (BUN > 25 mg/100 mL)
- Arterial hypertension (>140/90 mm Hg)
- Decreased glomerular filtration rate
- Ask patients to measure blood pressure frequently, but 10% develop it even in the absence of elevated blood pressure

These changes result from either vasospasm of arterioles or hypotension, which causes endothelial damage in arcuate arteries and arterioles.

Q.2. Define EULAR criteria.

Ans. The American College of Rheumatology/European League Against Rheumatism (EULAR) criteria for the classification of SSc **(Table 3)**.

TABLE 3: ACR/EULAR[2] criteria for classification of SSc.		
Eular	**Subitem**	**Weight/Score**
Skin thickening of the fingers of both hands extending proximal to the metacarpophalangeal joints (sufficient criterion)	–	9
Skin thickening of the fingers only (count the higher score)	• Puffy fingers • Sclerodactyly of the fingers (distal to the metacarpophalangeal joints but proximal to the proximal interphalangeal joint)	2 4
Fingertip lesions (only count the higher score)	• Digital ulcers • Fingertip pitting scars	2 3
Telangiectasia		2
Abnormal nailfold capillaries		2
Pulmonary arterial hypertension and/or interstitial lung disease (maximum score is 2)	Pulmonary arterial hypertension interstitial lung disease	2 2
Raynaud's phenomenon		3
Ssc-related autoantibodies (anticentromere, antitopoisomerase 1, anti-scl-70, anti-RNAP-III)	• Anticentromere • Antitopoisomerase • Anti-RNA polymerase III	3

These criteria are used to evaluate patients for inclusion in an SSc study. They do not apply to individuals with skin thickening that spares the fingers or those with a scleroderma-like condition that better accounts for their symptoms, such as nephrogenic sclerosing fibrosis, generalized morphea, eosinophilic fasciitis, scleroderma diabeticorum, scleromyxedema, erythromelalgia, porphyria, lichen sclerosus, graft-versus-host disease, or diabetic cheiroarthropathy. The total score is calculated by summing the highest score in each category. A total score of 9 or higher is used to classify a patient as having definite SSc.

Nailfold capillaroscopy: It is a very useful diagnostic tool in evaluating patients with Raynaud's phenomenon. During this procedure, a drop of immersion oil is applied to the base of the nail bed, allowing for microscopic examination of the nailfold capillaries. In cases of primary RP, the capillaries typically appear normal, whereas in connective tissue diseases (CTDs), capillaries may appear dilated and show signs of capillary loss or "drop-out." The presence of either positive antibodies or abnormal capillary findings is strongly indicative of CTD.

Systemic sclerosis diagnosis criteria: The diagnostic criteria for SSc have been established by the Scleroderma Criteria Subcommittee of the American College of Rheumatology and are widely accepted.

The patient should have either:
- *Major criteria*: Scleroderma or symmetric skin thickness proximal to the MCP joint or MTP joint, affecting limbs, face, neck, or trunk.
- *Minor criteria*:
    - Sclerodactyly
    - Digital pitted scars/loss of fingertip pulp
    - Bilateral basal pulmonary fibrosis (bilateral reticular pattern of linear or nodular densities mostly in the basal portion of the lung).
    - For diagnosis patient should have one major or two minor criteria. These criteria have 97% sensitivity and 98% specificity.

Classification of systemic sclerosis: The distinction is made principally on the basis of the extent of cutaneous involvement **(Table 4)**.

TABLE 4: Difference between diffuse and limited cutaneous systemic sclerosis.

dSSc	Limited cutaneous systemic sclerosis (lcSS)
<1 year interval between the onset of Raynaud's phenomenon and the development of skin changes	Long history of Raynaud's phenomenon
Truncal and peripheral skin involvement	Peripheral skin is involved mainly
Pulmonary fibrosis present	Late-onset pulmonary hypertension
Anti-topoisomerase antibody/SCL-70 antibody positive	Anticentromere antibody positive
Capillary dropout is visible in nailfolds	Capillary dilatation is visible in nailfolds
Tendon friction rub present	Absent
Renal failure, gastrointestinal tract, and myocardial involvement	Calcification and telangiectasias are more prominent

(dSSc: diffuse cutaneous systemic sclerosis; lcSS: limited cutaneous systemic sclerosis; SCL-70: anti-Scl-70 antibody)

Q.3. Define Raynaud's phenomenon and the difference between primary and secondary Raynaud's phenomenon.

Ans. Raynaud's phenomenon is characterized by an episodic reduction in blood flow to the fingers, triggered by cold or emotional stress. The condition is marked by a sequence of color changes in the affected digits, starting with white (pallor), followed by blue (cyanosis), and ending with red (rubor). Pallor is a key feature for diagnosis, although it may be brief in connective tissue disorders.

Evaluation of Raynaud's phenomenon **(Flowchart 1)**.

Primary Raynaud's phenomenon, also known as Raynaud's disease, is idiopathic and occurs as a standalone condition. Secondary Raynaud's phenomenon, or Raynaud's syndrome, is associated with an underlying disease or triggered by physical factors or medications.

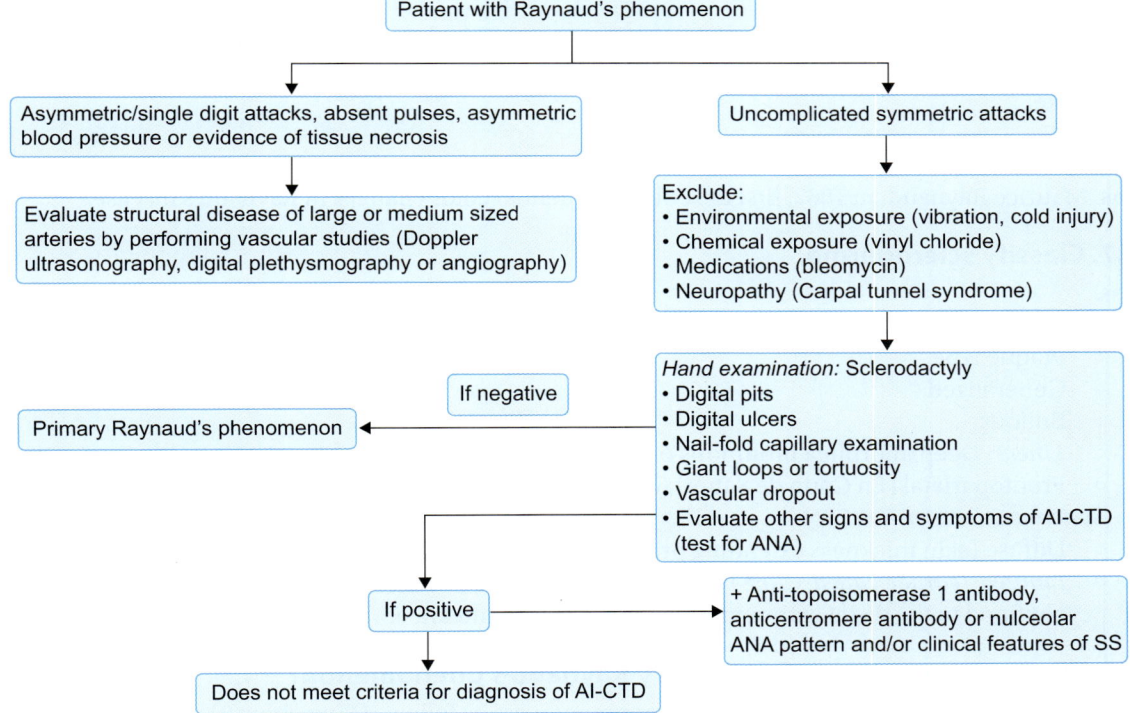

FLOWCHART 1: Raynaud's phenomenon evaluation.
(AI-CTD: autoimmune connective tissue disease; ANA: antinuclear antibody)

Q.4. What are the criteria for the diagnosis of primary Raynaud's phenomenon?

Ans. Vasospastic attacks are precipitated by exposure to cold or emotional stimuli.
- Bilateral involvement of extremities.
- Absence of evidence of organic peripheral arterial occlusion (normal peripheral pulses and nail-fold capillary microscopy).
- Absence of gangrene, and if present, limited to the skin of the fingertips. No evidence of underlying disease, drug, or occupational exposure that could precipitate vasospasm.

- Negative immunological abnormalities or antinuclear antibody (ANA) test.
- Normal ESR.
- Female sex of <25 years
- History of symptoms for at least 2 years.

Q.5. What is pterygium inversum unguis (PIU)?
Ans. Pterygium inversum unguis is a rare nail abnormality in which the distal nailbed adheres to the ventral surface of the nail plate, with obliteration of the distal groove. It is seen in:
- Systemic lupus erythematosus (SLE)
- SSc
- DM
- Raynaud's
- Neurofibromatosis
- Onychomycosis
- Stroke

Q.6. Who was Raynaud?
Ans. Maurice Raynaud, in 1862, first described sequential color changes in Raynaud's disease.

Q.7. Classify scleroderma.
Ans.
- *Localized (morphea)*:
  - Plaque type
  - Generalized
  - Bullous
  - *Linear*: Deep/morphea profundus or subcutaneous.
  - Frontoparietal (En Coup de Sabre) with or without hemiatrophy of the face.
- *Systemic scleroderma (SSc)*:
  - Diffuse (skin thickness extending proximal to elbows and knees)
  - *Limited (earlier called CREST syndrome or Thibierge–Weissenbach syndrome)*: Skin thickness confined to the distal extremities below the elbow and knee.

Q.8. What are the causes of secondary Raynaud's phenomenon?
Ans. The causes of secondary Raynaud's phenomenon are as follows **(Flowchart 2)**.
- Connective tissue disease
- Scleroderma
- SLE
- DM and polymyositis
- Mixed connective tissue disease
- Rheumatoid arthritis
- Polyarthritis and vasculitis.
- Sjögren's syndrome.
- *Obstructive arterial disease*:
  - Arteriosclerosis obliterans
  - Thromboangiitis obliterans
  - Arterial emboli

Chapter 4: Systemic Sclerosis, Dermatomyositis, and Other Connective Tissue Diseases

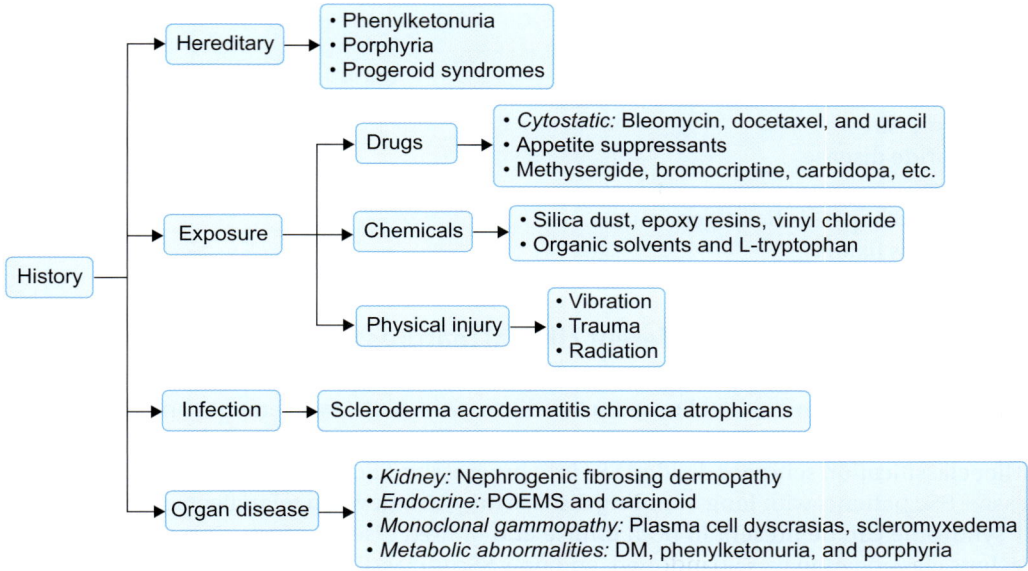

FLOWCHART 2: Causes of secondary Raynaud's phenomenon.
(DM: dermatomyositis; POEMS: Polyneuropathy, Organomegaly, Endocrinopathy, Monoclonal plasma cell disorder, and Skin)

Neurogenic disorders:
- Thoracic outlet syndrome
- Carpal tunnel syndrome
- Reflex sympathetic dystrophy.
- Hemiplegia
- Poliomyelitis
- Multiple sclerosis
- Syringomyelia

Drugs:
- Beta-blockers
- Ergot preparations
- Methysergide
- Bleomycin and vinblastine
- Clonidine
- Bromocriptine
- Cyclosporine

Trauma:
- Vibratory tools
- Hypothenar hammer syndrome
- Pianists and typists
- Meat cutters

Hematological causes:
- Cryoproteins
- Cold agglutinins

- Macroglobulins
- Polycythemia

Miscellaneous:
- Hypothyroidism
- Vinyl chloride disease
- Neoplasms
- Vasculitis and hepatitis B antigenemia
- Arteriovenous fistula
- Intra-arterial injections

Q.9. Give an overview of the different clinical features in CREST syndrome.

Ans. CREST stands for calcinosis cutis, Raynaud's phenomenon, esophageal dysmotility, sclerodactyly, and telangiectasia. It is now called limited scleroderma with skin involvement confined to areas distal to the elbows and knees (but involvement of the face and neck may be present).

Earlier classification schemes divided SSc into progressive SSc and CREST syndrome. But diffuse or progressive SSc patients with long-standing disease may also develop telangiectasia and calcinosis, so CREST syndrome can be present in both diffuse and limited disease of any duration. For this reason, the previous classification was abandoned, and now SSc is classified into diffuse and limited.

Q.10. Enumerate the diseases in which calcinosis cutis is found.

Ans. Disorders having calcinosis cutis may be categorized according to the type of calcification process. Dystrophic calcification—occurs in the setting of normal serum calcium and phosphate. It is seen in:
- Trauma
- Insect bite
- Varicose veins
- *Infections*: Onchocerciasis, histoplasmosis, andcryptococcosis
- *Tumors*: Pilomatrixoma, epithelial cysts or syringoma, basal cell carcinoma (BCC), hemangioma, trichoepithelioma, and pyogenic granuloma.
  - *Panniculitis*: Connective tissue disorders-DM, SSc, and SLE.

Q.11. What are the eye changes in SSc?

Ans.
- Tightness of lids
- Shallow fornices
- Decreased tear secretion
- Keratoconjunctivitis sicca
- Sjögrens syndrome
- Retinopathy with hemorrhage, exudates, and cytoid bodies due to vascular changes.

Q.12. How is the nervous system affected in SSc?

Ans. In SSc, the nervous system can be affected through several mechanisms, including:
- Thickening of the vessel walls in the white matter.
- Lymphocytic and granulomatous infiltration of the meninges.
- Malabsorption, leading to vitamin B12 deficiency, which can cause subacute combined degeneration of the spinal cord.
- Calcification, which may result in spinal cord compression

- Peripheral nerve involvement, marked by increased collagen deposition in the epineurium and perineurium.
- Intimal thickening of the vasa nervosa.

Q.13. What is a windmill maneuver?
Ans. An attack of Raynaud's may be broken at times by swinging the affected arm in a wide circle from the shoulder.

Q.14. How is childhood diffuse SSc different from adult SSc?
Ans. The following are characteristics of pediatric SSc:
- Raynaud phenomenon is less frequent.
- Cardiac wall involvement is more common, causing 50% deaths.
- Renal disease is uncommon
- Predominantly acrosclerotic
- Course is slower
- Visceral involvement is less common
- Involution of sclerosis may occur with minimal residue
- However, it can be rapidly progressive and fatal.

Q.15. What is pseudoscleroderma?
Ans. Sclerosis of skin in conditions other than morphea or SSc. Approaching a case based on clinical symptoms and physical examination—special emphasis is laid on the character and distribution of skin thickening and associated findings should be laid.

Q.16. Enlist common differential diagnosis of SSc.
Ans. The differential diagnosis includes the following **(Flowchart 3)**:

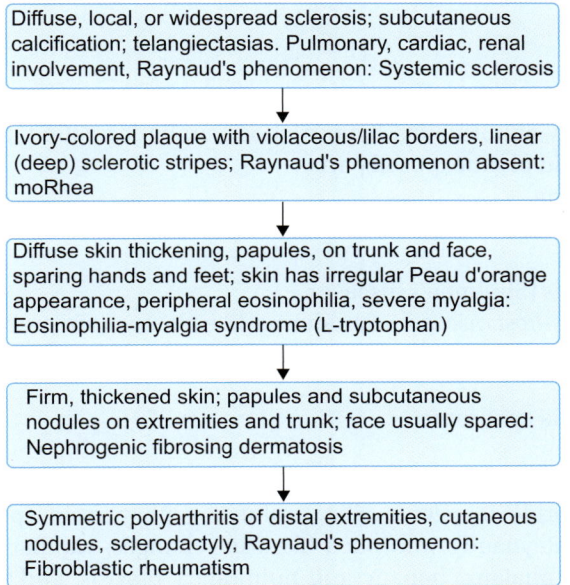

FLOWCHART 3: Approach to a case based on clinical symptoms and physical examination.

All other disorders within the scleroderma spectrum: Localized scleroderma, such as generalized morphea and multiple plaque morphea—no Raynaud's, no systemic involvement, acral part usually not involved, improves with years.
- **Acral vasospasm:**
    - *Raynaud's phenomenon*:
        - Primary Raynaud's—no systemic features and no sclerosis.
        - Other autoimmune connective tissue diseases like:
            - SLE
            - Rheumatoid arthritis
            - DM/Polymyositis
- *Other vascular disease*: Hematologic
- Cryoglobulinemia
- Cold agglutinins
- *Hyperviscosity syndrome*: Systemic vasculitis
- Buerger's disease (thromboangiitis obliterans)

Other causes for skin sclerosis (Pseudo-scleroderma)
- *Infiltrative disorders*:
    - Amyloidosis
    - *Scleromyxedema*: Thickening and hardening of skin with lichenoid papule forming confluent plaques and enlargement of body folds. Sclerodactyly, Raynaud's, and esophageal immotility may be present
    - *Scleredema of Buschke*: No vascular changes or Raynaud's seen, hands and feet pads, no immunological abnormality, wrinkling occurs on pinching involved skin. It has a rapid onset, non-pitting induration of the head, shoulder, trunk, and arms.
    - *Lichen sclerosus atrophicus*: Porcelain white atrophic/indurated plaque with follicular plugs.
    - Hansen's disease
- *Metabolic diseases*:
    - Diabetes mellitus
    - Myxedema
    - *Porphyria cutanea tarda*: Cutaneous induration present, induration is mingled with atrophy, mottled pigmentary abnormality, hypertrichosis, milia formation, and occasional bullae and erosion, especially in photoexposed parts.
    - Congenital porphyria
    - Phenylketonuria
- *Inflammatory diseases*:
    - Eosinophilic fasciitis (Shulman's disease)
    - *Chronic graft-versus-host disease*: Scleroderma-like changes are preceded by maculopapular or lichen planus-like eruption; joint contracture is present.
    - Sarcoidosis
    - Eosinophilia myalgia syndrome
    - Toxic oil syndrome
- *Scleroderma-like disorders-scleroderma like changes can be induced by*:
    - Solvents-vinyl chloride, benzene, silica, toluene, epoxy resin (produces unusual form of scleroderma with Raynaud's, morphea-like skin changes, capillary abnormality of nailfold, osteolysis of distal phalanx, hepatic and pulmonary fibrosis, and thickened walls of dermal arteries).

- ○ *Drugs causing pseudoscleroderma*:
  - Pentazocine
  - Bleomycin
  - L-tryptophan
  - Bromocriptine
  - Docetaxel
  - Isoniazid
  - Sodium valproate—vitamin K (Texier's disease)
  - Cocaine
  - Carbidopa
  - Nitrofurantoin
  - Interferon (IFN) alpha and interleukin-2 (IL-2)
- *Miscellaneous*:
  - ○ *Acrodermatitis chronica atrophicans*: It starts with bluish-red infiltrates on the distal part of one or both limbs, spreading proximally to the elbow in the upper limb, groin, and buttocks. Skin is thinned, wrinkled, and mottled in appearance with visible veins.
  - ○ *Nephrogenic fibrosing dermopathy*: Progressive cutaneous and systemic fibrosis involving extremities, trunk, with sparing of face and internal organs. Joint contractures and painful disability present.
  - ○ GEMSS (glaucoma, ectopia lentis, microspherophakia, joint stiffness, stocky short pseudoathletic build) syndrome is characterized by a patient with a stocky, pseudoathletic physique. In this condition, cutaneous sclerosis typically affects the upper back and limbs while sparing the face.
  - ○ *POEMS syndrome (also called Crow–Fukase-Takatsuki syndrome)*: Polyneuropathy, organomegaly, endocrinopathy, M protein, skin changes. Features resembling SSc are diffuse hyperpigmentation, scleroderma. Other features include hyperhidrosis, hypertrichosis, and lymphadenopathy.

Q.17. How do you manage SSc case?

Ans. *Management of a case of systemic sclerosis*:
Four facets of SSc—
1. Immunomodulators
2. Vascular component
3. Antifibrotic
4. Organ-based treatment

Immunomodulator:
- Cyclosporin A improves skin score.
- Methotrexate improves skin score and grip
- *Cyclophosphamide*: Significant improvement in skin and lung fibrosis, though minor effect on pulmonary function test.
- Immunoablation or stem cell transplantation.
- Extracorporeal photopheresis.
- Antithymocyte globulin-improve skin score.
- Mycophenolate mofetil
- Oral Acetretin, etanercept, and thalidomide.
- *Azathioprine*: 2 mg/day.

Therapy for Raynaud's and digital ischemia:
- *Calcium-channel blockers*:
    - Improve digital blood flow
    - Improve finger temperature
    - Induce healing of digital ulcer
        Side effect: Dilates the gastroesophageal junction, which leads to esophageal regurgitation.
        - Nifedipine—10 mg TDS or 10–20 mg QID
        - Amlodipine–diltiazem
        - *Other vasodilators*: Oral reserpine, guanethidine, ketanserin 20 mg BD to 40 mg TDS.
- *ACE inhibitors*:
    - Captopril 15–150 mg/day variable effect
    - Used in Raynaud's and scleroderma renal crisis.
- *Angiotensin receptor blocker*: Inhibits vascular remodeling
- Antioxidant agents
- Prostacyclin analogs-iloprost
- *Alpha-adrenergic blockers*:
    - Prazosin—oral 1 mg TDS decreases the frequency and severity of vasospasm
    - Effective only at high doses, which are orthostatic
- *Endothelin receptor blocker*:
    - Bosentan decreases the number of new digital ulcers
    - No effect on healing
- Anticoagulants may be used in cases of thrombosis and compromised vascular flow. Examples include tissue plasminogen activator, heparin (low molecular weight heparin), and urokinase.
- Selective serotonin reuptake inhibitors (SSRIs)
- *Phosphodiesterase 5 inhibitor*: Sildenafil and tadalafil for Raynaud's and digital ulcers.
- *Nitrate formulations*: Less useful due to increased vasodilatation
- *Surgery*:
    - Digital microarteriolysis
    - Avoid amputation, if possible
    - Lumbar sympathectomy is beneficial for lower limb Raynaud's/ulceration, improves circulation for a year or 2, but has long-lasting benefit.
- Topical glyceryl trinitrate therapy
- Pentoxifylline—400 mg TDS alone or in combination with nifedipine.
    - Improves capillary function.

Potential antifibrotic strategies:
- *D-penicillamine*:
    - 125 mg alternate day for 2 years.
    - 750 (500–1,000) mg/day for 2 years.
        Effects:
        - Decreased skin thickness.
        - Decreased further visceral involvement.
- Relaxin
- *IFN-gamma*: Influences fibroblast behavior; decreases skin score and improves blood gas analysis, but has no effect on systemic changes.
- Transforming growth factor (TGF-B) modulators
- Colchicine: 0.5 mg bd/TDS or 1 mg/day for 6 days/week.

Effects:
- Improve skin elasticity.
- Mouth opening
- *Isotretinoin*: 1 mg/kg helps in cutaneous sclerosis.

Organ-based treatment strategies:
- *Digital vasculopathy and its complications*:
  - *Digital ischemia*:
    - Paronychia
    - Finger pulp loss
      - IV Iloprost for Raynaud's and healing digital ulcers and prevents recurrent lesions.
        - Oral iloprost are not effective at low doses and side effects limit higher dose treatment.
        - Mainstay for critical digital ischemia and incipient gangrene.
        - *Mechanism of action*: Induces prolonged vasodilatation, decreases platelet aggregation, and promotes endothelial cell lining
      - *Antiplatelets*: Aspirin and clopidogrel, and dipyridamole-especially used in critical digital ischemia and infarction.
      - Warm hands for 5 min/4 hours in warm water.
      - *IV prostaglandins*: Prostaglandin E1 (PGE1) (alprostadil)—for refractory Raynaud's phenomenon.
      - Discourage smoking.
      - *Prostacyclin infusion*: 2.5–10 mg/kg/min continuous infusion over 72 hours produces improvement for 8 weeks.
        - *Side effects*: Hypertension, headache, facial flushing, nausea, vomiting, diarrhea, pain at the angle of law.
- *Kidneys*: Scleroderma renal crisis was the most common cause of mortality before the use of ACE inhibitors.
  - ACE inhibitors
  - Hemodialysis/renal transplantation has surprising improvement in kidney and skin manifestations
  - Recovery of renal function can occur after months of dialysis.
- *GI tract*:
  - *For esophageal dysmotility*: Metoclopramide 10 mg before each meal.
  - *To increase lower esophageal sphincter tone*: Domperidone.
  - *To augment gastric and small bowel motility*: Cisapride 10 mg TDS prior to each meal.
  - *For reflux esophagitis*: Ranitidine 150 mg BD or cap omeprazole 20–60 mg/day.
  - *For bacterial overgrowth-related hypomotility*: Erythromycin acts as a motilin receptor agonist; it stimulates gastric concentration and hastens gastric emptying and promotes intestinal mobility.
  - *Rectal prolapse*: Requires surgical intervention.

  Acute abdominal emergencies like acute pseudo-obstruction are better managed conservatively. Enzyme supplements are required for pancreatic insufficiency.
- *Lungs*: Earlier, the most common cause of death was scleroderma renal crisis, but now it is PAH.
  - *PAH*:
    - *Vasodilators*: Calcium channel blockers.
    - *Anticoagulant*: Like warfarin for moderate to severe pulmonary hypertension
    - *Prostaglandins and their analogs*: Intravenous iloprost for significant pulmonary hypertension.

- *Epoprostenol (prostacyclin)*: Continuous infusion in patients with primary pulmonary hypertension.
- Sildenafil; effective in PAH
- *Bosentan*:
    - *Sitaxsentan*: ILD/pulmonary fibrosis—
        - *Cyclophosphamide*: 1.5–2 mg/kg/day, improves forced vital capacity (FVC), improves skin scores. It should be combined with low-dose prednisolone.
        - *Carbocysteine*:
            - Drugs under evaluation-pirfenidone, etanercept, and IFN-α.
- *Calcinosis*: Anticoagulants, colchicine, intralesional steroid, bisphosphonates, chelation therapy, calcium channel blockers (CCB), surgical excision, CO_2 laser-effective in 6 weeks.
- *Articular pain*: Prednisolone and methotrexate.
- *Skin*:
    - *Topical tretinoin*: 0.025–0.05%—decreases perioral and facial tightening and creases.
    - Factor XIII given IV and isotretinoin 1 mg/kg help in cutaneous sclerosis
    - Intravenous 5-FU.
    - *Cyclosporin*: Improved skin induration but no visceral involvement.
    - Dexamethasone pulse therapy.
- *Cardiac*:
    - Antihypertensive-minoxidil, captopril-relieves encephalopathy and improves renal function.
    - Myocarditis may respond to immunosuppression.

Q.18. Classify pulmonary hypertension.
Ans.
Group (1) PAH:
- Idiopathic
- Familial
- *Related condition*: Connective tissue disease, congenital left-to-right shunt, portal hypertension, human immunodeficiency virus (HIV), toxins, and drugs.
- *Associated with significant venous/capillary involvement*:
    - Pulmonary venous occlusive disease
    - Pulmonary capillary hemangiomatosis
    - Persistent pulmonary hypertension of the newborn

Group (2) pulmonary venous hypertension:
- Left-sided atrial/ventricular disease
- Left-sided valvular heart disease

Group (3) pulmonary hypertension associated with hypoxemia:
- Chronic obstructive pulmonary disease (COPD)
- ILD
- High altitude

Group (4) pulmonary hypertension due to chronic thrombotic or embolic disease:
- Proximal pulmonary thromboembolic obstruction
- Distal thromboembolic obstruction

Group (5) miscellaneous:
- Sarcoidosis
- Vascular compression

Q.19. What are the central nervous system (CNS) changes in SSc?
Ans.
- Autonomic neuropathy
- Trigeminal neuropathy
- Carpal tunnel syndrome
- Meralgia paresthetica
- Subacute combined degeneration due to malabsorption, causing vitamin B12 deficiency.
- Soft tissue calcification causing spinal cord compression
- Prolonged sensory chronaxie (also occurs in tabes dorsalis)
- Impotence

Q.20. What is myocardial Raynaud's phenomenon?
Ans. Microvascular coronary vasospasm causing myocardial fibrosis is called myocardial Raynaud's phenomenon.

Q.21. What is the course of SSc in pregnancy?
Ans. SSc in pregnancy is usually unchanged, but the chances of postpartum renal failure and peripheral gangrene increase. The indications for termination of pregnancy include ACE inhibitors are given for hypertension, though they may risk the fetus.

Q.22. Name the diseases associated with SSc.
Ans. The diseases associated with SSc are:
- *Connective tissue disease*: SLE, DM, Sjögrens syndrome, polymyositis, myasthenia gravis, and muscle dystrophy.
- *Vascular disease*: Temporal arteritis, thrombophlebitis, Degos disease, cryofibrinogenemia.
- *Others*: Autoimmune hemolytic anemia, microangiopathic hemolytic anemia, autoimmune neutropenia, congenital agammaglobulinemia with IgA deficiency, monoclonal gammopathy, purpura, pemphigus vulgaris, urticaria pigmentosa, primary biliary cirrhosis, pseudoxanthoma elasticum, and celiac disease.

Q.23. What is the prognosis of SSc, and what factors affect prognosis?
Ans. Overall, there is a fourfold increase in mortality in a case of SSc.
- *Factors having poor prognosis are*:
  - Male gender
  - Extensive skin involvement
  - Visceral involvement
  - >60% decrease in diffusing capacity of the lungs for carbon monoxide (DLCO) (pulmonary diffusing capacity)
  - Patients with decreased CMI or T cells
  - HLA B-8 positive patients
- *Factors having a good prognosis*: Disease involving only the hands.

Q.24. What are the causes of death in SSc?
Ans. *Causes of death*:
- PAH (most common)
- Intercurrent infection
- Cardiac failure
- Renal failure
- Malignant hypertension
- Perforation of the gastrointestinal tract (GIT).

Q.25. What is lupoderma?
Ans. Patient with progressive SSC may have clinical features that resemble SLE and consist of fever, serositis, anemia, and positive LE cell test. This condition is called lupoderma.

Q.26. What is the scoring system of SSc?
Ans. *Hidebound/tethering skin score of Furst*: Sites examined—face, back, chest, abdomen, arms, forearm, hands, thighs, legs, and feet.
- *0*: Skin not tethered
- *1*: Mild tethering
- *2*: Moderate tethering
- *3*: Severe tethering
  Total score—total of all points for all sites. Maximum score = 30
  Modified Rodnan skin score based on the extent and severity of skin thickening. Sites examined—face, both right and left foot, leg, thigh, fingers, hand, forearm, upper arm. Anterior chest and abdomen—a total of 17 sites.

Grades:
- *0*: No skin involved
- *1*: Mild thickening
- *2*: Moderate thickening
- *3*: Severe thickening
  Maximum score = 51
  The higher the skin score, the worse the prognosis, and there is an increased risk of internal involvement.

Q.27. What is scleroderma sine scleroderma?
Ans. Presentation of pulmonary fibrosis or renal, cardiac, or GIT disease:
- No cutaneous involvement
- Raynaud's may be present
- *ANA*: Anti-Scl-70, anticentromere or anti-RNA polymerase I, II, III antibody present.

Q.28. What is prescleroderma?
Ans. Prescleroderma will have the following features:
- Raynaud's phenomenon.
- Nailfold capillary changes and evidence of digital ischemia.
- Specific circulating auto antibodies-antitopoisomerase (SC1-70), anticentromere antibody, anti-RNA polymerase I, II, and III.

Q.29. What is GAVE?
Ans. Watermelon stomach is the popular name for gastric antral vascular ectasia (GAVE)—a condition in which the lining of the stomach bleeds, causing it to look like the characteristic stripes of a watermelon when viewed by endoscopy. It can occur by itself, as a side effect of some medications, or in patients with diffuse SSc.

Q.30. What is scleroderma renal crisis (SRC) and its association with autoantibodies?
Ans. The cardinal features of SRC comprise a new onset of significant systemic hypertension (>150/85 mm Hg) and decreased renal function <30% reduction in estimated glomerular filtration rate (eGFR)]. The patient may also develop headaches, fever, malaise, hypertensive retinopathy, encephalopathy, and pulmonary edema. A strong association exists between SRC and ANA speckled pattern positive cases. Antifibrillarin or anti-U3-RNP antibodies may also identify young patients at risk of developing internal organ manifestations of SSc, including SRC. Conversely, SSc patients exhibiting anti-centromere antibody or anti-topoisomerase antibody are less likely to develop renal disease.

Q.31. What is peak age of onset of disease and F:M ratio in SSc?
Ans. Systemic sclerosis affects women more frequently than men, with a female-to-male ratio ranging from 3:1 to 6:1. The disease typically manifests in individuals during their fourth decade of life. Although SSc occurs across all racial groups, it is less common among Asians. African–American women with SSc tend to develop the diffuse form of the disease at a younger age and generally experience poorer survival rates compared to Caucasian women.

Q.32. What will happen if a graft of normal skin is placed on sclerodermatous skin?
Ans. Reciprocal skin grafting has shown that if sclerodermatous skin is placed in a normal bed, it remains sclerodermatous, and if clinically normal skin is placed in a sclerodermatous area, it becomes sclerodermatous.

Q.33. What are the causes of death in SSc?
Ans. Systemic sclerosis is associated with the highest case-specific mortality among systemic autoimmune CTDs. The leading causes of death are pulmonary hypertension, pulmonary fibrosis (ILD), and scleroderma renal crisis. Mortality due to scleroderma renal crisis has notably decreased in recent years with the use of ACE inhibitors. However, pulmonary complications, including ILD and pulmonary arterial hypertension, have emerged as the primary causes of death in individuals with SSc.

Q.34. Which is the recently approved drug for ILD in SSc?
Ans. Nintedanib (Ofev™) is a multiple tyrosine kinase inhibitor approved to slow the rate of lung fibrosis in ILD associated with SSc, approved by US FDA in 2019, dose is 150 mg BD.

Q.35. What are VEDOSS criteria?
Ans. VEDOSS refers to Very Early Diagnosis of SSc. It focuses on red flags like Raynaud's phenomenon, puffy fingers, and abnormal NFC findings, together with positive ANA. This criterion is considered sensitive to suspect SSc in the early edematous stage of SSc.

Q.36. Which are futuristic therapies in SSc?

Ans. Lenabasum (cannabinoid CB2 agonist), brentuximab vedotin (anti-CD30), and sarilumab (anti-IL6) are futuristics therapies in SSc, meant to slow down the fibrotic process.

Q.37. What is the relation between COVID-19 and SSc?

Ans. There are some intriguing similarities between Coronavirus disease 2019 (COVID-19) and SSc. Both diseases can cause high circulatory levels of IL-6 and can lead to endothelial damage and interstitial lung fibrosis. Theoretically, COVID-19 can unmask autoimmunity and even aggravate pre-existing SSc. The nucleolar pattern of ANA positivity has been described in many COVID-19 patients and is often associated with interstitial pneumonia and a poorer prognosis.

CASE 2: DERMATOMYOSITIS[3]

A 38-year-old married female, housewife, resident of Ahmedabad.

Chief Complaints

- Red raised itchy skin lesions over the face and neck associated with photosensitivity for last 1 year.
- History of swelling around the eyes for 1 year.
- History suggestive of proximal muscle weakness in lower limbs for the last 1 year.

Origin, Duration, and Progress

The patient was relatively asymptomatic 1 year ago when she started to develop reddish itchy skin lesions first over her face and neck, which aggravated on sun exposure. The lesions were initially transient, and gradually they turned persistent. She also developed swelling around her eyes that persisted throughout the day. She experienced difficulty in getting up from the sitting position and climbing stairs, which was preceded by recurrent episodes of pain in both thighs. She had lost around 3 kg of weight in the past 3 months.

Negative History

There was no history of fever, malaise, joint pain, recurrent oral lesions, Raynaud's phenomenon, headache, seizure, altered behavior, hair loss, chest pain, breathlessness, palpitation, post prandial pain in abdomen, difficulty swallowing, regurgitation, skin tightening, dryness of mouth, grittiness in eyes, joint pain, decreased urine output, blood in urine, and recurrent abortions.

Personal History

The patient experienced a decrease in her appetite and sleep. Bowel and bladder movements were unaltered. She had no addictions.

Past History

There was no past history of diabetes, hypertension, thyroid disorder, tuberculosis, blood transfusion, or surgical illness.

Family History

The patient was married for past 10 years. She had two children, an elder son, 7 years old, and a younger daughter, 5 years old. There was no history of similar illness in any family member.

Obstetric/Menstrual History

The patient had achieved menarche at 14 years of age. Her cycles were painless, regularly spaced at 28–30-day intervals, 3–5 days long.

General Examination

The patient was moderately built and nourished.
She was vitally stable. There was no evidence of jaundice, pallor, cyanosis, clubbing, edema, or lymphadenopathy.

Cutaneous examination revealed facial rash with eyelid edema with lilac-red border. Poikiloderma was noted over her upper chest, back, and the lateral aspect of her arms. Lichenified papules were seen over the meta-carpophalangeal and PIPs **(Figs. 4 to 7)**.

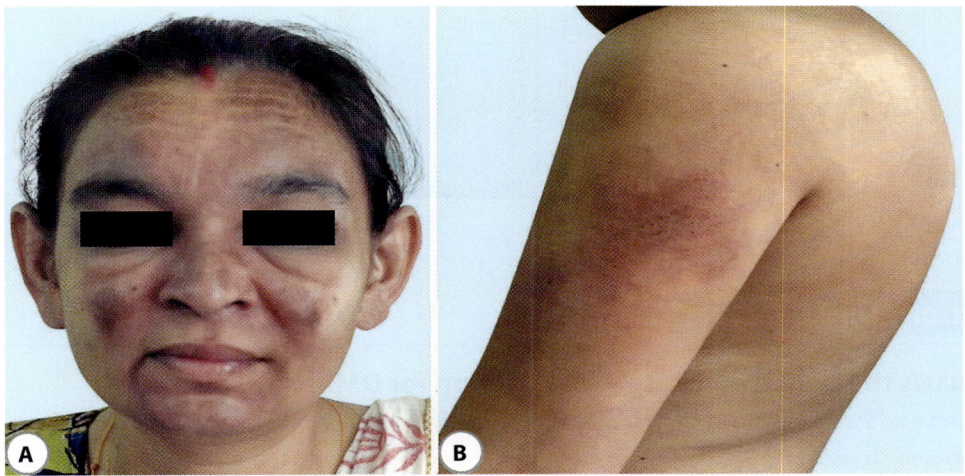

FIGS. 4A AND B: Heliotrope rash on face; erythema on upper arm.

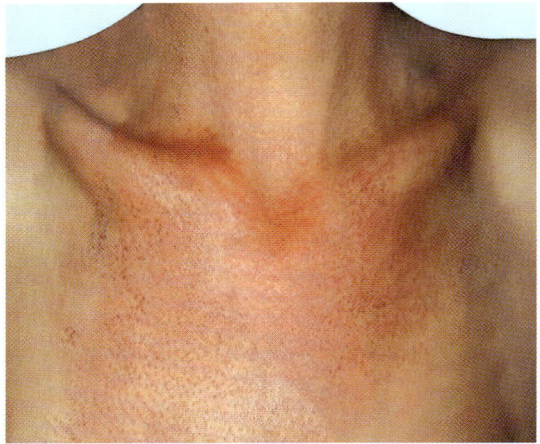

FIG. 5: V sign.

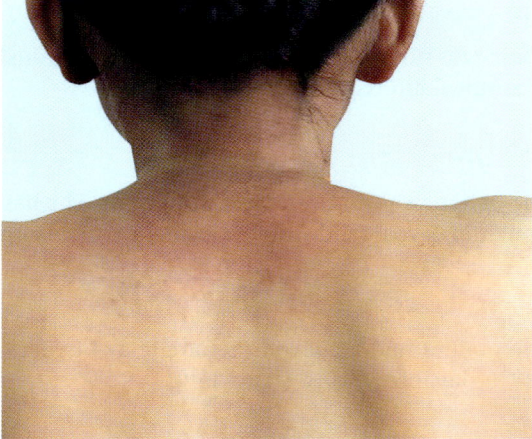

FIG. 6: Shawl sign.

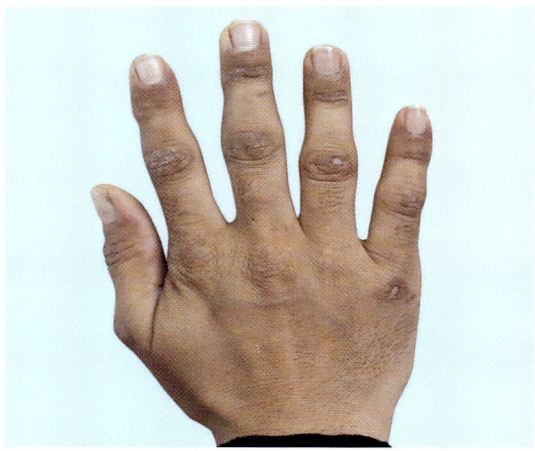

FIG. 7: Gottron's papules.

Questions and Answers

Q.1. Discuss the Bohan and Peter classification for DM.

Ans. Bohan and Peter classification for DM is discussed in **Table 5**.

TABLE 5: Bohan and Peter classification for dermatomyositis.[3]		
Features	**Polymyositis**	**Dermatomyositis**
Symmetrical proximal muscle weakness	*Definitive*: All of 1–4	*Definitive*: 5 plus any 3 of 1–4
Muscle biopsy evidence of myositis	*Probable*: Any 3 of 1–4	*Probable*: 5 plus any 2 of 1–4
Elevation in serum skeletal muscle enzymes	*Possible*: Any 2 of 1–4	*Possible*: 5 plus any 1 of 1–4
Characteristic electromyography (EMG) pattern of myositis		
Typical rash of dermatomyositis		

Q.2. What is DM sine myositis?

Ans. It is also known as amyopathic DM. When biopsy-confirmed hallmark skin signs of DM are observed without muscle weakness and with normal muscle enzyme levels for at least 6 months, a provisional diagnosis of DM sine myositis is considered. If these conditions persist for >24 months, a confirmed diagnosis of DM sine myositis can be made.

Q.3. Discuss the etiopathogenesis of DM.

Ans. It is an immune-mediated process triggered by external agents in genetically predisposed individuals. It is believed to be humorally mediated vasculopathic disease **(Table 6)**.

TABLE 6: Etiopathogenesis of dermatomyositis.	
Genetics	<ul><li>HLA-DR3 and -B8 (juvenile dermatomyositis)</li><li>HLA-DR52 (patients with anti-Jo-1 antibodies)</li><li>HLA-DR7 and -DRw53 (patients with anti-Mi-2 antibodies)</li><li>HLA-B14 and -B40 (adults with dermatomyositis overlap)</li><li>HLA-DRB1*15021 (Japanese with juvenile dermatomyositis)</li></ul>
Infectious precipitants	<ul><li>Picorna virus (substrate for aminoacyl-tRNA synthetases)</li><li>*Escherichia coli*</li><li>Coxsackie virus</li><li>Echovirus (in patients with hypogammaglobulinemia)</li></ul>
Drug and vaccine precipitants	<ul><li>Hydroxyurea</li><li>Lipid-lowering drugs (statins > gemfibrozil)</li><li>TNF-α inhibitors</li><li>Nonsteroidal anti-inflammatory drugs</li><li>Cyclophosphamide</li><li>Checkpoint inhibitors (e.g., ipilimumab)</li><li>D-penicillamine</li><li>BCG vaccine</li></ul>

(BCG: bacillus Calmette–Guérin; TNF-α: tumor, necrosis factor alpha)

Q.4. Discuss the demographic factors.

Ans.
- *Age*: Bimodal presentation: 50–60 years of age; 5–14 years.
- *Gender*:
  - Female:Male: 2:1 (adult)
  - Female:Male: 5:1 (child)
- *Ethnicity*: More common in African-american

Q.5. What are the proposed diagnostic criteria for cutaneous DM?

Ans. Sontheimer proposed the following diagnostic criteria for cutaneous DM:[3]
- The presence of two major criteria or one major and two minor criteria, along with skin biopsy findings characteristic of cutaneous DM **(Boxes 1 and 2)**.

BOX 1	Major criteria for cutaneous dermatomyositis.

- Heliotrope sign
- Gottron papules
- Gottron sign

> **BOX 2**   **Minor criteria for cutaneous dermatomyositis.**
>
> - Macular violaceous erythema involving (each area counts as a minor criterion)
> - Scalp/Anterior hairline
> - Malar eminences of face, forehead, or chin
> - V area of neck or upper chest (V sign)
> - Posterior neck or posterior shoulders (shawl sign)
> - Extensor surfaces of arms or forearms
> - Linear streaking overlying the extensor tendons of the dorsal hands
> - Periungual erythema
> - Lateral thighs or hips (Holster sign)
> - Medial malleoli
> - Nailfold capillary telangiectasia, hemorrhage-infarct
> - Poikiloderma
> - Mechanic's hands
> - Cutaneous calcinosis
> - Cutaneous ulcers
> - Pruritus

Q.6. Discuss in brief the classical signs of cutaneous DM.

Ans. Summary of cutaneous manifestations of DM **(Table 7)**.

TABLE 7: Summary of cutaneous manifestations of DM.	
Heliotrope sign **(Fig. 4)**	• A pink-violet (lilac) rash, predominantly affecting the eyelids and periorbital skin, • Waxing and waning course
Eyelid edema	May or may not be present
Lesions are more pronounced on extensor surfaces, including the elbows, knees, metacarpophalangeal joints, and both proximal and distal interphalangeal joints	
Gottron papules **(Fig. 7)**	• Pink-violaceous papules located over the interphalangeal and metacarpophalangeal joints • Secondary lichenification of papules over knuckles
Gottron sign **(Fig. 8)**	• Macular, pink-violaceous erythema involving joints, such as the elbows or knees • Involvement of elbows and/or knees
Photodistributed poikiloderma (telangiectatic erythema, epidermal atrophy, and dyspigmentation) **(Fig. 10)**	
V sign **(Fig. 5)**	Over the upper chest
Shawl sign **(Fig. 6)**	Over the upper back
Holster sign **(Fig. 9)**	Overphoto-protected areas, such as the lateral thighs
Calcinosis cutis [a sign of delayed diagnosis, postponed initiation of systemic corticosteroids, and/or advanced disease that is resistant to treatment **(Fig. 11)**]	Hard, irregular papules or nodules favoring sites of trauma (elbows/knees) ± pain ± limitation of function

Chapter 4: Systemic Sclerosis, Dermatomyositis, and Other Connective Tissue Diseases

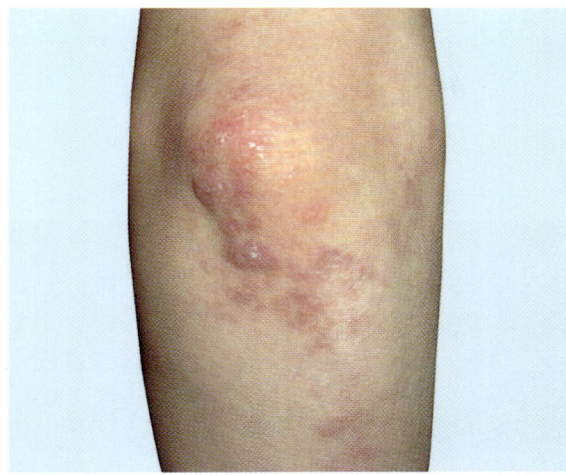

FIG. 8: Gottron sign.

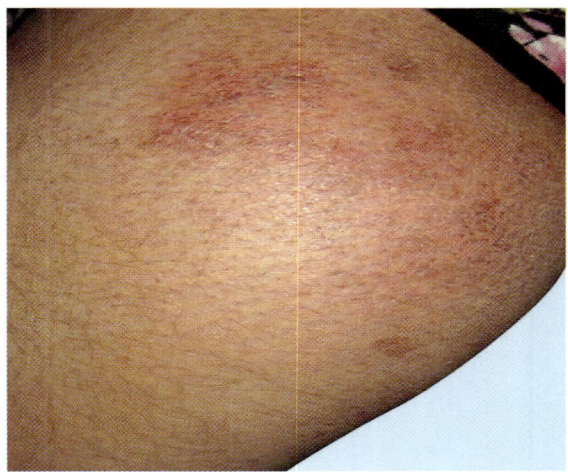

FIG. 9: Holster sign.

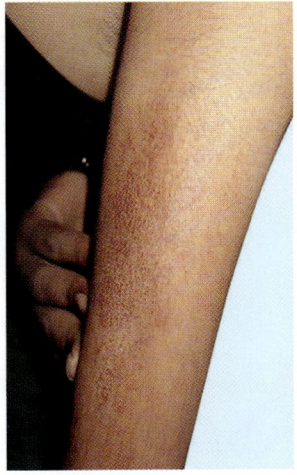

FIG. 10: Poikiloderma in extensor distribution.

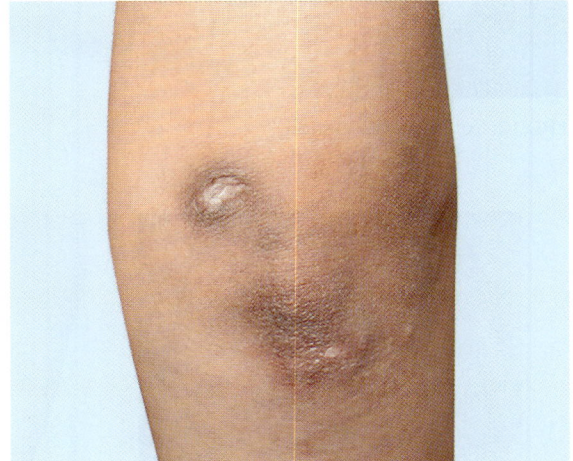

FIG. 11: Calcinosis cutis.

Q.7. Enumerate the uncommon presentations of cutaneous DM.
Ans.
- Cutaneous erosions or ulcerations **(Fig. 12)**
- Flagellate erythema **(Fig. 13)**
- Mechanic's hands (antisynthetase syndrome)
- Tender palmar papules
- Hyperkeratotic palmar papules
- Exfoliative erythroderma
- Cutaneous eruption that mimics pityriasis rubra pilaris (PRP) (Wong variant) **(Fig. 14)**
- Pustular eruption of the elbows and knees

- Vesiculobullous lesions
- Ovoid palatal patch **(Fig. 15)**
- Gingival telangiectasias
- Panniculitis
- Lipoatrophy (especially in juvenile DM)
- Small vessel vasculitis (especially in juvenile DM)

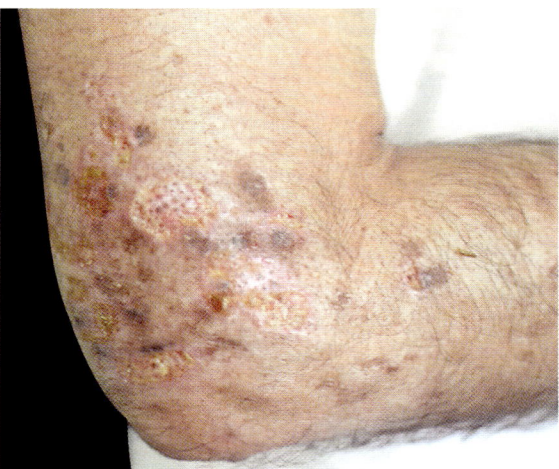

FIG. 12: Cutaneous ulceration.

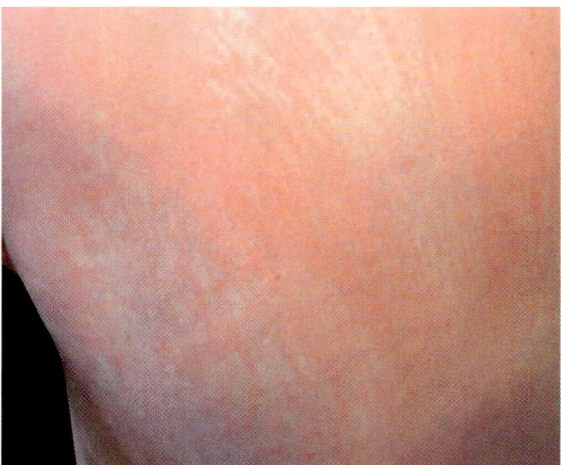

FIG. 13: Flagellate dermatitis.

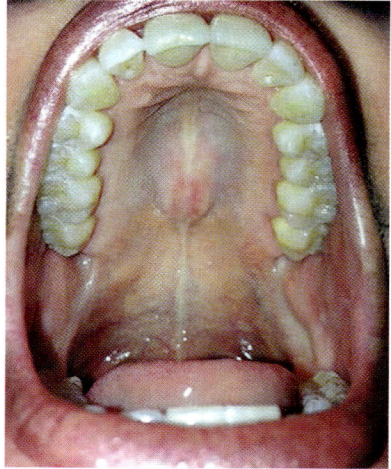

FIG. 14: Ovoid palatal patch.

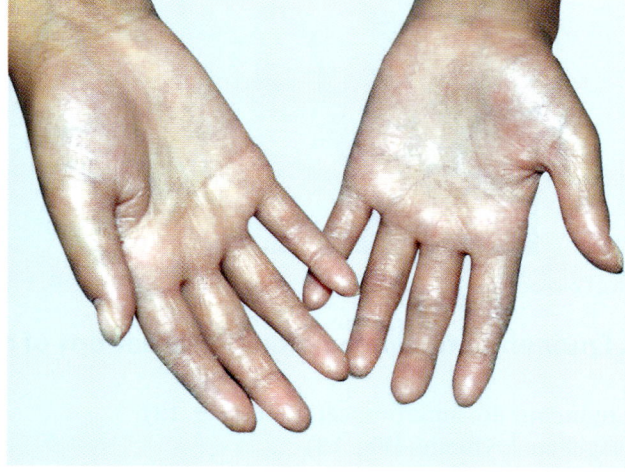

FIG. 15: Pityriasis rubra pilaris (PRP)-like presentation in WONG variant

Q.8. What is Samitz's sign?

Ans. The sign refers to thickening, roughness, hyperkeratosis, and irregularity of the cuticle with minimal or no redness or inflammation **(Fig. 16)**.

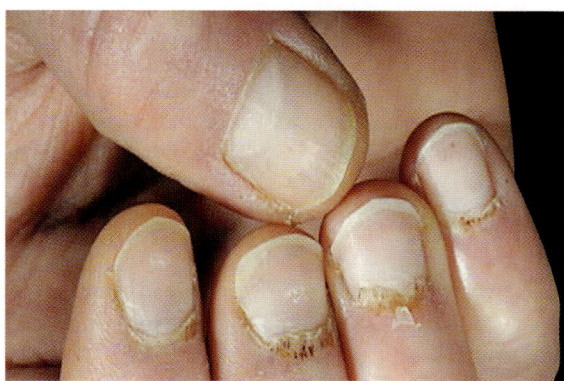

FIG. 16: Ragged cuticles.

Q.9. What is the antisynthetase syndrome?

Ans. This condition is marked by myositis, arthritis, Raynaud's phenomenon, ILD, fever, and acral skin changes, often referred to as "mechanic's hands." It is associated with the presence of autoantibodies, such as anti-Jo-1, anti-PL-7, anti-PL-12, anti-IJ, and anti-EJ.

Q.10. What do you mean by mechanic's hands?

Ans. It refers to non-inflammatory hyperkeratosis that typically develops on the hands or feet, commonly affecting the radial surfaces of the fingers and the outer edges of the feet **(Figs. 17A and B)**.

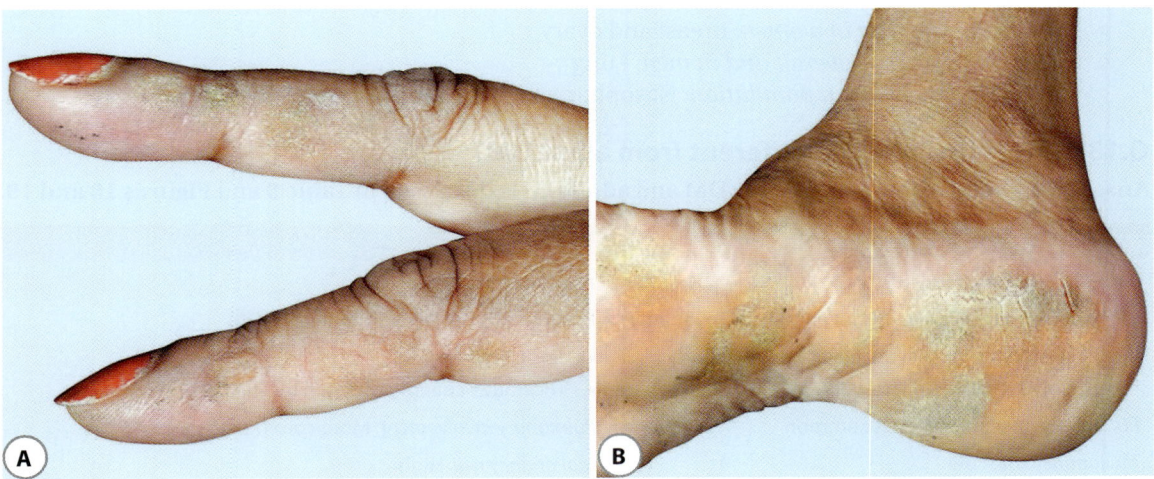

FIGS. 17A AND B: Mechanic's hands and feet.

Q.11. Discuss the systemic findings in DM.
Ans. Systemic findings in DM are discussed in **Table 8**.

TABLE 8: Systemic findings in dermatomyositis.

System	Symptom	Inference
Musculoskeletal	• Malaise • Difficulty in combing hair or getting up from a sitting position • Difficulty in initiating swallowing • Gastroesophageal reflux	• Symmetrical proximal muscle involvement, especially of the extensor groups (triceps and quadriceps) • Due to cricopharyngeal muscle dysfunction or possible overlap with systemic sclerosis • Due to distal esophageal muscle involvement
Respiratory	Dry cough and progressive breathlessness	• Diffuse interstitial fibrosis • ARDS
Cardiac	Chest pain, palpitations	Arrhythmias and conduction abnormalities
Joint	Multiple joint pain and swelling	Nonerosive inflammatory polyarthritis

Q.12. What is the association of DM with malignancies?
Ans.
Risk factors include:
- Advancing age
- Severe skin conditions with necrosis
- Difficulty swallowing (dysphagia)
- Weakness of the diaphragm
- Absence of extramuscular systemic involvement (such as ILD).
- Presence of antibodies to anti-transcription intermediary factor 1 gamma (anti-TIF1γ) or nuclear matrix protein 2 (NXP-2).
- Malignancies may be detected either before, at the time of, or following the onset of DM.
- The highest risk of malignancy occurs in the initial years after a DM diagnosis.
    - *Most common type in women*: Breast and ovary
    - *Most common type overall and in men*: Lung
    - *In the Southeast Asian population*: Nasopharyngeal carcinoma

Q.13. How is juvenile DM different from adult DM?
Ans. The difference between juvenile DM and adult DM is discussed in **Table 9** and **Figures 18 and 19**.

TABLE 9: Difference between juvenile and adult DM.

Juvenile dermatomyositis	Adult dermatomyositis
The most common idiopathic inflammatory myopathy	Polymyositis is more common than DM
• *Rash*: Atypical, can occur anywhere in the body • Ulcerative changes are frequently seen	• *Rash*: Typical of DM • Ulcerative changes are seen less frequently
Pulmonary involvement: Less common	*Pulmonary involvement*: More common
Malignancy risk: Low	*Malignancy risk*: High
Calcinosis: More common	*Calcinosis*: Less common
Anti-p155/140: Most common antibody	*Anti-Mi2*: The most common antibody

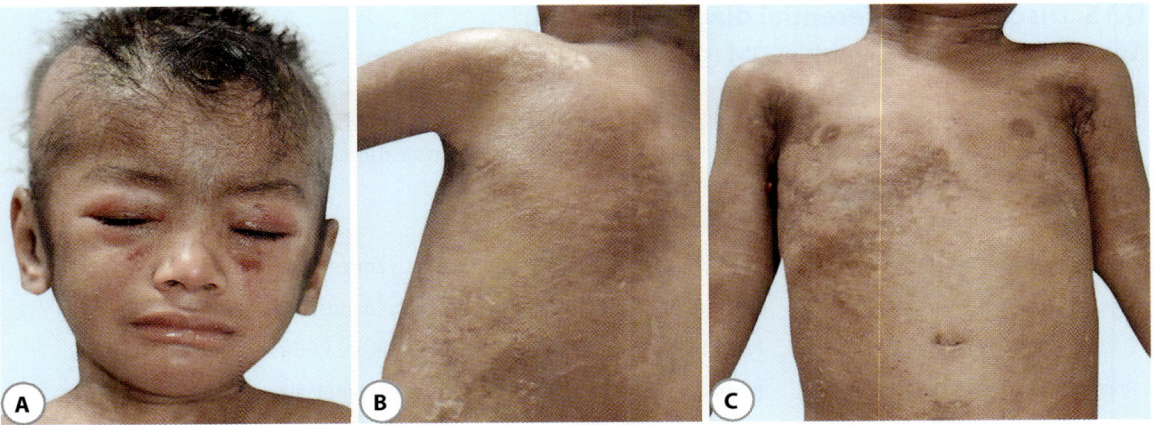

FIGS. 18A TO C: Poikilodermatous rash over face, trunk, and periorbital edema.

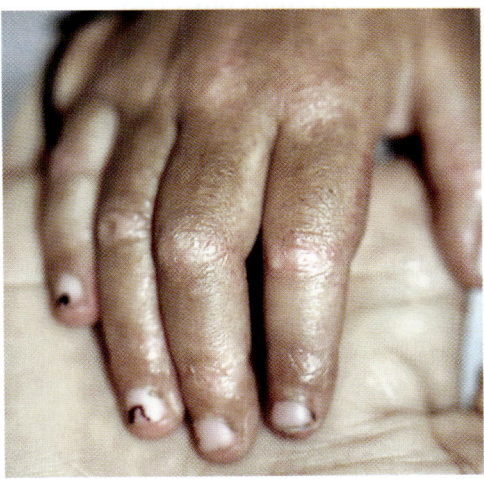

FIG. 19: Gottron papules: Juvenile DM.

Q.14. How do you differentiate the rash of SLE from that of DM?

Ans. A comparison of the rashes seen in SLE and DM is presented in the **Table 10** below:

TABLE 10: Difference between rash of SLE and DM.	
Dermatomyositis	**SLE**
Significant pruritus that affects quality of life	Less pruritic
Involves MCP, PIP, and DIP joints	Spares MCP, PIP, and DIP joints
Poikiloderma in the extensor distribution	Absent
Characteristic muscle weakness	Less characteristic muscle weakness (5–15%)

Q.15. Discuss the differential diagnosis of DM.

Ans. The differential diagnosis of DM is discussed in **Table 11** below:

TABLE 11: Differential diagnosis of DM.	
Psoriasis and seborrheic dermatitis	Poikiloderma, absence of characteristic psoriatic nail changes, and histopathology are conclusive
Phototoxic drug eruption	Only over photoexposed sites
Cutaneous T-cell lymphoma	Poikiloderma begins over intertriginous zones
Systemic sclerosis	Salt and pepper pigmentation, edema of hands in the early stage
Trichinosis	Periorbital edema and painful muscles without other features
Photodistributed form of MCRH	No nailfold changes and distinct histopathological features
Nephrotic syndrome	Anasarca, No heliotrope edema

(DM: dermatomyositis; MCRH: multicentric reticulohistiocytosis)

Q.16. How would you investigate a patient with DM?

Ans. A diagnosis of cutaneous DM[3] is suggested by the combination of typical skin manifestations, muscle weakness, and laboratory evidence of myositis. However, for patients presenting with unclear or ambiguous skin findings, or those with cutaneous features indicative of DM but without clinical signs of muscle involvement, a skin biopsy is recommended.[4]

For patients exhibiting cutaneous signs consistent with DM, an evaluation for associated muscle disease should be conducted. Since muscle disease may develop later, individuals without overt myositis should be monitored regularly with muscle exams and serum levels of creatinine kinase and aldolase every 2–3 months **(Table 12)**.

TABLE 12: Laboratory evaluation of DM.	
Baseline laboratory investigations	• CBC • Renal function test • Liver function test • Urine microscopic examination • Random blood sugar • Lipid profile
Skin	Biopsy
Muscle	• Serum creatine kinase, serum aldolase, and urine creatine • Electromyography • Muscle biopsy • MRI or USG (if EMG or biopsy are negative/declined)
Pulmonary	*PFT with DLCO if abnormal*: HRCT
Cardiac	• Echocardiogram • ECHO/Holter monitoring
Esophageal	Barium swallow/manometry

Continued

Continued

Malignancy screen	- Stool for occult blood - S. PSA - CA125, CA 19-9 - Mammogram - Pap smear - Transvaginal ultrasound - HRCT chest, abdomen, and pelvis - Colonoscopy, upper endoscopy
If chronic systemic corticosteroids are in the plan	DEXA bone density scan

(CBC: complete blood count; HRCT: high-resolution computed tomography; PFT: pulmonary function test; PSA: prostate-specific antigen)

Q.17. Discuss the various autoantibodies found in DM along with their implications.

Ans. Tables 13 and 14 below summarizes the key autoantibodies identified in dermatomyositis (DM) and their clinical implications.

TABLE 13: Various autoantibodies found in DM, along with their significance and function.

Autoantibody	Function	Significance
Anti-p155	Transcription intermediary factor 1	- Extensive cutaneous disease associated with malignancy - Ovoid palatal patch, red on white telangiectatic patches
Anti-NXP-2 (p140)	Nuclear transcription, RNA metabolism	Calcinosis (JDM > ADM), malignancy
Anti-Mi-2	Helicase-transcription	- Classic cutaneous disease (Good response to treatment) - They often present with a rapid and severe onset, accompanied by prominent cutaneous symptoms. However, they typically respond well to treatment and have a favorable long-term prognosis
Anti-Jo-1, anti-PL-7, anti-PL-12, IJ, and EJ	Intracytoplasmic protein synthesis	- Antisynthetase syndrome - Patients with anti-Jo-1 antibodies often show a partial response to treatment and have a poorer long-term prognosis
Anti-SRP	Protein translocation	- Fulminant and refractory myopathy (cardiac involvement) - Some patients with anti-signal recognition particle (SRP) antibodies may experience a rapid onset of severe proximal muscle weakness, significantly elevated serum CK levels, and muscle biopsies that reveal muscle fiber necrosis and regeneration with minimal to no inflammation
Anti-CADM-140 (MDA5)	Innate immunity	Clinically amyopathic DM, severe cutaneous ulcerations

TABLE 14: Various autoantibodies found in DM, along with their significance.

Autoantibody	Significance
ANA (speckled and nucleolar)	Clinically amyopathic DM
Antipolymyositis/Scl (PM-Scl)	DM/PM/SS overlap
Anti-Ku, anti-U2 RNP	DM-SS overlap
Anti-U1 RNP	Overlap with other AI-CTDs

Q.18. Discuss the principles of management of DM.
Ans.
Assess involvement of potentially affected organs: Skin, muscle, and lung.
- Screening for *malignancy*: As treatment of the cancer may reduce disease severity or even induce disease remission
- *Cutaneous* DM has a *discordant* treatment response with *muscle* disease, with recalcitrant skin disease continuing years after muscle disease is in remission
- *Collaborative management* under the rheumatologist, dermatologist, neurologist, and pulmonologist is critical for patients with multisystem involvement

Q19. Which topical agents are preferred for cutaneous lesions of DM?
Ans. *Photoprotection*: First step in management, though 60% of cases are minimally photosensitive

Topical corticosteroids: Class I or II creams and ointments with or without occlusion are used to treat areas such as the hands, extensor surfaces for short period, where the risk of corticosteroid-induced skin atrophy is lower. Whereas, lower-potency agents (e.g., groups 6–7) are preferred for areas more susceptible to atrophy, such as facial erythema and the heliotrope rash.
- Reduce pruritus, erythema, and scaling; can be tried to mitigate the problem of nailfold sensitivity
- Topical *calcineurin inhibitors* such as tacrolimus 0.1% ointment or pimecrolimus 1% cream can also be used; safe to use over the *face* without concern for atrophy or hypopigmentation

Q.20. What would be the management for skin-limited disease in DM?
Ans. Skin lesions in DM are often resistant to photoprotection and topical treatments alone, requiring the addition of antimalarial medications like HCQS and/or methotrexate. For patients who do not respond to these treatments, more aggressive immunosuppressive or immunomodulatory therapies may be necessary.

Topical treatment plus:
- *Antimalarials*: Hydroxychloroquine (200 mg twice daily) or chloroquine (250 mg daily) plus quinacrine (100 mg daily) is the first line of treatment
- Antimalarials also ameliorate mild symptoms of inflammatory arthritis

Q.21. What is the first-line systemic therapy for DM?
Ans. The aim of systemic treatment is to resolve pruritus and skin abnormalities or to achieve sufficient improvement, allowing mild, residual disease to be managed effectively with topical therapies.

Corticosteroids: There is no universally accepted glucocorticoid regimen for treating inflammatory myopathies, but two key principles are generally followed:
1. Begin treatment with high doses for the initial months to achieve disease control.
2. Gradually taper to the lowest effective dose, with a total treatment duration ranging from 9 to 12 months.

For severe, life-threatening cases, pulsed intravenous methylprednisolone (0.5–1 g/day) is typically administered over 3 consecutive days. This may be followed by monthly intravenous cyclophosphamide (0.5–1.0 g/m^2). After the initial treatment, oral prednisolone (0.5–1 mg/kg/day) is introduced.

DMARDs to be started to prevent steroid toxicity on long-term use.

The current first-line glucocorticoid-sparing agent is usually either azathioprine or methotrexate.
- Methotrexate (20–25 mg/week) unless ILD; azathioprine (2.5 mg/kg/day)
- Cyclosporine (3–3.5 mg/kg/day)

Treatment options for treatment refractory DM: Intravenous immune globulin (IVIG) and mycophenolate mofetil (MMF) are the preferred treatments for refractory cutaneous DM.[3]

Q.22. Is there any role of rituximab in the treatment of DM?

Ans. Rituximab is advocated as a third-line therapy for DM. It may be given as 4 weekly IV infusions of 375 mg/m^2/infusion.

It may be useful in myositis, especially with anti-Jo 1 and anti-Mi 2 autoantibodies.

Further research is needed to assess the effectiveness of rituximab for cutaneous DM,[3] establish the optimal treatment protocol, and identify the patient groups that may benefit most from this therapy.

Q.23. What is the role of intravenous immunoglobulin (IVIG) in the management of DM?

Ans. Intravenous immunoglobulin has shown effectiveness in treating refractory extracutaneous manifestations of DM and seems to offer benefits for patients with cutaneous symptoms who have not responded well to other treatments.

Relatively quick in action: Preferred in acutely ill or severely declining patients with *dysphagia* or respiratory involvement.

Dose: 2 g/kg body weight divided over 3–5 days.

REFERENCES

1. Efrimescu CI, Donnelly S, Buggy DJ. Systemic sclerosis. Part I: epidemiology, diagnosis, and therapy. BJA education. 2023;23(2):66-75.
2. Del Galdo F, Lescoat A, Conaghan PG, Bertoldo E, Čolić J, Santiago T, et al. EULAR recommendations for the treatment of systemic sclerosis: 2023 update. Ann Rheum Dis. 2025;84(1):29-40.
3. Sontheimer RD. Cutaneous features of classic dermatomyositis and amyopathic dermatomyositis. Curr Opin Rheumatol. 1999;11(6):475-82.
4. Marvi U, Chung L, Fiorentino DF. Clinical presentation and evaluation of dermatomyositis. Indian J Dermatol. 2012;57(5):375-81.

Erythroderma

INTRODUCTION

Erythroderma is an inflammatory skin disorder characterized by diffuse erythema and scaling involving >90% of body surface area (BSA). Etiology varies in children and adults. Any age group can be affected. Age of onset in adults is usually after 45 years while in children, the average age of onset is 3.3 years.

CLINICAL OUTLINE

Points to be covered in history:
- *Onset:* Rapid (drug reactions) insidious (pre-existing dermatoses); ask when the disease started and how was the clinical nature of the disease to start with.
- *Precipitating causes:* Ask if it was associated with any other cause likely to result in disease such as preceding history of sore throat and use of drugs aggravating the condition.

With specific consideration to psoriatic erythroderma:
- Fluctuations in disease course along with season
- Relation to sunlight
- Involvement of other body parts (see for nail and joint disease)

PSORIATIC ERYTHRODERMA

- History of localized disease
- Personal or family history of psoriasis
- Classic psoriasiform plaques on elbows, knees, sacrum, etc.
- Well circumscribed plaques at margin of erythroderma
- Large lamellar scales
- Collarettes of scales: Are suggestive of ruptured pustules of pustular psoriasis
- Psoriatic nail changes (coarse irregular pits, oil drop sign, etc.)
- Psoriatic arthritis

ERYTHRODERMA DEVELOPING FROM PRE-EXISTING ECZEMATOUS DERMATOSES (BOX 1)

- *Spongiotic dermatitis—atopic dermatitis*:
    - History of localized disease, often moderate to severe
    - Marked pruritus
    - Personal or family history of atopy
    - Classic atopic lesions in antecubital and popliteal fossae
    - Excoriations
    - Lichenification and prurigo nodularis
    - Focal skin atrophy from years of steroid use
- *Spongiotic dermatitis—other etiologies-like contact dermatitis*:
    - Distribution of original skin lesions
    - History of contactant
    - History of pre-existing venous disease
    - Chronic actinic dermatitis—photo-accentuation
- *Other pre-existing dermatoses—Pityriasis rubra pilaris (PRP)*:
    - *Initial lesion:* Seborrheic dermatitis-like eruption of the scalp
    - Cephalocaudal spread
    - Generalized salmon colored slightly infiltrated erythema
    - *Interspersed islands of sparing*: Nappy claires
    - Worsening postsun exposure
    - Palmoplantar keratoderma (PPK), often orange
    - Nutmeg-grater appearance of individual follicular pink hyperkeratotic papules
- *Drug reactions*:
    - Temporal correlation to a recently introduced drug
    - Rapid onset and progression to erythroderma
    - Fine scales
    - Lymphadenopathy
    - Organomegaly
    - Fever

BOX 1   **Adult-onset erythroderma frequency.**[1]

Pre-existing dermatoses: 52% (27–68%)
Psoriasis—Most common cause: 23% of all cases
Spongiotic dermatitis: 20% of all cases
- *Drug reactions*: 15%
- CTCL: 5%
- *Idiopathic*: 20% (7–33%)

(CTCL: cutaneous t-cell lymphoma)
Source: Sigurdsson V, Steegmans PH, van Vloten WA. The incidence of erythroderma: A survey among all dermatologists in Netherlands. J Am Acad Dermatol. 2001;45:675-8.

- *Cutaneous T-cell lymphoma*:
  - Severe debilitating pruritus
  - Fissured, painful keratoderma
  - Alopecia
  - Hepatosplenomegaly
  - Lymphadenopathy
  - Leonine facies
- *Idiopathic (Red man syndrome)*:
  - Elderly man
  - Chronic and relapsing course
  - Dermatopathic lymphadenopathy
  - Pruritus
  - PPK
- *Norwegian scabies*:
  - Down syndrome or nursing home patient
  - Burrows
  - Massively thickened nails
  - keratoderma

Take and describe complete treatment history: Ask relevant questions to obtain maximum information in a language understandable to the patient; e.g., to know of oral steroid use, ask whether patient was advised to take any medicine with the milk; to know of methotrexate use, ask if he was prescribed any tablets once weekly. However, answers to these questions are presumed so narrate it that way.

- *Relevant past medical history*:
  - Ask for history of hypertension, diabetes, tuberculosis, and hepatitis.
  - Psoriasis being a part of metabolic syndrome has associated hypertension and/or diabetes when occurring in adults. As treatment of psoriasis requires usage of immunosuppressive agents, history of tuberculosis becomes important.
- *Personal history*:
  - *Diet:* Omega-3 fatty acid rich diet offers protection in psoriasis.
  - *Appetite:* It can be reduced in debilitating state like erythroderma.
  - *Habits/Addiction:* Alcoholism is associated with increased disease severity and repeated attacks of psoriasis. Tobacco use also associated with psoriasis.
- *General examination:* Persistent, universal inflammation of the skin may have important consequences for thermoregulation, hemodynamics, intestinal absorption, protein, water, and other metabolism.
- *Temperature:* Patient can present with hypothermia (radiant and convective heat loss from the body surface is increased) or hyperthermia (an increase in metabolic activity provides compensatory increases in body heat production)
- *Pulse:* Blood volume and cardiac output may all be increased giving rise to pounding pulse and tachycardia.
- Blood pressure
- Respiratory rate
- *Nail changes:* Look for specific psoriatic nail changes such as nail pitting, oil-drop sign, and splinter hemorrhages. Usually, nails are shiny due to chronic rubbing associated with pruritus in cases of cutaneous t-cell lymphoma (CTCL)-induced erythroderma. Also look for pallor.

- *Sclera:* To see the signs of hepatitis
- *Pedal edema:* Hypoalbuminemia may contribute to the edema caused by skin inflammation itself, or cardiac failure.
- *Lymphadenopathy:* There can be firm, tontender enlargement of the inguinal and axillary lymph nodes. Fine needle aspiration cytology (FNAC) of the lymph node is required to differentiate dermatogenic lymphadenophy from malignant causes such as lymphoma.
- *Local examination*:
    - *Develop a logical and systemic approach to skin examination:* Approaching each patient in the same way, carefully examining the skin, and documenting your findings in a reproducible, legible fashion is the most reliable way to make correct diagnoses.
    - Try to examine the skin in a room with daylight.
    - Examine the entire skin surface during the first dermatologic examination.
    - *Appearance:* Generalized erythema (90%) BSA with a shiny appearance, fine white or yellow scaling, arises classically in the flexures, progresses and skin becomes dull red. Induration appears later.
    - *Scalp and body hair*: These may shed if erythroderma is present for long duration.
    - *"Nose sign of exfoliative dermatitis":* Complete absence of erythema and scaling of the nasal and perinasal skin in patients of psoriatic erythroderma.
    - Deck-chair sign
    - Areolar sparing
    - PPK
    - *Nail changes:*
        – Onycholysis, subungual hyperkeratosis, splinter hemorrhages, paronychia, beau's lines, occasionally, onychomadesis,
        – *Shore line nails:* All nails, transverse line of nail plate discontinuity preceded by transverse line of leukonychia; defective nail matrix keratinization followed by total nail matrix arrest.[2]

ERYTHRODERMA IN CHILDREN

History

- Age of onset
- *Intrauterine*: Graft-versus-host disease (GVHD)
- *A congenital onset*:
    - Ichthyosis
    - Immunodeficiency
    - Infections
- Sex
- *Consanguinity for autosomal recessive disorders*:
    - Autosomal recessive (AR) congenital icthyosiform erythroderma
    - Netherton syndrome
    - Other AR conditions
- Family history of similar complaints
- Term/preterm/low birth/acquired disseminated cutaneous candidiasis/harlequin ichthyosis
- History of seizures/lethargy/hypotonia—metabolic cause
- History of intake of drugs/topical medications—drug induced

- History of hypotension/wheezing/diarrhea/flushing—mastocytosis
- Malnutrition/Cystic fibrosis
- History of isomorphic phenomenon/joint pain or swelling
- Family history of similar complaints

Muco-cutaneous Examination
- Collodion baby
- *Primary skin lesion:* Macule, papules, pustules, vesicles, and bullae
- *Vesiculobullous:* Bullous ichthyosiform erythroderma, staphylococcal scalded skin syndrome (SSSS), and mastocytosis
- *Pustules:* Congenital candidiasis/psoriasis/staphylococcal
- Scales-fine/lamellar/polycyclic with double edge (ichthyosis linearis circumflexa)/swirled pattern
- *Skin induration:* Leathery skin—Omenn syndrome, lichenification–atopic ds
- Eczema
- *Pruritis:* Constant and severe in atopic and immunodeficiency; associated AD cases; mastocytosis, moderate in Netherton syndrome (NS), and Sjögren–Larsson syndrome
- *Lichenification*: Sjögren–Larsson/Atopic/NS
- Mucosa-involved/not involved and cheilitis
- Scalp alopecia (scarring/nonscarring), brittle hair/short hair
- Ichthyosis (scarring), metabolic disease (holocarboxylase synthetase deficiency, biotinidase deficiency, and citrullinemia), NS, and Omenn syndrome
- *Nails*: Paronychia, dystrophy, pitting, salmon patch, shinny, beau's line, onychomadesis, onycholysis, shoreline nails, and splinter hemorrhage
- *Palms and soles*: PPK (PRP, ichthyosiform erythroderma, and scabies)
- Eclabium/Ectropion
- *Focus of infection*: Conjunctivitis, rhinitis, and omphalitis
- Nikolsky sign would be positive in SSSS.
- Darier's sign/doughy skin
- *Islands of sparing*: PRP
- *Fissuring, contractures*: Ichthyosiform erythroderma, psoriasis, and scabies
- *General physical examination*: Anthropometry
- Protein–energy malnutrition (PEM)
- Lymphadenopathy
- Edema pedal/generalized
- *Characteristic faces*:
  - Cleft lip/palate
  - Low set ears, hypertelorism, antimongoloid slant, micrognathia, and short philtrum

Systemic Examination
- *Eye*: Keratitis/conjunctivitis/cataract/retinopathy/xerophthalmia
- *Auditory*: Deafness
- *Central nervous system (CNS)*: Spastic paralysis/mental retardation/deafness/seizures
- *Cardiovascular system (CVS)*: Anomalies/Cardiomyopathy/Valve anomalies
- *Musculoskeletal*: Kyphosis/scoliosis/dislocated hips/myopathy/stature
- *Per abdomen*: Hepatosplenomegaly
- *Genitalia*: Cryptorchidism/Hypogonadism

Questions and Answers

Q.1. How do you investigate a case of erythroderma?

Ans.
- *To establish the diagnosis*:
  - Multiple serial punch biopsies are taken simultaneously and repeated over months to increase the diagnostic yield. Preferred site should be discrete small lesion. Nonspecific in one-third to half cases—hyperkeratosis, parakeratosis, and acanthosis. Chronic inflammatory infiltrate may mask the features of underlying etiology.
  - It is especially important to differentiate benign inflammatory erythroderma from Sézary syndrome given the aggressive course of this lymphoma. Distinguishing histopathological features of Sézary syndrome include Pautrier microabcesses, atypical lymphocytes, basilar lymphocytes and dense dermal infiltrate.[1] Identification of numerous dilated blood vessels favor a diagnosis of benign inflammatory erythroderma.[1]
  - Direct immunofluorescence, if PF suspected.
- *Baseline investigations*:
  - Complete blood count (CBC), peripheral smear (PS), erythrocyte sedimentation rate (ESR), renal function test (RFT), liver function test (LFT), serum electrolytes, blood sugar, and urine and stool routine and microscopic examinations
  - Mild anemia with hematocrit values between 35 and 38% are thought to be due to folic deficiency, iron deficiency, and a chronic inflammatory state. More severe anemia is unusual.
  - Leukocytosis of greater than 20,000 leukocytes/mm^3 is seen in both benign and malignant forms of erythroderma.
  - Eosinophilia and increased IgE are frequently observed findings in erythroderma secondary to atopic dermatitis and drug reactions but are not diagnostic of these conditions.
  - Griffiths et al.[7] observed transient CD+ T cell lymphopenia in HIV negative patients with acute erythroderma as a consequence of T-cell sequestration in the skin.
  - Increased ESR, hypoalbuminemia, and hyperglobulinemia are frequent findings
  - Lymphoma workup if clinical suspicion

For diagnosis of Sézary syndrome, Sézary cell count analysis can be helpful.
- In current practice, greater than 20% or absolute count of at least 100/mm^3 Sézary cells is diagnostic for Sezary syndrome **(Box 2)**.

BOX 2	<10% circulating Sézary cells is nonspecific and is seen in a variety of benign dermatosis.
• Contact dermatitis • Atopic dermatitis • Psoriasis	• Lichen planus • Discoid lupus • Parapsoriasis

- Immunophenotyping, flow cytometry, and particularly, B- and T-cell gene rearrangement analysis
- Differentiating Sézary syndrome from erythrodermic actinic reticuloid can be difficult since the two diseases can have similar clinical presentations and high levels of circulating Sézary cells in the peripheral blood. However, immunophenotyping and nuclear contour index (NCI) of blood phenotypes can help differentiate the two since actinic reticuloid has increased CD8+ T cells and decreased NCI as compared to Sézary syndrome.
- *Leukemia workup:* Peripheral blood smears and bone marrow examination
- *Skin scrapings:* Hyphae or scabies mites

- Human immunodeficiency virus (HIV) test in right setting; use polymerase chain reaction (PCR) for viral detection, rather than enzyme-linked immunosorbent assay (ELISA) (exfoliative dermatitis has been reported to predict seroconversion in HIV infection)
- *Other:* If the cause in doubt, evaluate patients for occult tumors/malignancies
- Chest X-ray (CXR) and routine cancer screenings appropriate for age and sex (e.g., mammogram, stool occult blood test, sigmoidoscopy, prostate examination, serum prostate specific antigen level, and cervical smear)

Imaging:
- Computed tomography (CT), magnetic resonance imaging (MRI), CXR, and mammography, if clinical features indicate
- Patch test to detect contact allergens (test only during remission)

Q.2. How to treat a patient with erythroderma?

Ans. Serious medical threat, requires hospitalization

Regardless of underlying disease, initial management:
- Nutritional assessment and correction
- Correction of fluid, electrolyte, and protein imbalances
- Prevention of hypothermia
- Treatment of secondary infections

Principles of management:
- Maintain skin hydration
- Avoid scratching
- Avoid precipitating factors
- Topical steroids and antihistamines
- Ascertain and treat the underlying cause and complications
  (First generation sedating oral antihistamines may ease the often-severe pruritus)
  Drug-induced erythroderma **(Table 1)**.

TABLE 1: Drug-induced erythroderma.

Commonly observed	Recorded with
Sulfonamide	Ayurvedic
Isoniazid	Unani
Streptomycin	Homeopathic
NSAIDS	Indigenous medication
Antiepileptic	Topical medications

When the implicated drugs are withdrawn and symptomatic treatment given, *excellent prognosis* is recorded.
Only vancomycin and ceftriaxone have been described to cause erythroderma in neonates.
Vancomycin causes generalized erythema and hypotension due to histamine release.

Treatment of erythroderma:
- If drug reaction has not been ruled out, all nonessential medications should be discontinued if possible.
- Oatmeal baths and wet dressings to weeping or crusted sites followed by bland emollients and low-potency topical corticosteroids can help reduce inflammation and pruritus. High potency

corticosteroids should be avoided due to increased systemic absorption from the extensive surface area involvement and increased permeability of erythrodermic skin.
- Sedating oral antihistamines can enhance this effect and relieve anxiety.
- Patient require warm and humidified environment to increase comfort, prevent hypothermia, and increase moisture to the skin.
- Diuretics may be needed to treat edema and systemic antibiotics may be required for secondary bacterial infections.
- Patients who are refractory to topical therapy should receive systemic therapy directed at the unerlying etiology.
- Antibiotics will be required to control secondary infection. Heng[3] has suggested that colonization of the skin by *Staphylococcus aureus* may actually cause erythroderma, which will clear with appropriate antibiotic therapy.
- There is some evidence that the use of systemic steroids or potent topical steroids in psoriatic erythroderma may provoke the development of pustule formation.[4] In such cases, low dose methotrexate, acitretin, or ciclosporin[5] may be safer alternatives.
- Topical tar and UV therapy should also be avoided on erythrodermic psoriasis.
- The optimum treatment of erythrodermic cutaneous lymphoma is still debated. Options include systemic steroids, psoralen and ultraviolet A (PUVA), total body electron-beam irradiation, topical nitrogen mustard, and systemic chemotherapy.[6]

Q.3. Define acute skin failure.
Ans. It is defined as "loss of normal temperature control with inability to maintain the core body temperature and failure to prevent percutaneous loss of fluid, electrolyte and protein, with resulting imbalance, and failure of the mechanical barrier to prevent penetration of foreign materials".

Q.4. What is the normal requirement of proteins and how many proteins and scales are lost in erythroderma?
Ans. The normal requirement is 1 gm/kg/day approximately; 20–30 g of scales and 200 g of proteins per day.

Q.5. Why does patient experience edema in this condition?
Ans.
- Vasodilatation resulting in fluid seeping from intracellular compartment to the extracellular compartment
- Proteins are lost in scales resulting in hypoalbuminemia
- High-output cardiac failure
- Inflammation resulting from primary skin disease
- Renal involvement

Q.6. Enumerate different types of scales seen in various disorders.
Ans.
- *Micaceous scales:* Psoriasis
- *Branny (furfuraceous) scales versicolor*: Pityriasis
- *Collarette of scales:* Pityriasis rosea
- *Wafer-like scale:* Pityriasis lichenoides chronica
- *Fish-like scales:* Ichthyosis

- *Double edged scale:* Nethertons syndrome
- *Carpet tack-like scales:* Discoid lupus erythematosus
- *Trailing scales:* Erythema annulare centrifugum

Q.7. Enlist complications of erythroderma.
Ans.
- *High output cardiac failure:* The blood flow through the skin is markedly increased and there is fluid loss by transpiration, with consequent tachycardia and a risk of high-output cardiac failure, especially in elderly patients.
- *Hypothermia and hyperthermia:* Increased skin perfusion leads to thermoregulatory disturbances. Shivering and hypothermia may occur even though the skin feels deceptively warm, also known as concealed pyrexia.
- *Hypoalbuminemia:* Causes include increased plasma volume, decrease in protein synthesis, increase in metabolism, and protein loss via scaling and exudation.
- *Altered immune responses:* Increased gamma globulins, increased serum immunoglobulin E (IgE); CD4 T-cell lymphocytopenia.
- Dehydration
- *Infections:* Colonization of the skin with *Staphylococcus aureus* is common, and this can lead to secondary cutaneous infections. Respiratory infections are also common, and the majority who die, do so from pneumonia.
- Fluid electrolyte imbalance
- Altered immune function
- Pulmonary complications
- Peripheral edema

Q.8. What is concealed pyrexia?
Ans. In erythroderma, due to increased peripheral skin perfusion, body feels warm and so even if patient gets fever, it is not noticed. This is concealed pyrexia. Therefore, rectal temperature must be taken.

Q.9. What is the triad of Sézary syndrome?
Ans. Erythroderma, generalized lymphadenopathy, and presence of neoplastic T-cells.

Q.10. What is Sézary cell?
Ans. An atypical lymphocyte with a moderately to highly infolded or grooved nucleus (e.g., a cerebriform lymphocyte with nuclear contour index of 6.5 or more). Sézary cells, mycosis cells, Lutzner cells, and cerebriform lymphocytes are synonymous terms.

Q.11. Which are the types of Sézary cell?
Ans.
- *Small Sézary cell:* Cell diameter <12 microns, i.e., the size of a normal lymphocyte
- *Large Sézary cell:* Cell diameter of 12 microns, i.e., larger than a normal lymphocyte
- *Very large Sézary cell:* Cell diameter >14 microns, clearly neoplastic

Differentiating Sézary syndrome from erythrodermic actinic reticuloid[3] can be difficult since the two diseases can have similar clinical presentations and high levels of circulating Sézary cells in the peripheral blood. Differentiating Sézary syndrome from erythrodermic actinic reticuloid[3] can be difficult. In actinic reticuloid there is increased peripheral CD8+ T cell count and decreased NCI. However, immunophenotyping and nuclear contour index (NCI) of blood phenotypes can help to diagnose Sézary syndrome.

Q.12. Why barrier nursing is important in erythroderma?
Ans. Scales harbor bacteria, which thus serve as a source of infection to others.

Q.13. What is the drug of choice for pustular psoriasis?
Ans. Acitretin is considered a treatment of choice for pustular psoriasis.

Acitretin is an oral retinoid (vitamin A derivative) commonly used to treat severe psoriasis, typically prescribed at a dose of 0.25–1 mg/kg body weight per day. It should be taken with food to enhance absorption, as it requires fat for optimal uptake through the intestinal wall. Available in 10 mg and 25 mg capsules, acitretin is a metabolite of the earlier retinoid etretinate. Its mechanism of action in psoriasis involves reducing the proliferation of skin cells.

Acitretin is contraindicated during pregnancy due to its teratogenic effects, and strict birth control measures must be followed during treatment and for 3 years after discontinuation. As a result, acitretin is rarely prescribed to individuals of childbearing potential. If prescribed, they are required to undergo a blood pregnancy test before starting treatment and regularly during the course of therapy.

The most common side effects are mucocutaneus effects such as cheilitis and hair loss, which are dose dependent. Acitretin is not immunosuppressive, is generally safe for long-term use, and has no time limit restrictions.

REFERENCES

1. Ram-Wolff C, Martin-Garcia N, Bensussan A, Bagot M, Ortonne N. Histopathologic diagnosis of lymphomatous verses inflammatory eryhtroderma: A morphologic and phenotypic study on 47 skin biopsies. Am J Dermatopathol. 2010;32(8):755-63.
2. Shelley WB, Shelley ED. Shoreline nails: sign of drug-induced erythroderma. Cutis. 1985;35(3):220-4.
3. Heng MCV, Kloss SG, Chase DG. Erythroderma associated with mixed lymphoendothelial cell interactions and Staphylococcus aureus infections. Br J Dermatol. 1986;115(6):693-705.
4. Boyd AS, Menter A. Erythrodermic psoriasis. Precipitating factors, course, and prognosis in 50 patients. J Am Acad Dermatol. 1989;21:985-91.
5. Studio Italiano Multicentrico Nella Psoriasi. Management of erythrodermic psoriasis with low-dose cyclosporin. Dermatology. 1993;187(Suppl. 1):30-7.
6. Marsden JR. Cutaneous T-cell lymphomas. In: Lebwohl M, Heymann WR, Berth-Jones J, Coulson I (Eds). Treatment of Skin Disease: Comprehensive Therapeutic Strategies. London: Mosby; 2002. pp.131-7.
7. TW Griffiths, SR Stevens, KD Cooper. Acute erythroderma as an exclusion criterion for idiopathic CD4+ T lymphocytopenia Arch Dermatol. 1994;130(12):1530-3.

CHAPTER 6

Lepra Reactions

INTRODUCTION

Lepra reactions constitute one of the most common causes requiring admission in a dermatology ward, and good understanding of diagnosis and management of lepra reactions is mandatory for dermatology residents and consultants.

CASE 1: TUBERCULOID LEPROSY WITH TYPE-1 REACTION

History of Presenting Illness

A 22-year-old married female, resident of Ahmedabad, working as housewife, presented to the outpatient department (OPD) with chief complaints of reddish, raised non-itchy lesion over face associated with decreased sensations for 2 months. She gave history of taking medicines for the same past 1 month. Recently, the lesion has increased in size along with formation of raw areas over the lesion since last 10 days. She also had tingling and numbness over bilateral extremities since last 2 months.

There was no history of:
- Bleeding from nose and nasal stuffiness
- Joint pain
- Swelling over feet
- Slippage of footwear unknowingly
- Fever with evanescent crops of lesions
- Loss of eyebrows/eyelashes
- Inability to close eyes completely
- Recent onset reduced vision associated with or without painful red eye, excess lacrimation from eye, and reduced blinking rate
- Sharp shooting pain across elbow, wrist, at back of the knee and/or ankle
- Impaired grip, difficulty in buttoning and unbuttoning the shirt, slippage of things out of the hand, painless repeated blisters, wounds or burns on hands and feet
- Multidrug therapy (MDT) intake in family or neighborhood
- No history of diabetes mellitus (DM), hypertension (HTN), tuberculosis (TB) or any other major surgical or medical illness
- Family history was not significant.
- No history of tobacco chewing or alcohol intake or any addiction

Treatment History

The patient was diagnosed as borderline tuberculoid leprosy (BT) and was on World Health Organization (WHO) multibacillary (MB) adult MDT for 2 months.

Physical Examination

On general examination:
- The patient was fairly built and nourished, conscious, cooperative, and well oriented to time, place, and person
- *Temperature:* 97.8°F by digital thermometer
- *Pulse rate:* 84 beats/min with normal force, volume, and tension in right radial artery
- *Respiratory rate:* 16 breaths/min
- *Blood pressure:* 122/80 mm Hg
- There was no evidence of icterus, clubbing, cyanosis, pedal edema, or lymphadenopathy
- Systemic examination was normal

Cutaneous Examination

There was a single, well defined, erythematous ulcerated plaque present over right cheek, nose, and upper lip along with approximately 4 × 2 cm sized ill-defined ulcer present below eye on right cheek **(Figs. 1A and B)**.

Sensory Examination

- *Temperature examination (hot and cold differentiation):*
  - Intact on plaque
  - Intact over bilateral extremities

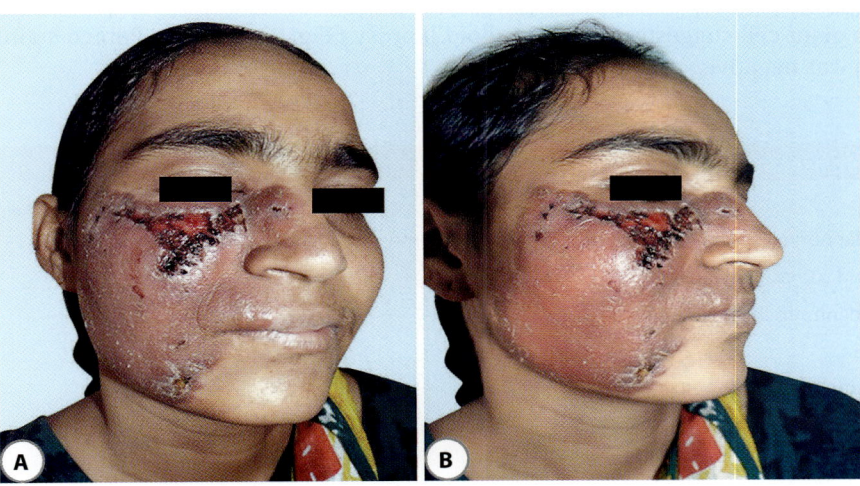

FIGS. 1A AND B: A single, erythematous, plaque with well-defined margins and sloping edge over right cheek, nose, and upper lip; (B) Ulceration and crusting just below right eye and on nose.

- *Touch (fine and crude)*:
  - Intact on plaque
  - Intact over bilateral extremities
- *Pain (superficial and deep)*:
  - Intact on plaque
  - Intact over bilateral extremities

Nerve Examination

Nerve examination is given in **Table 1**.

Motor Examination

Motor function of facial muscles and hand muscles were normal.

Investigations

- *Hemoglobin (Hb):* 10.4 g%
- *Total leukocyte count*: 9,800/mm^3
- *Differential leukocyte count:* Neutrophils 64% and lymphocytes 36%
- *Platelet counts:* 2,20,000/mm^3
- *Fasting blood sugar:* 76 mg%
- *Serum bilirubin:* 0.98 mg%
- *Serum glutamic oxaloacetic transaminase (SGOT)*: 36 IU/mL
- *Serum glutamic pyruvate transaminase (SGPT)*: 31 IU/mL
- Renal function tests were within normal limits.
- Slit smear examination from both eyebrows and earlobes—acid fast-bacilli resembling lepra bacilli not seen
- Biopsy from the facial lesion showed thinned epidermis along with presence of granulomas in the superficial and deep dermis located primarily around neurovascular and adnexal structures consisting of epithelioid cells, lymphocytes, and occasional polymorphonuclear cells and Langhans giant cell suggestive of tuberculoid leprosy **(Fig. 2)**. The Fite Faraco staining of biopsy specimen was negative.

TABLE 1: Nerve examination findings in the given case.		
Nerve	Right	Left
Greater auricular nerve	++ Tenderness: Grade I	+
Supraorbital and supratrochlear	–	–
Infraorbital and infratrochlear	–	–
Supraclavicular	–	–
Ulnar, radial cutaneous, and median	–	–
Lateral popliteal	–	–
Anterior and posterior tibial	–	–

Management

As per the severity grading, ulcerated plaque and facial plaque categorize as severe type 1 reaction (T1R), which needs to be managed aggressively with systemic corticosteroids. Hence, the patient was started on prednisolone (30 mg) once daily with milk in the morning along with continuation of standard WHO MB MDT. Topical fusidic acid cream was given to apply over ulceration on face. The patient showed significant improvement in the skin lesions after 1 month **(Figs. 3A and B)**.

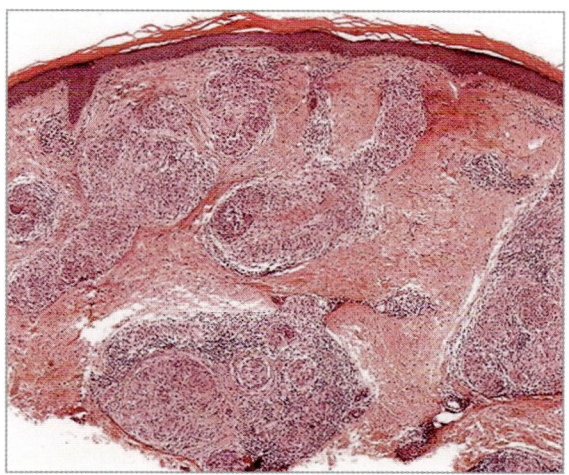

FIG. 2: Histology of borderline tuberculoid leprosy lesion.

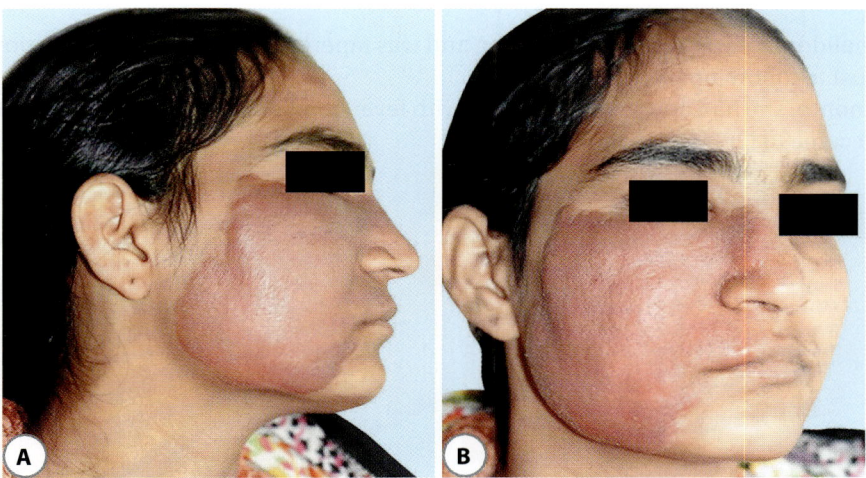

FIGS. 3A AND B: Follow-up after 1 month treatment—Ulcers healed, infiltration is significant.

CASE 2: CLINICAL HISTORY

A 42-year-old female patient, resident of Uttar Pradesh, farm laborer by occupation, coming from lower socioeconomic group, was admitted in the dermatology ward with chief complaints of sudden eruption of multiple, painful, reddish skin lesions over outer aspect of thighs, legs, and face. Initially, the lesions were pink in color gradually becoming red and then brownish over a period of 2–3 weeks. Patient also complained that some of the lesions over forearms progressed to form ulcers. Appearance of skin lesions was associated with fever, malaise, headache, joint pain more over both legs, and swelling over both hands and feet.

Origin, Duration, and Progress

Patient was clinically asymptomatic 3 years back when he gradually developed multiple skin lesions with change in color of the skin. The lesions were red in color and were distributed symmetrically over all limbs, chest and upper back **(Fig. 4A)**. As lesions were asymptomatic, patient did not seek medical advice for them. The lesions then became gradually thickened and elevated over last year. Patient also noticed thickening of ear lobes and deepening of facial ridges with red nodular lesions. For these complaints, patient visited a dermatologist and was put on blister pack therapy to be taken monthly for 3 months, which initially lead to improvement in clinical condition. Patient developed current clinical picture associated with high-grade fever and joint pains for last 2 weeks.

Patient also had complaint of reduced sensations on hands and feet with history of repeated trauma and development of ulcer over the sole of right foot. Patient experienced bouts of epistaxis and edema feet. History of accidental slippage of footwear was present.

There was no history of any ocular complaints.

Past treatment history was reviewed: She used to develop recurrent red lesions on all four limbs for past 2 years. Was treated with high doses of prednisolone (60 mg). On tapering the dose to 20 mg, she used to experience flare of the evanescent lesions accompanied with constitutional symptoms.

Thalidomide in the dose of 300 mg was added which was giving her day time sedation and severe constipation.

Dose of thalidomide was reduced to 200 mg and was tapered to 100 mg after resolution of ENL.

She was lost to follow-up.

Before 1 month, she had another flare of ENL with fever, joint pains, necrotic lesions on her forearm **(Fig. 4B)** and came to OPD for management.

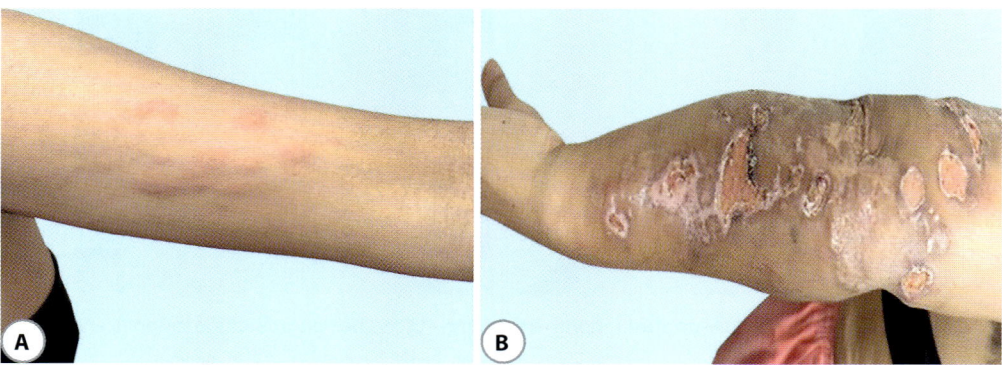

FIGS. 4A AND B: (A) Erythema nodosum leprosum; and (B) ENL necroticans.

Chapter 6: Lepra Reactions

Questions and Answers

Q.1. Describe leprosy reaction and mention the types of lepra reaction.
Ans. During the course of leprosy, acute and intermittent episodes of sudden inflammatory exacerbation of pre-existing lesions or sudden development of crops of new lesions along with systemic symptoms may occur, which is described as "leprosy reactions". It may occur during the treatment or sometimes patients may present to health facilities directly in reaction.

Although any type of leprosy may undergo leprosy reactions, predominantly those patients with borderline type of disease experience more reactions. Relatively stable/or polar forms and indeterminate form undergo leprosy reactions very rarely.
- *Precipitating factors:* Borderline forms of leprosy, intercurrent infections (viral, malaria, etc.), anemia, mental and/or physical stress, puberty, pregnancy, parturition, or surgical interventions.
- *Types:*
  - Type-1 reaction (T1R), also known reversal leprosy reaction, is an example of type-IV hypersensitivity (allergic) reaction (Coombs and Gell) and it is defined as "an inflammatory episode in leprosy patients characterized by sudden and abrupt appearance of erythema, swelling, and tenderness in the pre-existing lesions with or without neuritis".
  - Type-2 leprosy reaction or [erythema nodosum leprosum (ENL)] occurs due to humoral immunity and it is an example of type-III hypersensitivity (allergic) reaction (Coombs and Gell). The alteration in the cell-mediated immunity to antigens specific to leprosy without generalized reduction in the cell-mediated immunity (CMI) is noted.

Q.2. What is the difference between type 1 and type 2 leprosy reactions?
Ans. The differences are summarized in **Table 2**.

TABLE 2: Differences between type-1 and 2 leprosy reactions.		
Signs	**Type 1**	**Type 2**
Pathogenesis	Type IV delayed hypersensitivity	Type III immune complex mediated hypersensitivity
Skin involvement	• Pre-existing skin lesions suddenly becomes reddish, swollen, warm, painful/tender but the rest of the skin is normal • If very severe may undergo ulceration	• Fresh, evanescent crop of reddish, tender, cutaneous/subcutaneous papulonodules lesions appear (not associated with leprosy patches) • ENL lesions commonly occur on extensor surfaces of arms and legs
Nervous system	Nerves close to patch/plaque may be enlarged and become tender due to neuritis, which may result into loss of nerve function (loss of sensation and muscle weakness) and may appear suddenly/rapidly	Nerve involvement is not as severe as T1R
Constitutional symptoms	• Good, with little or no fever or other constitutional symptoms • Moderate grade of T1R have fever as a component	Poor, with prominent fever and general malaise
Eye involvement	Weakness of eyelid muscles leading to incomplete closure may occur (nerve involved) if lesions is around eye	Internal eye disease (iritis, iridocyclitis) occurs, lepromatous nodules are seen
Systemic involvement	Not affected	May be affected

(ENL: erythema nodosum leprosum; T1R: type-1 reaction)

Q.3. How do you differentiate between relapse and late reversal reaction?

Ans. Occurrence of late reversal reaction in a patient who has been released from treatment may lead to suspicion of "relapse". It is important to remember that late reversal reactions present within 1–2 years of being released from treatment and they present with symptoms of T1R while for patients to be labelled as having relapse, they must fulfill criteria of developing new leprosy patches after completion of surveillance period [2–5 years from release from treatment (RFT)].

Q.4. What is difference between mild and severe type 1 reactions?

Ans. Type 1 leprosy reactions are classified into mild and severe type based on **Table 3**.

TABLE 3: Classification of type-1 leprosy reaction.	
Mild	• Few skin lesions with features of reaction clinically; erythema and/or pain (except over face) • Absence of any nerve pain or loss of function
Severe	• Nerve pain or paresthesia • Development of loss of nerve function or increasing nerve function impairment • Fever and edema of hands, feet, and face • If mild reaction persists for >6 weeks • Involvement of face • Ulcerative skin lesion

Q.5. Discuss different types of type 2 leprosy reactions (ENL).

Ans. ENL can be categorized into acute, recurrent, or chronic as follows:
- *Acute type:* When a single episode lasts <24 weeks
- *Recurrent:* When a new subsequent episode of ENL occurs 28 days or more after stopping treatment for ENL
- *Chronic:* When new subsequent episodes keep on occurring for 24 weeks or more while patient has been on ENL treatment either continuously or where any treatment-free period had been 27 days or less.

Q.6. Classify ENL based on the severity.

Ans. ENLIST scoring system has been validated to classify the severity of ENL. It is based on following parameters; pain rating on the visual analogue scale, fever, number—inflammation and extent of skin lesions, peripheral edema, bone pain, inflammation of joints and/or digits due to ENL, lymphadenopathy, and nerve tenderness due to ENL. Each item is graded by giving scores from 0–3 and the score for each item should be *added* together to obtain the ENLIST ENL severity scale score.

Mild ENL is categorized as an ENLIST ENL severity scale score of *8 or less*.

Q.7. Describe the management of lepra reaction.

Ans. *Type-1 lepra reactions:* The objective of treatment is to restore normal nerve function and to prevent further inflammation-mediated neural damage. MDT should be started if patient is newly diagnosed with reaction or it should be continued if patient is already on MDT along with the appropriate T1R treatment.
- *Mild (limited to skin lesions and without ulceration/neuritis):* Reassurance and nonsteroidal anti-inflammatory drugs (NSAIDs) (aspirin or paracetamol)

- *Severe reactions (facial lesions, markedly inflamed skin lesions/ulceration/neuritis/impending or recent paralysis):* Steroids + splinting of affected nerves in the acute stage or surgical decompression
- The current evidence suggests that individuals should be treated with 0.5–1 mg/kg/day of prednisolone (or equivalent), reduced gradually to zero over the course of 20 weeks.

Other immunosuppressants that can be used are methotrexate, cyclosporine, azathioprine, mycophenolate mofetil, and topical tacrolimus (0.1%).

Type-2 lepra reactions
- *Mild/moderate reaction (fever with few skin lesions only):* Rest, NSAIDS like aspirin, colchicine
- *Severe ENL (fever, large numbers of ENL lesions/pustular lesions with or without neuritis, arthritis, orchitis, uveitis, ENL necroticans):* Rest + analgesics + steroids/thalidomide, clofazimine in larger doses. Oral and parenteral corticosteroids rapidly control the symptoms of ENL. Doses of 1–2 mg/kg body weight are usually required.

Thalidomide should be given, especially in cases of chronic recurrent ENL and steroid dependence.

Q.8. What is current leprosy situation in India?
Ans. With various intervention introduced under National Leprosy Eradication Programme (NLEP) in the last few years, number of new leprosy cases detected have come down to 75,394 in 2021–2022 from 1,25,785 in 2014–2015, accounting for 53.6% of global new leprosy cases. The prevalence rate is 0.4 per 10,000 population.

Q.9. What is WHO disability Grading for leprosy disabilities?
Ans. WHO disability grading:
- *Hands and feet*
    - *Grade 0:* No anesthesia, no visible deformity or damage
    - *Grade 1:* Anesthesia present, but no visible deformity or damage
    - *Grade 2:* Visible deformity or damage present
- *Eyes*
    - *Grade 0:* No eye problem due to leprosy; no evidence of visual loss
    - *Grade 1:* Eye problems due to leprosy present, but vision not severely affected as a result of these (vision: 6/60 or better; can count fingers at 6 m)
    - *Grade 2:* Severe visual impairment (*vision:* worse than 6/60; inability to count fingers at 6 m) also includes lagophthalmos, iridocyclitis, and corneal opacities

Q.10. What are the risk factors for development of deformities?
Ans. Risk factors for deformity are:
- *Age:* More frequent in 20–50-year age group
- *Sex:* Male sex
- *Occupation:* Laborers working on daily wedges
- *Type of leprosy:* Bacillary index >3 carry a high risk if not treated early
- *Number of nerve trunk involved:* >3 nerve trunk involvement increases the risk manifold.
- History of recurrent reactions
- *Duration of active diseases:* Longer the disease remains untreated, greater the risk of disability

Types of deformities:
- *Primary deformities:* Directly caused by tissue reaction to infection with *Mycobacterium leprae*
    - *Face:* Loss of eyebrows and eyelashes, facies leonine, lagophthalmos, depressed nose, and ear deformities

- *Hands:* Claw hand and wrist drop
- *Feet:* Foot drop and clawing of toes
- *Other:* Gynecomastia, perforation of palate
- *Secondary deformities:* These occur as a result of damage to anesthetic parts of the body—corneal ulcers, hand and foot ulceration, and mutilation.

Q.11. Name reconstructive surgeries for deformity in leprosy.
Ans.
- *Ulnar claw hand*:
  - Modified Stiles–Bunnell transfer flexor digitorum superficialis four tail or (FDS-4T) procedure
  - Zancolli's lasso procedure—flexor digitorum superficialis transfer
- *Foot drop:* Tibialis posterior tendon transfer and tendoachilles lengthening
- *Lagophthalmos*:
  - Lateral tarsorrhaphy,
  - McLaughlin's tarsorrhaphy

Q.12. What is National Strategic Plan (2023–2027) for Leprosy?
Ans. Central Leprosy Division, WHO, and International Federation of Anti-Leprosy Associations (ILEP) along with participation of the NLEP partners, experts, and representatives of persons affected by leprosy have drafted the National Strategic Plan and Roadmap for Leprosy 2023–2027 for moving toward achieving interruption of transmission of leprosy in India.

This roadmap aims to provide a clear path and guidance to all key stakeholders and provide a blueprint for focused interventions to achieve the goals of NLEP for the period 2023–2027.

Vision: Leprosy free India with zero infection and disease, zero disability, zero stigma, and discrimination

Goal: Accelerate toward achieving interruption of leprosy transmission in India

Specific objectives:
1. Strengthen leadership, commitment, and partnerships
2. Acceleration of case detection
3. Provision of quality services
4. Enhanced measures for prevention of disease, disabilities, stigma, discrimination and violation of human rights
5. Digitalization of surveillance systems
    These five are the strategic pillars of the national strategic plan 2023-2027.

CHAPTER 7

Cutaneous T-cell Lymphoma

INTRODUCTION

Cutaneous T-cell lymphoma (CTCL) can present as widespread nodules, plaques, fungating/ulcerated nodules or as erythroderma requiring inpatient management in the dermatology ward. CTCL refers to a diverse group of skin-related cancers originating from skin homing T cells. These neoplasms exhibit significant differences in their clinical features, histological characteristics, immunophenotypic profiles, and prognoses.

Extranodal lymphomas are cancers that arise in tissues or organs outside the lymphatic system. When lymphoma is confined to the skin with no signs of disease elsewhere at the time of diagnosis, it is referred to as "primary" cutaneous lymphoma. These lymphomas can be classified into two main categories: (1) CTCL and (2) cutaneous B-cell lymphomas. Approximately, 75–80% of primary cutaneous lymphomas are T-cell in origin, while 20–25% are B-cell types. In 1975, studies revealed that most lymphoid[1] infiltrates in the skin were of T-cell origin, leading Edelson to introduce the term CTCL.[2]

Mycosis fungoides (MF) is the most prevalent form of CTCL, making up nearly 50% of all primary cutaneous lymphomas. It is known for its slow progression and distinctive clinical and pathological characteristics. The second most common category of CTCL consists of primary cutaneous CD30+ lymphoproliferative disorders.

APPROACH TO A CASE

History

A 60-year-old male, presented with chief complaints of generalized itching along with discrete reddish plaques and nodules over face, trunk and limbs since last 3 years, which gradually progressed to involve all of his trunk, face, and limbs in the last 7 months. Patient gave history of significant weight loss in last 3 months.

On examination, erythematous and scaly plaques were seen on face and limbs. Few lesions were showing ulceration/crusting at places. Ulcerated nodules/tumors **(Figs. 1 to 3)** were present at various sites, especially on the abdomen. Multiple nontender enlarged lymph nodes were palpable in groin, axillae, submental, and submandibular region.[3]

Serial biopsies were taken in the past, but all were showing changes of chronic dermatitis. Recent biopsy confirmed the diagnosis of CTCL.

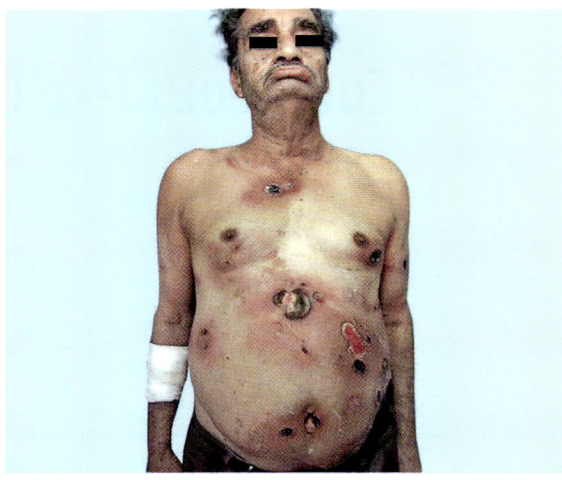

FIG. 1: Multiple, erythematous plaques with crusting and one plaque over abdomen having erosion.

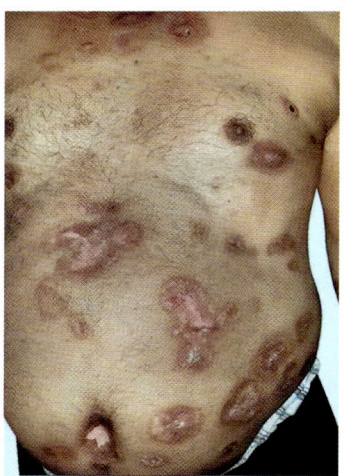

FIG. 2: Multiple, well-defined plaques of irregular shapes and sizes, with center of some lesions showing hypopigmentation (The same lesions shown in **Fig. 1** after healing).

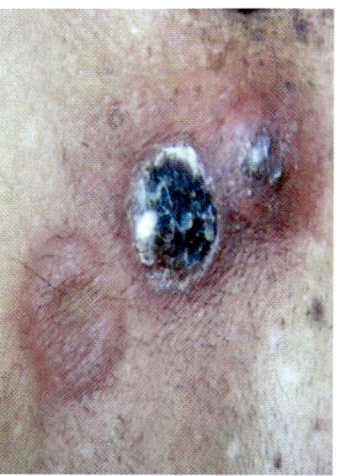

FIG. 3: Close-up view of the lesions in **Figure** 1 showing crusting at the center and some arcuate-shaped lesions.

Physical Examination

Physical examination involves determination of types of skin lesions.
- In the patch or plaque stage, lesions display significant variation in color, with varying degrees of scaling and borders. Few patients can have predominantly poikilodermatous changes **(Figs. 4 and 5)**. In the erythrodermic stage (Sézary syndrome), assess the percentage of the body surface area affected and observe any ulceration present on the lesions. In the tumoral stage, record the total number of lesions, their largest size, and the aggregate of affected body areas.

- Physical palpation of the lymph node to identify palpable lymph node, especially those >1.5 cm in largest diameter and check for firm consistency, regularity, if any clustering is found, or if they are mobile/fixed
- Look for any organomegaly.

Histopathological Findings

Histopathological findings are given in **Figure 6**.
- Epidermotropism
- Dense lymphocytic infiltrate
- Skin biopsy should be taken from most indurated area that is the most developed part of the lesion; mostly the center, if single biopsy is to be taken.
- A skin biopsy is crucial for confirmation. The primary diagnostic feature is the presence of abnormal lymphoid cells in the epidermis, i.e., epidermotropism. The dermis is infiltrated with atypical lymphoid cells **(Fig. 6)**.

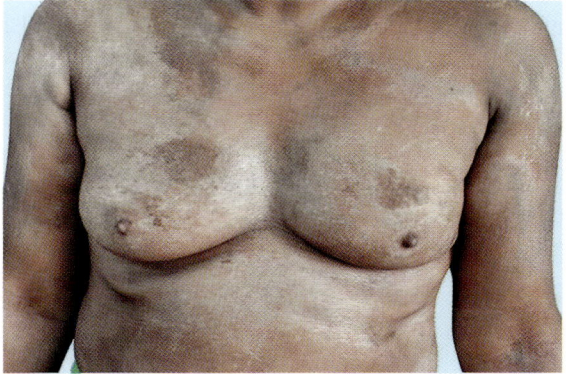

FIG. 4: Multiple, plaques over chest and abdomen showing hypo as well as hyperpigmentation.

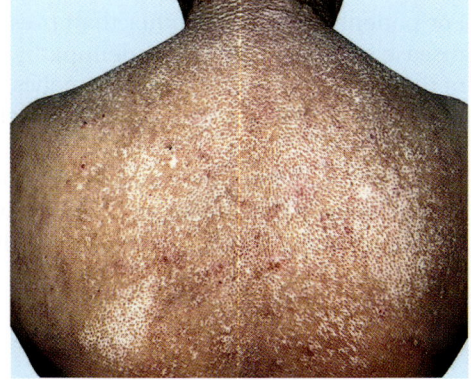

FIG. 5: Reflecting salt-pepper hypopigmentation and some degree of erythema and crusting over upper back.

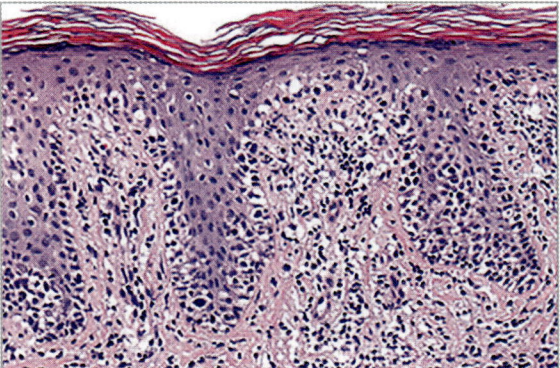

FIG. 6: Epidermotropism, dense dermal infiltrate of atypical lymphocytes.

- Immunophenotyping should be performed to evaluate Pan-T cell markers (CD2, CD3, CD4, CD5, CD7, and CD8) and a B-cell marker such as CD20.
- CD30 testing may also be necessary in cases where lymphomatoid papulosis, anaplastic lymphoma, or large-cell transformation are suspected.

Blood Test
- Complete blood count (CBC) with differential, liver function tests, renal function test, lactate dehydrogenase (LDH), comprehensive chemistries is recommended.
- Abnormal lymphocytes can be analyzed through Sézary cell count, which involves determining the absolute number of Sézary cells, by flow cytometry. This may include assessing markers such as CD4+/CD7- or CD4+/CD26-12, along with calculating the CD4:CD8 ratio.
- Ideally, T-cell receptor gene analysis of peripheral blood mononuclear cells should be done.

Radiological Test[1]
In early stages (T1N0M0 and T2N0MO) with limited skin involvement, only X-ray or ultrasonography screening of peripheral lymph nodes are done.
- For patients with stages other than presumed stage IA, or in selected individuals with limited T2 disease and no evidence of adenopathy or blood involvement, computed tomography (CT) scans of the neck, chest, abdomen, and pelvis, along with fluorodeoxyglucose (FDG)-positron emission tomography (PET) scan, are recommended to assess potential lymphadenopathy or visceral involvement.
- PET scans may improve the detection of systemic disease, and the level of PET activity is often correlated with the histological grade of lymph nodes.
- In cases where CT scans cannot be safely performed, magnetic resonance imaging (MRI) can be used as an alternative.

Lymph Node Biopsy
Excisional biopsy is recommended for patients with a lymph node that is either >1.5 cm in diameter and/or is firm, irregular, clustered, or fixed.

Biopsy site:
- The preferred site for biopsy is the largest lymph node draining the affected skin area, or if FDG-PET scan data is available, the node with the highest standardized uptake value (SUV).
- In the absence of additional imaging information, and when multiple lymph nodes are enlarged and similar in size or consistency, the biopsy should be performed in the following order of preference: Cervical, axillary, and inguinal regions.

Differential Diagnosis[4]
Differential diagnosis is as follows:
- Allergic contact dermatitis
- Parapsoriasis
- Atopic dermatitis

- Pemphigus foliaceus
- Plaque psoriasis
- Pustular psoriasis
- Infections such as tinea corporis, leishmaniasis, leprosy, and coccidioidomycosis
- Lymphomatoid papulosis
- Adult T-cell leukemia/lymphoma (ATLL)

Treatment for cutaneous T-cell lymphoma is given in **Table 1**—it depends on correct characterization of the stage of the disease.

Stage IA disease: It refers to patients with patches, plaques, or papules covering <10% of the total skin surface, without any involvement of lymph nodes or internal organs. Treatment for stage IA disease typically involves skin-directed therapies.

Skin directed therapies include:
- *Topical corticosteroids:* The selection of steroid strength is based on the affected body area and the severity of skin symptoms and signs. Typically, high-potency or super-high potency corticosteroids are used.
- Topical chemotherapy (nitrogen mustard or carmustine)
- Topical retinoids
- Topical imiquimod
- Local radiation (X-ray or electron beam)
- Phototherapy [ultraviolet B (UVB) or psoralen and UVA (PUVA)]

TABLE 1: Treatment of cutaneous T-cell lymphoma (CTCL) according to stage of disease.

Stage prognostic group	First-line	Second-line	Experimental
Stage IA–IIA: Good prognosis	• Expectant or SDT • SDT • PUVA + IFN-α • PUVA + Bexarotene • TSEBT	• SDT • HDACi (vorinostat/depsipeptide) • Denileukin diftitox	
Stage III: Intermediate prognosis	• Methotrexate • ECP/IFN-α/bexarotene combination	• Alemtuzumab • TSEB • Single agent chemotherapy • HDACi • Denileukin diftitox	RicAlloSCT
Stage IIB/IV*: Poor prognosis	• Radiotherapy (TSEB) • Chemotherapy (single/multiagent)	• HDACi • Denileukin diftitox • Palliative therapy	RicAlloSCT

*Maintenance therapy with SDT alpha-interferon/bexarotene for residual skin disease.

Note: SDT consists of treatment with emollients, topical steroids, PUVA or UVB, and topical chemotherapy.

(ECP: extracorporeal photopheresis; HDACi: histone deacetylase inhibitors; IFN-α: interferon alpha; PUVA: Psoralen + UVA; RicAlloSCT: reduced-intensity conditioned allogeneic stem cell transplant; SDT: skin directed therapy; TSEBT: total skin electron beam therapy)

Stage IB/IIA disease: Stage IB disease refers to patients with patches, plaques, or papules covering 10% or more of the total skin surface, with no involvement of lymph nodes or internal organs. Stage IIA disease includes patients with any size of patches, plaques, or papules, along with reactive palpable lymph nodes (N1) or isolated, scattered neoplastic cells in the lymph nodes (N2) on histological examination, while maintaining the nodal architecture and with no visceral involvement.

Treatment

Treatment is given in **Table 1**.
- Topical corticosteroids
- *Topical chemotherapy:* Mechlorethamine (nitrogen mustard), carmustine (BCNU), and peldesin (BCX-34, an inhibitor of the purine nucleoside phosphorylase enzyme)
- *Radiotherapy:* Total skin electron beam (TSEB)
- *Phototherapy/Photochemotherapy:* PUVA, broadband and narrowband UVB, UVA1, and extracorporeal photopheresis.

Systemic Therapies

- *Immunotherapy:* Interferon-α, interferon-γ, and cyclosporine
- *Retinoids:* Bexarotene
- *Toxin therapy:* Denileukin diftitox
- *Histone deacetylase inhibitors:* Vorinostat, romidepsin, and depsipeptide
- Biologics like CD-25 (daclizumab), CD-52 (alemtuzumab), and CD-4 antagonist (zanolimumab)
- Proteasome inhibitors such as bortezomib

Systemic Chemotherapy

Cyclophosphamide, hydroxydaunomycin, oncovin, and prednisolone—CHOP.

Rigorous "treat-to-cure" regimen: This includes total skin electron beam (TSEB) therapy at 3,000 cGy, combined with cyclophosphamide, daunorubicin, etoposide, and vincristine.

"Gentle palliative" regimen: A sequential treatment plan using topical therapies such as nitrogen mustard, superficial radiotherapy, and TSEB, with progression to PUVA therapy, if necessary, is recommended.

Allogeneic Hematopoietic Stem Cell Transplantation

Treatment for MF should be stage-specific, with an emphasis on palliative care rather than aggressive attempts to cure the disease.

Questions and Answers

Q.1. Classify CTCL.

Ans. World Health Organization (WHO) and European Organization for Research and Treatment of Cancer Classification (EORTC) reached a consensus classification for cutaneous lymphomas, and it was revised by WHO in 2008; CTCLs are broken down into the following classifications **(Table 2)**.

TABLE 2: European Organization for Research and Treatment of Cancer Classification (EORTC)/ World Health Organization (WHO) 2008 classification of CTCL.

Indolent (low-grade/slow growing) clinical behavior	Aggressive clinical behavior
<ul><li>Mycosis fungoides (MF)</li><li>*MF variants and subtypes*:<ul><li>Folliculotropic MF</li><li>Pagetoid reticulosis</li><li>Granulomatous slack skin</li></ul></li><li>Primary cutaneous CD30+ lymphoproliferative disorders</li><li>Primary cutaneous anaplastic large-cell lymphoma</li><li>Lymphomatoid papulosis</li><li>Subcutaneous panniculitis-like T-cell lymphoma (histiocytic cytophagic panniculitis), in which there is no involvement of superficial parts of the skin (epidermis and dermis). T-cells usually have a–ß phenotype, CD3+, CD4-. Patients present with nodules on lower extremities and trunk and with systemic symptoms such as fever and malaise. Hemophagocytosis may be seen on histology (blood cells are found within phagocytes)[5]</li><li>Primary cutaneous CD4+ small/medium pleomorphic T-cell lymphoma usually presents with a single lesion and progresses slowly</li></ul>	<ul><li>Sézary syndrome</li><li>Adult T-cell leukemia/lymphoma</li><li>Extranodal natural killer (NK)/T-cell lymphoma, nasal type; this is associated with Epstein–Barr virus and is aggressive</li><li>Primary cutaneous peripheral T-cell lymphoma, unspecified</li><li>Primary cutaneous aggressive CD8+T cell lymphoma</li><li>Cutaneous γ/δ T-cell lymphoma</li></ul>

Q.2. What is the TNMB classification of MF?

Ans. The TNMB classification of MF is given in **Table 3**.

TABLE 3: TNMB staging of mycosis fungoides (MF).

TNMB stage	Description
Skin	
T1	Limited patches, papules and plaques covering <10% of the skin surface; may further stratify into T1a (patch only) versus T1b (plaque ± patch)
T2	Patches, papules, and plaques covering ≥10% of the skin surface; may further stratify into T2a (patch only) versus T2b (plaque ± patch)
T3	One or more tumors (≥1 cm diameter)
T4	Confluence of erythema covering ≥80% body surface area
Node	
N0	No clinically abnormal peripheral lymph nodes; biopsy not required
N1	Clinically abnormal peripheral lymph nodes; histopathology Dutch grade 1 or NCI LN0–2
N1a	Clone negative
N1b	Clone positive
N2	Clinically abnormal peripheral lymph nodes; histopathology Dutch grade 2 or NCI LN3
N2a	Clone negative
N2b	Clone positive
N3	Clinically abnormal peripheral lymph nodes; histopathology Dutch grades 3–4 or NCI LN4; clone positive or negative
NX	Clinically abnormal peripheral lymph nodes; no histological conformation

Continued

Continued

TNMB stage	Description
Visceral	
M0	No visceral organ involvement
M1	Visceral involvement (must have pathology confirmation and organ involved should be specified)
Blood	
B0	Absence of significant blood involvement; ≤5% of peripheral blood lymphocytes are atypical (Sézary cells)
B0a	Clone negative
B0b	Clone positive (identical to skin T-cell clone)
B1	Low blood tumor burden; >5% of peripheral blood lymphocytes are atypical (Sézary cells) but does not meet the criteria of B2
B1a	Clone negative
B1b	Clone positive (identical to skin T-cell clone)
B2	High blood tumor burden; ≥1,000/μL Sézary cells with positive clones

Q.3. What are the differential diagnoses of nodular stage of MF?
Ans. B-cell lymphoma, sarcoidosis, leprosy, carcinoma cutis, and leishmaniasis.

Q.4. What are the histopathological findings of MF?
Ans.
- Hyperconvoluted (cerebriform) lymphocytes of approximately the same width as the basal keratinocytes.
- Early lesions show diffuse lymphocytic infiltrate in papillary dermis with a tendency of lymphoid cells to line up close to the epidermis (toy soldier sign)
- Disproportionate exocytosis
- *Pautrier's microabscesses:* Intraepidermal clusters of atypical lymphocytes
- Epidermotropism is an important clue to the diagnosis apparent in well-developed plaques.
- If the number of the large cells exceeds 25% of whole infiltrate, it indicates transformation/progression into a secondary large cell lymphoma.

Q.5. What is toy soldier sign?
Ans. Linear aggregates of neoplastic lymphocytes along the dermoepidermal junction in MF.

Q.6. What is the other name for Pautrier's microabscess?
Ans. Darier nest.

Q.7. Which are the poor prognostic factors for MF?
Ans.
- Higher age at onset (over 60 years)
- Skin stage (thick plaques are an independent poor prognostic factors)
- Presence of nodal (IVA) or visceral (IVB) disease
- Presence of T-cell clone
- Absence of CD7, high LDH, large cell size, periodic acid-Schiff (PAS) inclusions, and number of circulating Sézary cells

Q.8. What are the other names of Sézary cell?

Ans. Mycosis cells, Lutzner cell, monster cell, cerebriform lymphocyte, and atypia cellules monstreuses are the other names of Sézary cell.

Q.9. What are the stains used to identify Sézary cell?

Ans. Periodic acid–Schiff (PAS) and Wright–Giemsa stain are the stains used to identify Sézary cells.

Q.10. What are the other causes of Sézary cell in blood?

Ans.
- Sézary syndrome
- Actinic reticuloid
- Erythroderma secondary to psoriasis

Q.11. What is photodynamic therapy?[6-8]

Ans. The photodynamic reaction involves the activation of photosensitizers, primarily porphyrins, by visible light in the presence of oxygen. This leads to the production of reactive oxygen species, especially singlet oxygen. Light sources commonly used in photodynamic therapy (PDT) include lasers, xenon arc or discharge lamps, incandescent filament lamps, and solid-state light-emitting diodes (LEDs).

Q.12. What are the indications of PDT?

Ans.
- Nonhypertrophic actinic keratosis of face and scalp [Food and Drug Administration (FDA) approved]
- Basal cell carcinoma
- Acne vulgaris
- Squamous cell carcinoma
- Photoaging
- Morphea
- Sebaceous hyperplasia

Q.13. What are the topical agents used in PDT?

Ans. Aminolevulinic acid (ALA) and methyl aminolevulinate (MAL).

Q.14. What is the difference between ALA and MAL?

Ans. Difference between ALA and MAL is given in **Table 4**.

TABLE 4: Difference between aminolevulinic acid (ALA) and methyl aminolevulinate (MAL).		
	ALA	MAL
Formulation	Hydroalcoholic solution	Cream
Structure	More hydrophilic	Less hydrophilic
FDA-approved light source	Blue	Red
Application	No occlusion	Occlusion
Device	Blue-U	Aktilite
Energy	10 J/cm^2	37 J/cm^2

(FDA: Food and Drug Administration)

Q.15. What is the mechanism of action of PDT in CTCL?

Ans. The accumulation of protoporphyrin IX (PpIX) is believed to occur due to enhanced penetration of ALA through the abnormal epidermis over tumor sites. This leads to the preferential accumulation of PpIX in proliferating, iron-deficient tumor cells. Porphyrins produced from ALA are primarily localized near the mitochondria, where they can induce apoptosis or necrosis in malignant cells. The Soret band, at a wavelength of 410 nm, is the key excitation peak for PpIX.

Q.16. What are the side effects of PDT?

Ans. Side effects include a burning sensation, pain, and, less commonly, pruritus during light exposure following ALA application. Additionally, hyperpigmentation and hypopigmentation can occur.

Q.17. What is extracorporeal photochemotherapy (ECP)?

Ans. Extracorporeal photochemotherapy, also known as photopheresis, a type of pheresis, is a procedure where a portion of the patient's blood is withdrawn, treated with a photosensitizing agent, exposed to UVA light, and then reinfused into the patient. This outpatient treatment typically follows a 2-day cycle, repeated every 2–4 weeks, and may continue for months or years depending on the patient's response. Each session lasts about 4 hours and is carried out through a peripheral vein.

Q.18. What is the mechanism of action of ECP?

The mechanism of action of ECP involves several key processes:
- Induction of dendritic cell differentiation, leading to the internalization and presentation of tumor-associated antigens
- Enhancement of immune responses targeting tumor cells through T-cell activation
- Promotion of apoptosis in activated or autoreactive T cells
- Facilitation of shifts in the production of immunoregulatory cytokines
- Stimulation of antigen-specific regulatory T cells to modulate immune responses

Q.19. What are the indications of ECP?

Ans.
- Cutaneous T-cell lymphoma (FDA-approved)
- Scleroderma
- Pemphigus vulgaris
- Pemphigus foliaceus
- Epidermolysis bullosa acquisita
- Acute graft-versus-host disease (GVHD)
- Chronic GVHD
- Prevention of GVHD

Q.20. What are the indications of ECP in CTCL?

Ans. Stage III or IV MF with evidence of blood involvement, either by presence of a T-cell clone by *TCR* gene rearrangement analysis, a circulating Sézary cells count of >10% of total lymphocyte or peripheral CD4:CD8 ratio of >10.

Treatment is delivered every 2–4 weeks with response typically seen at 3–6 months. Bexarotene or interferon alpha has been combined in cases where response is poor.

Q.21. How to monitor the disease activity in CTCL following ECP?

Ans. Tumor burden should be assessed before treatment and then every 4–8 weeks during treatment through the following measures:
- *Skin:* Monitor clinical skin involvement using a skin map for documentation.
- *Blood:* Evaluate lymphocyte count, CD4/CD8 ratio, and percentages of CD4+/CD7- and/or CD4+/CD26- cells.
- *Lymph nodes:* Use CT or PET/CT scans to assess lymph node size and metabolic activity.
- *Molecular analysis:* For patients in clinical remission, molecular testing can be performed every 3–6 months for more sensitive detection of tumor presence.

Q.22. What are the side effects of ECP?

Ans.
- *Associated with 8-methoxypsoralen:* Nausea and photosensitivity
- *Cardiovascular effects:* Hypotension, congestive heart failure, flushing, and tachycardia
- *Venipuncture-related issues:* Possible loss of venous access with repeated use and hematoma formation at the intravenous access site.

Q.23. Comment on photochemotherapy in CTCL.

Ans. The clinical effectiveness of photochemotherapy (psoralen + UVA, PUVA) has been recognized for over 20 years, with response rates ranging from 79–88% in stage IA and 52–59% in stage IB disease. To minimize risks, it is recommended to limit the total number of PUVA treatment sessions to fewer than 200 or to ensure that a cumulative dose does not exceed 1,200 J/cm^2.

Q.24. What is the mechanism of action of photochemotherapy?

Ans.
- Psoralen cross-links with epidermal deoxyribonucleic acid (DNA), inhibiting DNA replication and inducing cell cycle arrest.
- Psoralen photosensitization leads to changes in the expression of cytokines and their receptors.
- PUVA treatment can restore abnormal keratinocyte differentiation patterns and decrease the number of proliferating epidermal cells.

Q.25. What are the indications of photochemotherapy in CTCL?

Ans.
- Stage IB/IIA disease that are intolerant or fail to respond to topical therapies.
- Flexural sites ("sanctuary sites")

Q.26. Role of radiotherapy in MF.

Ans. Mycosis fungoides is a highly radiosensitive malignancy. Individual thick plaques, eroded plaques, or tumors can be effectively treated with low-dose superficial orthovoltage radiotherapy.

Total skin electron beam therapy is typically reserved for patients who do not respond to first- and second-line treatments. TSEB, using 4–6 MeV energy, is particularly effective for patients with skin-limited MF. The standard total dose is 36 Gy, delivered in fractions of 1.5–2 Gy over an 8–10-week period. Recently, lower total doses of 10–12 Gy have been used, offering shorter treatment durations, fewer side effects, and the potential for retreatment.

Total skin electron beam is most beneficial for patients with tumor-stage MF, where complete response rates of approximately 40% have been observed. For patients with plaque-stage disease and single tumors, local radiotherapy using X-rays or preferably electron beams can be considered. This can be done in combination with other treatments (such as PUVA) as an alternative to TSEB or for new tumors after TSEB. A dose of at least 8 Gy is usually sufficient for these cases.

For patients with unilesional MF, local radiotherapy may provide a curative outcome.

Adverse effects of TSEB may include temporary hair loss, telangiectasia, and an increased risk of skin malignancies.

Q.27. Role of chemotherapy in CTCL.

Ans. Chemotherapy is not recommended for patients with early-stage disease (IA, IB, or IIA).

For patients with stage IIB–IVB disease, single-agent chemotherapy has been shown to produce clinical responses. Agents used include oral chlorambucil (administered for 4–6 cycles at 0.15–0.2 mg/kg for 2–4 weeks), methotrexate, etoposide, and intravenous purine analogs such as 2-deoxycoformycin, 2-chlorodeoxyadenosine, and fludarabine.

Pentostatin, a potent adenosine deaminase inhibitor, is another emerging cytotoxic agent for use in MF.

Combination chemotherapy regimens including cyclophosphamide, doxorubicin, vincristine, prednisolone (CHOP).
- CHOP is widely used but is frequently associated with neutropenic sepsis. Risk is more in patients with ulcerated tumors and erythrodermic MF where T-cell number is markedly reduced. Risk can be minimized by reducing dose to one-third.

Q.28. What are the various systemic therapies for CTCL other than chemotherapy?

Ans. IFN-α, denileukin diftitox, histone deacetylase inhibitors, and retinoids are the various systemic therapies for CTCL other than chemotherapy.

Q.29. What is denileukin diftitox?

Ans. Denileukin diftitox is a recombinant fusion protein made up of the receptor-binding domain of interleukin-2 (IL-2) fused with the cytotoxic A-chain and the translocation B-chain from diphtheria toxin.

Q.30. Enumerate various types of MF.

Ans. Clinical variants of MF:
- Folliculotropic/Pilotropic
- Poikiloderma
- Hypopigmented
- Capillaritis-like
- Verrucous/Hyperkeratotic
- Psoriasiform
- Subcutaneous panniculitis-like T-cell lymphoma
- Bullous
- Ichthyosiform
- Erythrodermic MF

Tumor d'emblee: MF in which there is occurrence of tumor stage without prior formation of patch or plaque stage

Folliculotropic MF: It is seen in 10% of MF patients.

Folliculotropic MF is a variant characterized by the presence of follicular infiltrates, often with sparing of the epidermis. The head and neck areas are commonly affected.

Mucinous degeneration of the hair follicles is frequently observed and is typically referred to as MF-associated follicular mucinosis. In some cases, without follicular mucinosis, the condition is described as folliculocentric or pilotropic MF.

A key feature of this variant is the deep, follicular, and perifollicular distribution of neoplastic infiltrates, which makes them less responsive to skin-directed therapies.

Pagetoid Reticulosis (Woringer–Kolopp Disease/Unilesional MF)[9]:
This rare variant of MF is characterized by localized patches or plaques with intraepidermal proliferation of neoplastic T-cells, primarily found on the extremities, especially the feet. The typical histologic appearance shows a hyperplastic epidermis with significant infiltration of large, atypical pagetoid cells, which are arranged either singly or in clusters or nests. This form of MF generally has a favorable prognosis.

Granulomatous slack skin disorder: It is characterized by the evolution of circumscribed erythematous loose skin masses, especially in the body folds like axillae and groin. Some patients have underlying Hodgkin's lymphoma. Histopathological findings include multinucleated giant cells with intracellular leukocytes, surrounded by a dense leukocytic infiltrate. It usually has an indolent clinical course.

Lymphomatoid papulosis (LyP): It is a chronic, recurrent skin disorder marked by self-healing papulonecrotic or papulonodular lesions, with histological features suggestive of CD30-positive malignant lymphoma. LyP represents about 15% of all cases of CTCL. The typical skin manifestations are red-brown papules and nodules that may develop central hemorrhage, necrosis, and crusting, but typically resolve spontaneously within 3–8 weeks. Skin lesions in various stages of development are often present simultaneously. Following resolution, the lesions may leave behind temporary areas of hypopigmentation or hyperpigmentation or occasionally superficial atrophic (varioliform) scars. In some cases, the lesions heal without any sequelae or ulceration.

Subcutaneous panniculitis-like T-cell lymphoma (SPTCL)[10]: This condition is a type of CTCL characterized by subcutaneous infiltration of small, medium, or large pleomorphic T-cells with an a/B+ T-cell phenotype, often accompanied by a significant presence of macrophages. Patients typically present with one or more nodules or deeply seated plaques ranging in size from 1 to 20 cm in diameter. The skin lesions primarily affect the extremities and trunk, with the face being less commonly involved. As the nodules and plaques resolve, they may leave behind areas of lipoatrophy. Extracutaneous spread is rare.

REFERENCES

1. Jaffe ES, Harris NL, Stein H, Vardiman JW (Eds). World Health Organization Classification of Tumours. Pathology and Genetics of Tumours of Haematopoietic and Lymphoid Tissues. Lyon: IARC Press; 2001.
2. Lange-Asschenfeldt S, Babilli J, Beyer M, Ríus-Diaz F, González S, Stockfleth E, et al. Consistency and distribution of reflectance confocal microscopy features for diagnosis of cutaneous T cell lymphoma. J Biomed Opt. 2012:17(1): 016001.

3. Cheung MM, Chan JK, Lau WH, Foo W, Chan PT, Ng CS, et al. Primary non-Hodgkin lymphoma of the nose and nasopharynx clinical features, tumor immunophenotype, and treatment outcome in 113 patients. J Clin Oncol. 1998:16(1):70-7.
4. Gutte R, Kharkar V, Mahajan S, Chikhalkar S, Khopkar U. Granulomatous mycosis fungoides with hypohidrosis mimicking lepromatous leprosy. Indian J Dermatol Venereol Leprol. 2010;76(6):686-90.
5. Chan IK, Sin VC, Wong KF, Ng CS, Tsang WY, Chan CH, et al. Nonnasal lymphoma expressing the natural killer cell marker CD56: A clinicopathologic study of 49 cases of an uncommon aggressive neoplasm. Blood. 1997:89(12): 4501-13.
6. Herrmann JJ, Roenigk HH Jr, Hönigsmann H. Ultraviolet radiation for treatment of cutaneous T-cell lymphoma. Hematol Oncol Clin North Am. 1995;9(5):1077-88.
7. Zackheim HS. Cutaneous T cell lymphoma: Update of treatment. Dermatology. 1999:199(2):102-5.
8. Sinha AA. Heald P. Advances in the management of cutaneous T-cell lymphoma. Dermatol Clin. 1988:16(2):301-11
9. Haghighi B, Smoller BR, LeBoit PE, Warnke RA, Sander CA, Kohler S. Pagetoid reticulosis (Woringer-Kolopp disease): An immunophenotypic molecular and clinicopathologic study. Mod Pathol. 2000;13(5):502-10.
10. Willemze B, Jansen PM, Cerroni L, Berti E, Santucci M, Assaf C, et al. Subcutaneous panniculitis-like T-cell lymphoma: Definition, classification and prognostic factors: An EORTC Cutaneous Lymphoma Group Study of 83 cases. Blood. 2008:111(2):808-45.

CHAPTER 8

Short Cases: Infantile Hemangioma and Bullous Pyoderma Gangrenosum

INTRODUCTION

This chapter includes two different short clinical cases, namely, infantile hemangioma and pyoderma gangrenosum (PG). They are included here with brief history followed by frequently asked questions during objectively structured clinical examination (OSCE) and viva voce.

CASE 1: INFANTILE HEMANGIOMA

Chief Complaint

A 7-month-old infant was brought with swelling over face, which was bleeding oft-repeatedly since 6 months.

Origin, Duration, and Progress

Patient was relatively asymptomatic at birth. At 1 month of age, his parents noticed a reddish, raised, nonitchy skin lesion about the size of a pea on the right side of his cheek below his right eye. Gradually, the lesion increased in size over the past 6 months. The parents complained of bleeding off and on from the lesion (especially, after trauma) **(Fig. 1)**.

There was no history of pus discharge from the lesion. There was no history of convulsions, and parents did not notice any abnormality in eye movements.

Antenatal, Intranatal, and Postnatal History

- Child was born preterm by caesarean section necessitated due to placenta previa abnormality.
- *Birth weight*: 2.8 kg
- No complications at/after birth.

Family History

There was no history of similar complaints in any family member. The infant is younger of two siblings born out of a non-consanguineous marriage. Elder brother is 3 years old.

On Examination

Approximately 4 × 4 cm sized, nonpulsatile, erythematous swelling with overlying hemorrhagic crust present over the right side of face below the right eye.

Investigations

Baseline investigations such as complete blood count (CBC), liver function test (LFT), renal function test (RFT), random blood sugar (RBS), urine routine microscopy, and electrocardiography (ECG) were performed. Special tests such as 2D echo, ultrasonography (USG) of the local area, and magnetic resonance imaging (MRI) brain with MR angiography were undertaken to rule out PHACES (*P*osterior fossa brain malformations, *H*emangiomas, *A*rterial anomalies, *C*ardiac defects, *E*ye abnormalities, and sometimes, *S*ternal clefting) syndrome.

Treatment

The patient was admitted. After physical examination and sugar level estimation, tablet propranolol (1 mg/kg) was given in two divided doses 9 hours apart after feeds. Blood pressure, pulse rate, and sugar charting was done immediately before giving the dose; 30 minutes and 2 hours after giving the dose. The dose was skipped if the infant did not take feed. Topical mupirocin application and Jelonet dressing were advised. Within a week, syrup prednisolone (5 mg/5 mL) in 0.5 mg/kg dosing was also added. The dose was gradually tapered and stopped with complete clinical response **(Fig. 2)**.

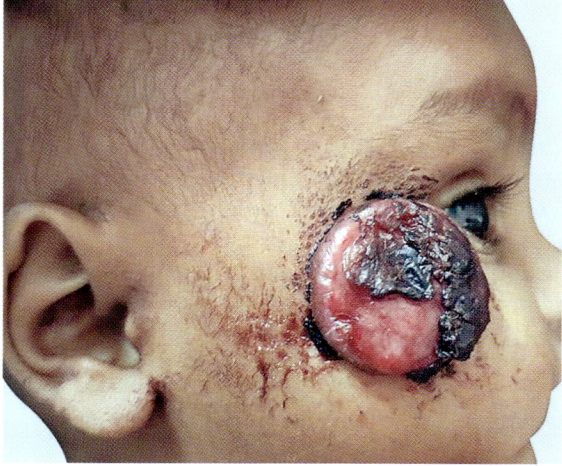

FIG. 1: Well-defined vascular swelling with hemorrhagic crusting.

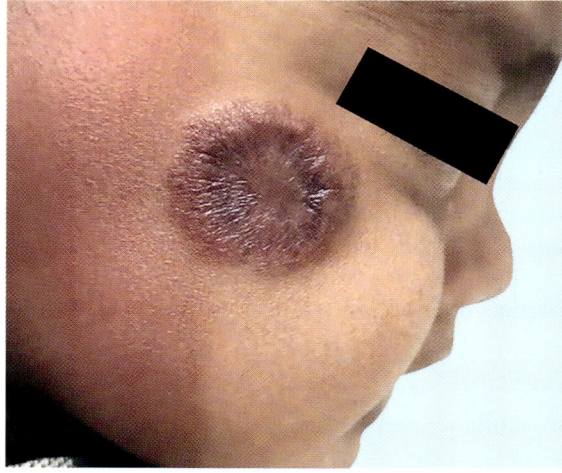

FIG. 2: Postinflammatory hyperpigmentation and scarring after 5 months of treatment.

Questions and Answers

Q.1. What are infantile hemangiomas (IH)?

Ans. Infantile hemangiomas are the most common type of soft-tissue tumors in infants.

Q.2. What are the risk factors for IH?

Ans.
- A retrospective study conducted in India reported a female predominance with a ratio of 2.3:1.[1]
- Additional risk factors identified include preeclampsia, placenta previa, placental disruption (such as from chorionic villus sampling), multiple gestation pregnancies, and advanced maternal age.[2]

Q.3. How to differentiate IH from vascular malformations?[1]

Ans. Difference between IH and vascular malformations are given in **Table 1**.

TABLE 1: Difference between infantile hemangiomas and vascular malformations.[4]	
Infantile hemangiomas	**Vascular malformations**
Infantile hemangiomas are more commonly seen in: • Girls (with a ratio of 2–5:1) • Premature or low-birth-weight infants • Infants born to older mothers or those who had chorionic villus sampling during pregnancy	No gender or gestation predilection
Infantile hemangiomas are typically not present at birth or may present as subtle precursor lesions; well-formed hemangiomas are seen less frequently	Typically, noticeable at birth, these lesions expand gradually in proportion to the child's growth and can persist into adulthood
They undergo rapid growth followed by spontaneous regression over the course of several years	
During the proliferating phase, there is endothelial cell hyperplasia, lobule formation, an increase in mast cells, and a prominent basement membrane. In the involuting phase, fibrofatty tissue gradually replaces the hemangioma with a noticeable reduction in mast cells once it has fully regressed	Dependent upon type, often irregular vascular channels
Negative for GLUT1, Lewis Y antigen, merosin, FcγRII, and Wilms tumor protein 1 (WT1)	Positive for GLUT1, Lewis Y antigen, merosin, FcγRII, and Wilms tumor protein 1 (WT1)

(GLUT1: glucose transporter-1)

Q.4. Discuss the theories of origin for IH.[3]

Ans. Research investigating the pathogenesis of IH has identified the following theories:
- Cells of placental origin
- Multipotent stem cells
- Mutations in vascular endothelial growth factor (VEGF) signaling
- Several theories have been proposed to explain the development of infantile hemangiomas, including the Folkman–Klagsbrun placental theory, endothelial progenitor cell theory, hypoxia theory, and angiogenesis theory, which are most widely accepted.

Placental theory:
- Hemangioma progenitor cells, including hemangioma stem cells (HemSC), are found in proliferating IH.
- When HemSC are grafted into immunodeficient mice, they form glucose transporter 1 (GLUT1)-positive vessels that resemble those of IH. In addition, IH lesions show positive staining for GLUT1, Lewis Y antigen, FcRII, and merosin, which are markers commonly associated with the placenta.
- This distinctive staining pattern, combined with the epidemiological links between IH and placental disruption, lends support to the theory that IH may have a placental origin.

Stem cell origin:
- Hemangioblasts are the progenitor cells that give rise to both endothelial and hematopoietic lineages.
- In vivo, the counterpart of hemangioblasts is believed to be the hemogenic endothelium, a primitive endothelial phenotype with the potential to differentiate into hematopoietic cells.
- This hemogenic endothelium expresses both endothelial markers, such as CD34 and vascular endothelial growth factor receptor 2 (VEGFR-2), and hematopoietic markers, including Tal-1, GATA-2, and Runx-1, indicating its dual differentiation potential.
- Additionally, angiotensin-converting enzyme (ACE) (also referred to as CD143) has been identified as a marker for primitive hematopoietic stem cells during human hematopoietic development.

Mutations in VEGF signaling: Heterozygous germline mutations in VEGFR2 and ANTXR1 (which encodes an integrin-like receptor on endothelial cells) have been found in a small group of individuals with IH. These mutations may contribute to a predisposition to developing hemangiomas.

Q.5. Discuss the clinical subtypes.
Ans.
- *Based on depth*:
  - Superficial plaque type
  - Deeper subcutaneous type
  - Mixed (both superficial and deep type)[5]
- *Based on extent of involvement*:
  - Localized (77%)
  - Segmental (18%)
  - Multifocal (5%)
  - Indeterminate[1]
- *Growth pattern type*:
  - Minimum or arrested growth
  - *Congenital hemangiomas*:[6]
    - Rapidly involuting infantile hemangioma (RICH)
    - Non-involuting infantile hemangioma (NICH)
    - Partially involuting infantile hemangioma (PICH)

Q.6. How to approach IH based on their morphology and color?
Ans. Approach to IH based on their morphology and color are given in **Flowchart 1**.

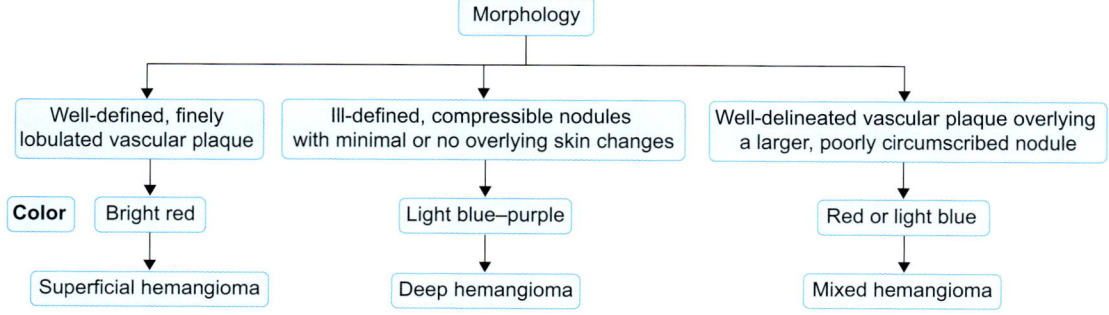

FLOWCHART 1: Approach to infantile hemangiomas based on their morphology and color.

Q.7. What is the natural course of resolution of IH?

Ans. Classic studies on the progression of untreated hemangiomas have shown that 30% of lesions completely involute by age of 3 years, 50% by age of 5 years, 70% by age of 7 years, and >90% by age of 9 years **(Table 2)**.[7]

TABLE 2: Highlighting features of infantile hemangioma according to stages of evolution.	
Clinical phase	**Features**
Prodromal phase	*Premonitory lesions*: Circumscribed telangiectasia, anemic, blue macule, or blurred swelling
Initial phase	Loss of typical skin structures with increasing thickness and induration
Proliferation phase (6–8 weeks)	• Bright red cutaneous infiltration with spreading of lesion • Exophytic or endophytic subcutaneous growth or thickness is seen • Firm and noncompressible
Maturation phase	• Raised, bosselated crimson red lesions • Maximum size is reached by 12–15 months • Surface complications such as ulceration may occur
Regression (involution phase)	• 50% have normal skin at the site of lesion • At times may leave fibro-fatty residuum, telangiectasia, yellow hypoelastic patches or may rarely scar • Involution is usually complete by 5 years of age in 50% of children, 7 years in 70%, and most by 10–12 years

Q.8. What are the various complications associated with IHs?

Ans. Complications **(Table 3)**:[8]
- *Local complications:* Ulceration, necrosis, hemorrhage, and infection
- *Multiple hemangiomas:* >5 indicate visceral involvement [liver and gastrointestinal tract (GIT)]
- *Large hemangiomas:* High output cardiac failure

TABLE 3: Complications associated with infantile hemangioma according to their location.	
Location	**Associated complication**
Periorbital and retrobulbar **(Fig. 3)**	Visual axis obscuration, amblyopia, and optic nerve compression
Auricular	EAC obstruction, hearing loss, and otitis externa
Nasal tip and large facial hemangiomas **(Figs. 3 to 5)**	"Cyrano nose" and permanent scarring and deformity
Beard or mandibular areas	Airway obstruction
Perioral	Feeding difficulties, ulceration, and disfigurement
Subglottic	Stridor and respiratory failure due to laryngeal involvement
Perineal	Ulceration

(EAC: external auditory canal)

Greater risk of ulceration if:
- Large, mixed, or segmental hemangiomas
- *Sites*: Lip, anogenital region, or skin folds (neck)
- *Whitish discoloration of hemangiomas*: Early sign of ulceration **(Fig. 6)**
- *Median age at ulceration*: 4 months

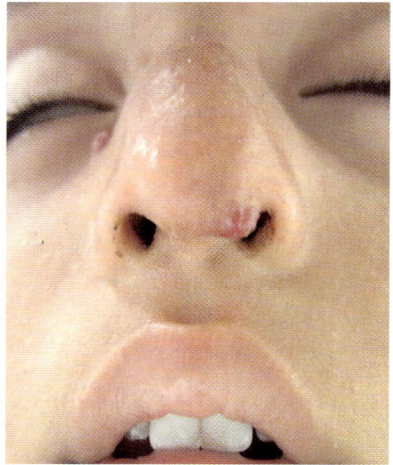

FIG. 3: Hemangioma involving nose, below right eye.

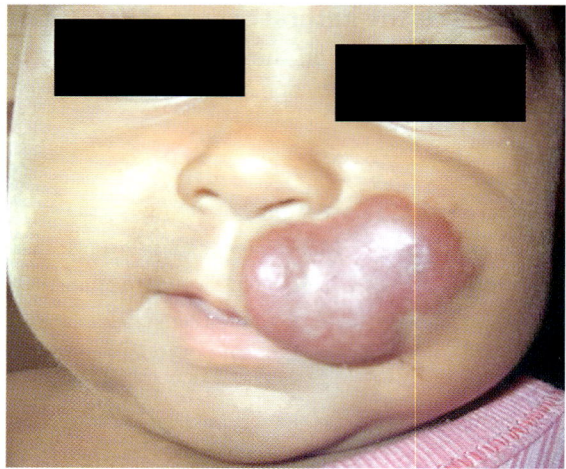

FIG. 4: Infantile hemangiomas (IH) deforming face.

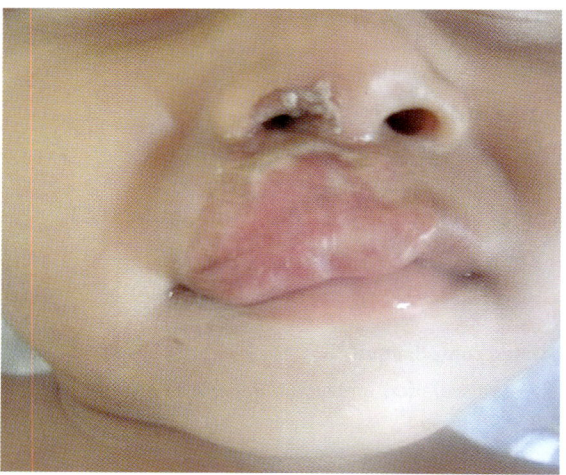

FIG. 5: Infantile hemangiomas (IH) on upper lip and right Ala nasi.

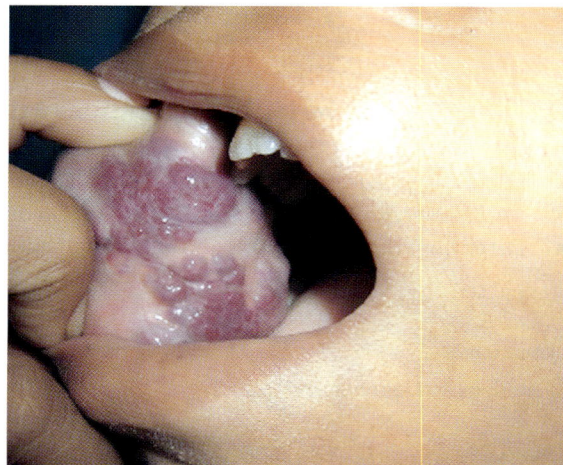

FIG. 6: Hemangioma in oral cavity.

Q.9. Name the syndromes associated with infantile hemangiomas?

Ans. Associated syndromes:
- PHACES syndrome *(Fig 7)*:[9]
    - Brain malformations, including posterior fossa abnormalities such as Dandy–Walker malformation and cerebellar hypoplasia
    - Segmental infantile hemangiomas, commonly located on the face and/or neck
    - Arterial abnormalities, such as aplasia, dysplasia, and aneurysms in the cervical and cerebral vessels

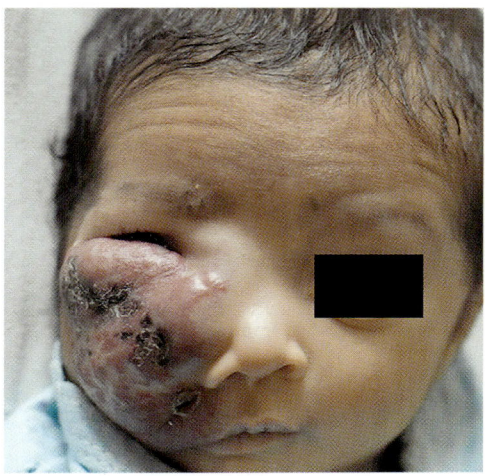

FIG. 7: PHACES syndrome.

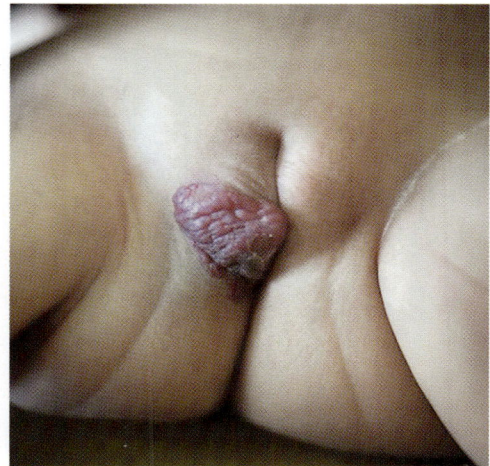

FIG. 8: LUMBAR syndrome.

- Cardiac defects, including ventricular septal defect, atrial septal defect, and coarctation of the aorta
- Eye abnormalities, such as retinal vascular issues and optic nerve hypoplasia
- Sternal defects and supraumbilical raphe
- *LUMBAR syndrome*[9] (**Fig. 8**):
    - Lower body segmental infantile hemangioma; lipoma; other cutaneous anomalies, e.g., "skin tag"
    - Urogenital anomalies, e.g., of the bladder, ureters, or genitalia
    - Myelopathy, e.g., tethered spinal cord and lipomyelomeningocele
    - Bony deformities, e.g., sacral anomaly, hip dysplasia, scoliosis, and leg length/width discrepancy
    - Anorectal anomalies, e.g., imperforate anus, fistula; arterial anomalies of the lower limb, e.g., stenosis and dysplasia
    - Renal anomalies, e.g., hypoplastic, single, or pelvic kidney
- *PELVIS syndrome:*[10]
    - *P*erineal hemangioma
    - *E*xternal genital malformations
    - *L*ipomyelomeningocele
    - *V*esicorenal abnormalities
    - *I*mperforate anus
    - *S*kin tags

Q.10. How would you manage a child with multiple hemangiomas?

Ans. *Found in 10–25% of infants* (**Fig. 9**):[1]
- It may be associated with *visceral hemangiomas.*
- *Liver:* It is the most common site of visceral hemangiomas.
- Evaluation for hepatic involvement is recommended when ≥5 *skin lesions* are present.
- *Consumptive hypothyroidism:* ↑ level of iodothyronine deiodinase in large cutaneous hemangiomas (proliferative phase), *hepatic hemangiomas* → deactivates thyroid hormone[11]

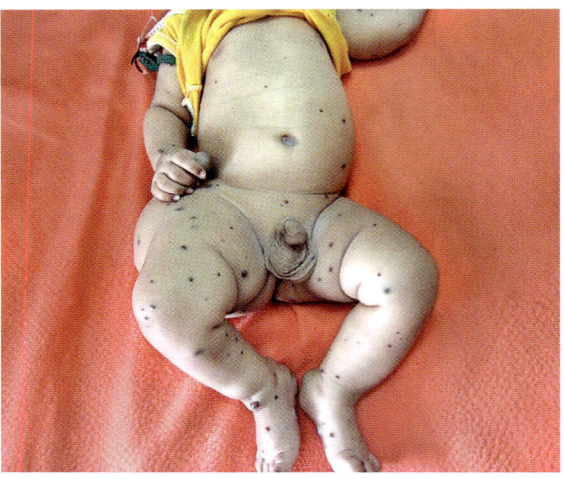

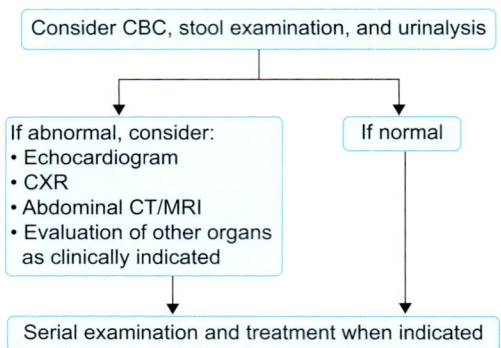

FLOWCHART 2: Approach to management.
(CT: computed tomography; CXR: chest X-ray; MRI: magnetic resonance imaging)

FIG. 9: Multiple hemangiomas in an infant.

Management **(Flowchart 2)**:
- Monitor for signs and symptoms of visceral involvement.
- Periodic physical examination
- Abdominal ultrasound

Q.11. What are the goals of treatment?

Ans.
- Prevention or reversal of complications that could threaten life or normal function
- Prevention of permanent disfigurement and reduction of psychosocial stress for both the patient and their family
- In lesions that may have a very good prognosis without treatment, aggressive or detrimental interventions should be avoided.
- Prevention or treatment of ulceration to minimize scarring, infection, and pain[12]

Q.12. What is the rationale behind conservative management?

Ans. *Active nonintervention:*[13] Most cases are self-limiting; for uncomplicated cases—
- Assure and educate the parents on the natural course of IH, its heterogeneity and need for follow ups.
- *Advocate regular follow-ups:* Serial photographs and hemispheric measurements need to be recorded to assess the course of the lesions.
- Apply bland ointments over the lesion to keep it soft and trim the patient's nails regularly.
- Address emotional and psychosocial issues arising from cosmetic appearance and social reaction.
- Alert–identify existing or impending sequelae, which can necessitate intervention.

Q.13. Enumerate the available treatment options.

Ans.
Treatment modalities **(Box 1)**[14]

> **BOX 1** Various treatment modalities available for infantile hemangioma.
>
> *Medical modalities*
> - *Systemic:*
>   - Corticosteroids
>   - Propanolol
>   - Interferon alpha
>   - Vincristine
>   - Cyclophosphamide
>   - Bleomycin
> - *Topical:*
>   - Corticosteroids
>   - Beta blockers
>   - Becaplermin
>   - Imiquimod
>
> *Surgical modalities*
> - Surgical excision (elliptical intralesional resection)
> - Laser (pulsed dye, Nd:YAG)
> - Cryotherapy
> - Sclerotherapy (polidocanol)
> - Noncontact, low-frequency ultrasound therapy
> - Embolization
> - Radiotherapy
>
> (Nd:YAG: Neodymium-doped Yttrium Aluminum Garnet)

Q.14. When would you consider medical management?

Ans. Indications for medical management:[15]
- *Function-threatening* hemangiomas (e.g., ocular, auricular, nasal tip, and genitalia)
- *Life-threatening* hemangiomas (impending respiratory distress)
- *Disfiguring* hemangiomas (e.g., large facial hemangioma)
- Ulceration
- Associated systemic involvement (>5 hemangiomas)

Q.15. What is considered the first-line therapy for IH?

Ans.
Systemic beta blockers:
- First line of management[16]
- *Mechanism of action:*
  - Vasoconstriction
  - Decreases *VEGF* and beta-fibroblast growth factor (*β-FGF*) genes
  - Blocks G protein-coupled receptor (GPCR)-kinase Leu41
  - Reduces matrix metalloproteinase-9 (MMP-9) and effects mesenchymal cells

Approach for propanolol therapy:
- *Step 1:* Patient selection and baseline investigations:
  - Establish the indication
  - Rule out contraindications:
    - Bronchial asthma
    - Heart failure
    - Sinus bradycardia
    - Hypoglycemia
    - Hypothermia
    - Heart block
    - Known allergy to propranolol

TABLE 4: Vital sign monitoring guidelines based on patient weight and clinical status.	
Weight >3.5 kg and no comorbidities	BP and HR immediately before first dose and every 30 minutes for 2 hours
Weight <3.5 kg and/or comorbidities	BP and HR immediately before first dose and every 30 minutes for 4 hours or longer

(BP: blood pressure; HR: heart rate)

TABLE 5: Clinical guidelines for propranolol use in infantile hemangiomas.	
Reviews	4–6 weeks after starting treatment, then 3–4 monthly
Increments	Increments greater than 0.5 mg/kg/day should include 2 hours post dose monitoring of HR and BP
Treatment discontinuation	• Usually at 12–14 months of age but can be later • Gradual dose reduction over 2–4 weeks

- *Step 2:* Regimens to give propranolol **(Tables 4 and 5)**:[17]
  - Two regimens are used in practice:
    1. 0.33 mg/kg/dose given 8 hourly for 1 week; thereafter, doubled to 0.67 mg/kg/dose to get desired 2 mg/kg/day
    2. 1 mg/kg/day and increased to 2 mg/kg/day after 1 week
- *Step 3:* Watch for complications:
  - Hypoglycemia (may manifest up to 6 months after therapy)
  - Hypotension (<50/30 mm Hg)
  - Bradycardia (<60 beats/min)
  - Sleep disruption
  - Acrocyanosis
  - Diarrhea

  Safety instructions for patients:
  - Only daytime dosing, exact dosing at least 6 hours apart
  - Frequent feeding
  - Skip the dose if refusal to feed
  - *If missed/spurted:* Wait till next dose
  - *If sick/not feeding:* Stop and consult
- *Step 4:* Monitor
  - Blood pressure (BP), pulse rate, and sugar charting every 1–3 hourly initially and after dose escalation and 2–3 monthly while on maintenance
  - Weight for dose modification
  - *Monitor progress:* Serial photography, color, texture, and growth
  - *For ulcerated hemangiomas:* Combine with barrier creams, antibiotics and pulsed dye therapy
  - *For PHACES syndrome:* Lowest dose, slow titration, and neurological follow-up **(Table 4)**

Topical timolol:[18]
- Safer alternative to propranolol
- 0.5% solution, 1 drop contains 0.25 mg
- *Dosage:* 1 drop/kg/day or 0.25 mg/kg/day
- Preferred for small thin cutaneous IH

Q.16. Discuss the role of corticosteroids.
Ans.
Systemic corticosteroids:[13]
- For severe life-threatening hemangiomas
- Initial oral dose of prednisone is 3–5 mg/kg/day.
- If the tumors stop growing or become smaller, it is tapered down gradually and ceased after 4–8 weeks **(Figs. 10 and 11)**

Intralesional corticosteroids:[19]
- Small focal lesions in locations such as *lip*
- *Triamcinolone acetonide*—total dose should not exceed *3–5 mg/kg* per treatment session, at monthly interval

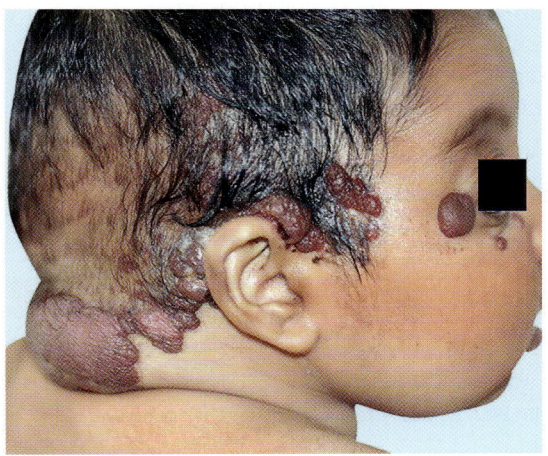

FIG.10: Pretreatment.

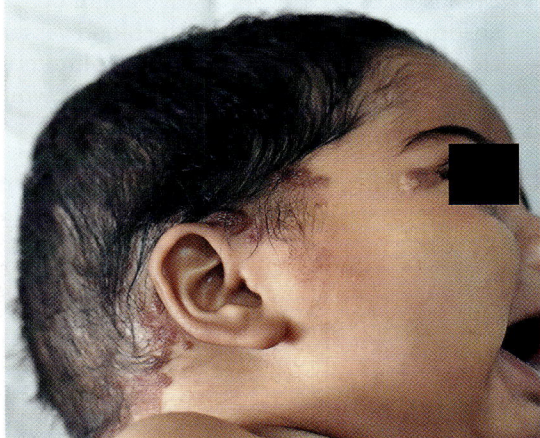

FIG.11: Post-treatment.

Q.17. Give an overview of novel treatment modalities.[14]
Ans.
- *ACE inhibitors:*[20]
  - Infantile hemangioma results from abnormal proliferation and differentiation of a primitive mesoderm-derived hemogenic endothelium, a process that is regulated by the renin–angiotensin system (RAS).
  - *Captopril:* Explored for infantile hemangiomas
  - Test dose *0.1* mg/kg
  - *0.15* mg/kg TDS over 24 hours
  - *0.3* mg/kg TDS for another 24 hours
  - *0.5* mg/kg TDS 1 week later, if a noticeable involution had not already occurred
  - Monitor for BP, renal function
- Imiquimod 5%
- *Radiation therapy and radioisotopes:* Kasabach–Merritt syndrome
- Intralesional interferon-alpha (IFN-α)
- *Becaplermin:*
  - Human platelet derived growth factor
  - 0.01% gel is used in ulcerated hemangiomas to promote healing

Q.18. What is the role of laser therapy in IH?

Ans. *Lasers:*[21] Target intravascular oxyhemoglobin and cause vascular injury.
- Argon laser (488–514 nm)
- Flashed light-pumped pulsed dye laser (PDL) (585–595 nm)
- Neodymium-doped Yttrium Aluminum Garnet (Nd:YAG) laser (1,064 nm)
- Potassium titanyl phosphate (KTP) laser (532 nm)

Pulsed dye laser:
- *Mechanism:* Selective photothermolysis, which targets blood vessels through heat transfer
- The goal of laser therapy for hemangiomas is to maximize thermal damage to the vascular components while minimizing harm to the surrounding epidermis and dermal tissues.
- To reduce the risk of damage to the epidermis and papillary dermis, flash lamp-pumped pulsed dye laser (LP-PDL) with a wavelength of 575–600 nm is used, as it emits light that is preferentially absorbed by hemoglobin in the blood vessels.
- However, the effectiveness of PDL is limited by its depth of vascular injury (1–2 mm), meaning that subcutaneous or mixed hemangiomas, which extend beyond this depth, do not benefit from PDL treatment.

Q.19. How will you manage ulcerated hemangiomas?[22]
Ans.

TABLE 6: Management of ulcerated hemangioma

Goal of therapy	Comment
Wound care	- Gentle debridement of crust with warm water irrigation or compress - Occlusive wound dressing with bland emollients (to help prevent drying and to reduce trauma and infection) - Topical antibiotics such as bacitracin, mupirocin, metronidazole, and silver sulfadiazine - Systemic antibiotics - Becaplermin
Pain control (ulcerated lip and perineal IH impeding feeding and voiding/stooling)	- Oral acetaminophen, occasionally opioids - Cautious application of topical 2.5% lidocaine ointment
Prevention of proliferation	- Intralesional or systemic corticosteroids and topical or systemic beta blockers - Pulsed dye laser (to accelerate re-epilthelialization) - Surgical excision if refractory to medical therapy

CASE 2: BULLOUS PYODERMA GANGRENOSUM[23]

Chief Complaints

Painful, fluid filled lesions that ruptured to form deep, painful raw areas over both leges and back for 2 months.

History of Present Illness
- A 2-year-old female child presented with chief complaint of 3–4 large blood-stained blisters and with few painful raw areas, which are nonhealing in nature for last 2 months on legs. The first lesions started over back then single large blister followed by development of raw area developed over both lower legs with surrounding redness. In the next 3–4 days, bullae ruptured on their own to leave behind superficial raw areas over bilateral legs and back.
- History of fever, mild grade, on and off, was present for 1.5 months. Fever was not associated with chills and rigors or evening rise of temperature and relieved by medications.

No history of:
- Joint pain
- Weight loss
- Abdominal pain
- Dryness of mouth or eyes.
- Prior drug intake
- Recent vaccinations
- Recent infection
- History of trauma at site of lesions
- Topical application over lesions
- No history of diabetes mellitus (DM), hypertension (HTN), tuberculosis (TB) or any other major surgical or medical illness.
- Family history was not significant

General Examination
- The child was conscious and was accompanied by mother and had an asthenic and pale look and appeared moderately nourished.
- *Temperature:* 100°F
- *Pulse rate:* 102 beats/min
- *Respiratory rate:* 20 breaths/min
- *Blood pressure:* 100/68 mm Hg (taken with help of pediatric colleague)
- There was no evidence of icterus, clubbing, cyanosis, and pedal edema.

Systemic Examination
Nothing significant was found.

Cutaneous Examination
Cutaneous examination showed multiple ulcers of varying size from 5 to 8 cm present over back and bilateral legs. Borders were well defined, elevated, and hyperpigmented. Edges were undermined. Floor was covered with slough and bloody discharge. Few vesicles were present over right leg **(Figs. 12A to C)**.

Investigations
Investigations are given in **Table 7**.

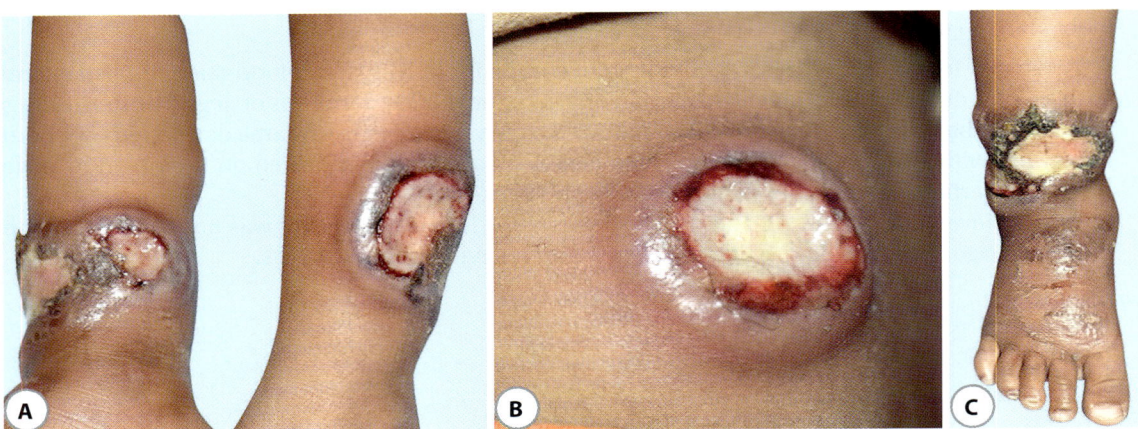

FIGS. 12A TO C: (A) Ulcers with slough and surrounding violaceous elevated border on both legs; (B) Single ulcer with slough on back; and (C) Ulcer and few vesicles on right leg and dorsum of foot.

TABLE 7: Investigation profile of patient.

Hemoglobin	11 g%
Total leukocyte counts	16,300 mm³
Differential leukocyte counts	Normal (N-69% and L-31%)
Platelet counts	2,76,00 mm³
Erythrocyte sedimentation rate (ESR)	72 mm in first hour
Fasting blood sugar	76 mg%
Total serum protein and albumin level	5.6 and 2.4 g%
Serum bilirubin	1.0 mg%
Serum glutamate oxaloacetate transaminase (SGOT)	34 IU/mL
Serum glutamate pyruvate transaminase (SGPT)	45 IU/mL
HIV and HBSAg	Negative
Urine routine and microscopy	Normal
Mantoux and pathergy test	Negative
Tzanck smear	Negative
ANA, RA factor, ASO, anticardiolipin antibody, p-ANCA and c-ANCA titers	Negative
Chest X-ray	Normal
Pus and stool culture	Negative for organisms
Skin biopsy (taken from the edge of the ulcer)	Lymphocytic vasculitis, extravasation of RBCs and neutrophilic abscess formation in the dermis consistent with pyoderma ganagrenosum (PG)

(ANA: antinuclear antibody; ASO: antistreptolysin O; c-ANCA: cytoplasmic antineutrophil cytoplasmic antibody; p-ANCA: peripheral ANCA; HIV: human immunodeficiency; HBSAg: hepatitis B surface antigen; RA: rheumatoid factor; RBC: red blood cell)

Management

Patient was started on syrup prednisolone (5 mg/5mL) 5 mL twice in a day and syrup cyclosporine (100 mg/mL) 0.5 mL once a day along with oral antibiotics.

Local care of ulcers with topical antimicrobial agents and paraffin gauze dressing was done.

The ulcers started healing within 4 weeks of initiating treatment. The dose of prednisolone and cyclosporine was gradually tapered. All ulcers healed 3 months after starting treatment **(Figs. 13A to C)**.

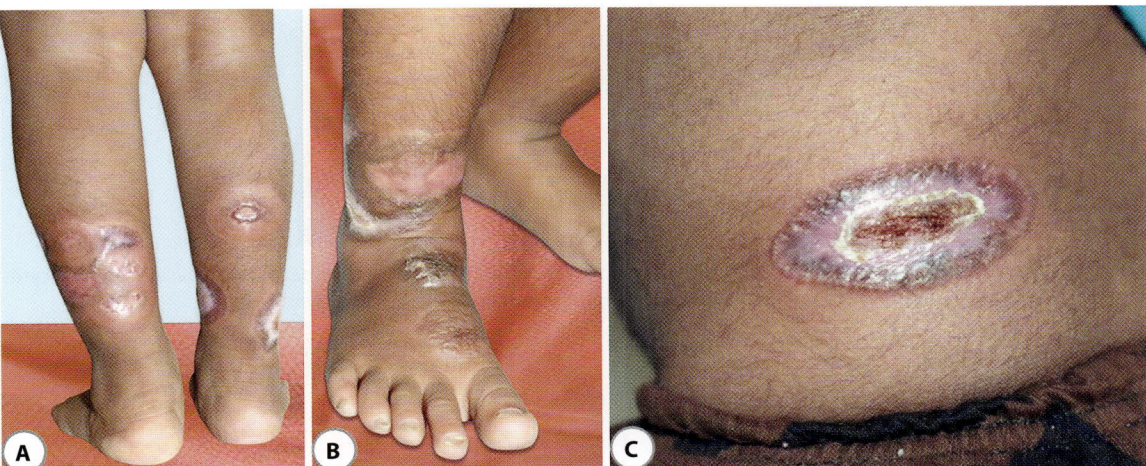

FIGS. 13A TO C: Post-treatment: Postinflammatory changes with cribriform scarring.

Questions and Answers

Q.1. Enlist and describe the clinical variants of PG.
Ans.
- *Ulcerative:*
  - Most common variant
  - Presents as intensely painful erythematous papule, pustule or nodule that ulcerates with a violaceous undermining edge and purulent necrotic base
  - Histopathology *(Fig. 14)*
- *Bullous/Atypical:*
  - It presents as painful, rapidly expanding vesicle/bulla.
  - It is most often associated with hematologic disease.
  - It may show overlap with Sweet syndrome.
  - Histopathogy *(Fig. 15)*
- *Pustular:*
  - It presents as pustules in generalized distribution.
  - Acute inflammatory bowel disease (usually ulcerative colitis) is associated with it.
- *Vegetative/Superficial granulomatous*: It presents as single, gradually enlarging nodule/abscess/plaque.

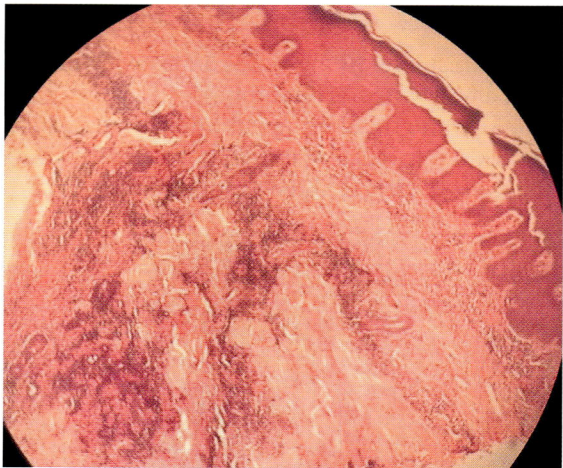

FIG. 14: Epidermal ulceration overlying granulation tissue, with subepidermal edema, numerous extravasated erythrocytes within the superficial dermis, and a marked inflammatory infiltrate, mainly composed of neutrophils.

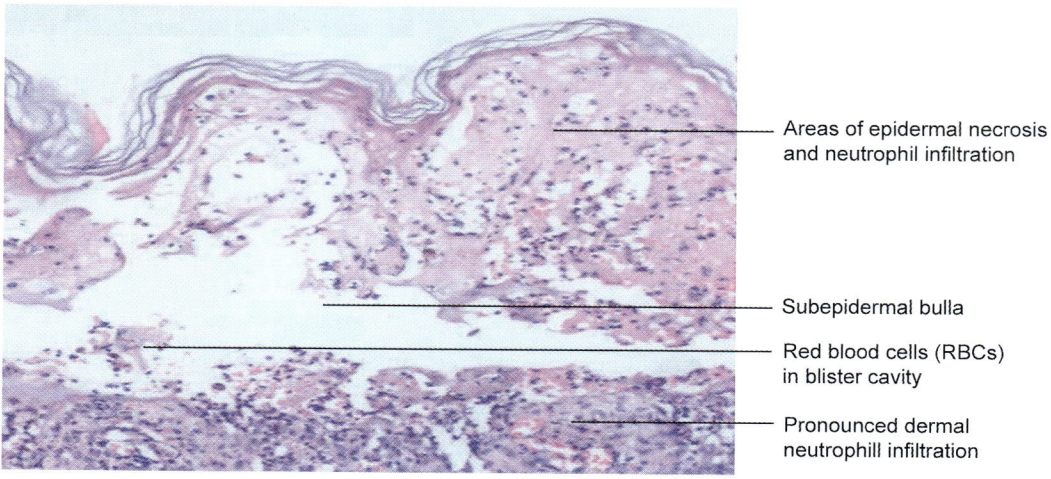

FIG. 15: Histopathology of bullous PG.

Q.2. Mention the diagnostic criteria for classic ulcerative PG?

Ans. Diagnostic criteria proposed by Daniel et al. are illustrated in **Box 2**. If both of the major criteria and at least two minor criteria are met, the diagnosis is confirmed.

> **BOX 2** **Major and minor diagnostic criteria for classic ulcerative PG.**
>
> *Major*:
> - Rapid progression of a painful, necrolytic cutaneous ulcer with an irregular, violaceous, and undermined border
> - Other causes of cutaneous ulceration have been excluded
>
> *Minor*:
> - History suggestive of pathergy or clinical finding of cribriform scarring
> - Systemic diseases associated with pyoderma gangrenosum
> - Histopathologic findings (sterile dermal neutrophilia, mixed inflammation, and lymphocytic vasculitis)
> - Treatment response (rapid response to systemic corticosteroids)

Q.3. What is the difference between classical and bullous PG?

Ans. Differences between classical and bullous PG are given in **Table 8**.

TABLE 8: Difference between classical and bullous pyoderma gangrenosum (PG).

Clinical pearls	Classical pyoderma gangrenosum	Bullous pyoderma gangrenosum
Bulla	Occasional	Frequent, can be hemorrhagic
Ulceration	Deep, destructive, and penetrating ulcer	Superficial ulceration and border can show vesicles and bullae
Spread of lesion	Undermining lesional spread	Concentric bullous areas spreading rapidly and centrifugally
Border	Violaceous or bright red	Blue–grey halo
Association with malignancy	Approximately 7% cases	• Two-thirds of cases: Hematological malignancy • AML, MDS, G-CSF therapy

(AML: acute myeloid leukemia; MDS: myelodysplastic syndromes; G-CSF: granulocyte-colony stimulating factor)

Q.4. How will you investigate a case of PG?

Ans.
- Detailed history and general examination
- *Baseline tests:*
  - Full blood count and differential blood count
  - Erythrocyte sedimentation rate
  - Metabolic profile
  - Autoantibody screen
  - Antineutrophilic cytoplasmic antibodies
  - Antiphospholipid antibodies
  - Rheumatoid factor
  - Chest radiography
- *Specific tests:*
  - Skin biopsy
  - Tissue culture
- *Other tests:*
  - Blood culture
  - Coagulation profile

- Human immunodeficiency virus (HIV), hepatitis B surface antigen (HBSAg)
- Computed tomography (CT) scan
- Gastrointestinal (GI) endoscopy
- Viral cultures
- Cryoglobulins

Q.5. Which differential diagnosis is to be considered in a case suspected of PG?
Ans.
- *Ulcerative PG:*
  - Traumatic nonhealing ulcer
  - Vascular [vasculopathy, venous stasis, vasculitis, and antiphospholipid antibodies (APLA)] ulcer
  - Ecthyma gangrenosum
  - Mycobacterial/atypical mycobacterial infection
  - Deep fungal infection (sporotrichosis)
- *Bullous PG:*
  - Bacterial infection (cellulitis/impetigo)
  - Viral infection
  - Fungal infection (mucormycosis)
  - Sweet syndrome, Behçet's disease
  - Erythema multiforme
- *Pustular PG:*
  - Bacterial/viral/fungal infection
  - Hidradenitis suppurativa
  - Pustular psoriasis
  - Pustular vasculitis
  - Pustular drug eruption
- *Vegetative PG:*
  - Infection (bacterial/viral/fungal)
  - Mycobacterial/atypical mycobacterial infection
  - Leishmaniasis
  - Malignancy
  - Factitious dermatitis

Q.6. Which systemic conditions are associated with PG frequently?[23]
Ans. Associated systemic diseases reported are:
- Crohn's disease
- Ulcerative colitis
- Collagen vascular diseases
- Wegener's granulomatosis
- *Arthritis:* Including rheumatoid and seronegative arthritis
- Hematologic malignancies such as chronic myeloid leukemia
- Monoclonal gammopathy
- Hepatic and pancreatic diseases
- Other neutrophilic dermatoses

Q.7. What are the syndromes associated with PG?
Ans.
- *PASH syndrome:* PG, Acne, Suppurative Hidradenitis
- *PAPA syndrome:* Pyogenic Arthritis, PG, Acne
- *PAPASH syndrome:* Pyogenic Arthritis, PG, Acne, Suppurative Hidradenitis

Q.8. How will you manage a case of PG?
Ans. If there is an associated disease, treatment of underlying disease can lead to improvement. But in vast majority of cases, such association may not be found in every case. Various treatment modalities have been tried with varying outcomes. These include
- Oral corticosteroids, preferably prednisone → 0.5–1 mg/kg/day *or* methylprednisolone, 1 g daily for 3–5 days (IV pulse)
- *Cyclosporine:* It has been reported as a very effective drug. Dose ranges from 2.5 to 5 mg/kg/day.
- *Colchicine:* 0.6 mg per oral TID
- *Dapsone*: 50–150 mg PO OD
- *Cyclophosphamide:* 50–200 mg daily or IV pulse (500–1,000 mg)
- *Azathioprine:* 50–100 mg daily
- *Thalidomide:* 50–150 mg daily
- *Methotrexate:* 2.5–25 mg orally, subcutaneously (SC) or intramuscularly (IM) weekly
- *Minocycline:* 100–200 mg/day
- *Biologics:*
  - *Infliximab:* 5 mg/kg/day intravenous (IV) at week 0, 2, and 6
  - *Etanercept:* 50–100 mg SC weekly (in 1 or 2 doses)
  - *Adalimumab:* 80 mg SC Injection as initial dose followed by 40 mg SC weekly or every other week
  - *Ustekinumab:* 45–90 mg SC
- *IV immunoglobulin:* 2 g/kg IV monthly given over 3–5 days every month

Other supportive treatments:
- Oral and topical antibiotics
- Topical and intralesional corticosteroids

REFERENCES
1. Zaenglein AL, Thiboutot DM. Infantile hemangiomas. In: Bolognia JL, Schaffer JV, Cerroni. Dermatology, 4th edition. Amsterdam, Netherlands: Elsevier; 2017. pp. 1786-802.
2. Ding Y, Zhang JZ, Yu SR, Xiang F, Kang XJ. Risk factors for infantile hemangioma: A meta-analysis. World J Pediatr. 2020;16(4):377-84.
3. Lo K, Mihm M, Fay A. Current theories on the pathogenesis of infantile hemangioma. Semin Ophthalmol. 2009;24(3):172-7.
4. Chiller KG, Passaro D, Frieden IJ. Hemangiomas of infancy: Clinical characteristics, morphologic subtypes, and their relationship to race, ethnicity, and sex. Arch Dermatol. 2002;138(12):1567-76.
5. Mulliken JB, Burrows PE, Fishman SJ. Diagnosis and natural history of hemangiomas. Mulliken and Young's Vascular Anomalies: Hemangiomas and Malformations. Oxford: Oxford University Press; 1988;4:68-110.
6. Krol A, MacArthur CJ. Congenital hemangiomas. Arch Facial Plast Surg. 2005;7(5):307-11.
7. Rotter A, Samorano LP, Rivitti-Machado MC, Oliveira ZN, Gontijo B. PHACE syndrome: Clinical manifestations, diagnostic criteria, and management. An Bras Dermatol. 2018;93:405-11.

8. Periocular IH, Lip IH. Infantile hemangiomas, complications and treatments. Seminars in Cutaneous Medicine and Surgery. Amsterdam, Netherlands: Elsevier;2016. pp. 108-16.
9. Yu X, Zhang J, Wu Z, Liu M, Chen R, Gu Y, et al. LUMBAR syndrome: A case manifesting as cutaneous infantile hemangiomas of the lower extremity, perineum and gluteal region, and a review of published work. J Dermatol. 2017;44(7):808-12.
10. Girard C, Bigorre M, Guillot B, Bessis D. PELVIS syndrome. Arch Dermatol. 2006;142(7):884-8.
11. Simsek E, Demiral M, Gundoğdu E. Severe consumptive hypothyroidism caused by multiple infantile hepatic haemangiomas. J Pediatr Endocrinol Metab. 2018;31(7):823-7.
12. Soliman YS, Khachemoune A. Infantile hemangiomas: Our current understanding and treatment options. Dermatol Online J. 2018;24(9).
13. Maguiness SM, Frieden IJ. Current management of infantile hemangiomas. Semin Cutan Med Surg. 2010;29(2):106-14.
14. Chen ZY, Wang QN, Zhu YH, Zhou LY, Xu T, et al. Progress in the treatment of infantile hemangioma. Ann Transl Med. 2019;7(22):692.
15. Moyakine AV, Herwegen B, van der Vleuten CJ. Use of the hemangioma severity scale to facilitate treatment decisions for infantile hemangiomas. J Am Acad Dermatol. 2017;77(5):868-73.
16. Hoeger PH, Harper JI, Baselga E, Bonnet D, Boon LM, Atti MC, et al. Treatment of infantile haemangiomas: Recommendations of a European expert group. Eur J Pediatr. 2015;174(7):855-65.
17. McGee P, Miller S, Black C, Hoey S. Propranolol for infantile haemangioma: A review of current dosing regime in a regional paediatric hospital. Ulster Med J. 2013;82(1):16-20.
18. Khan M, Boyce A, Prieto-Merino D, Svensson Å, Wedgeworth E, Flohr C. The role of topical timolol in the treatment of infantile hemangiomas: A systematic review and meta-analysis. Acta Derm Venereol. 2017;97(10):1167-71.
19. Chantharatanapiboon W. Intralesional corticosteroid therapy in hemangiomas: Clinical outcome in 160 cases. J Med Assoc Thai. 2008;91(Suppl 3):S90-6.
20. Itinteang T, Davis P, Tan S. Treatment of infantile hemangioma with an ACE inhibitor: A paradigm shift. ACE Inhibitors: Medical Uses, Mechanisms of Action, Potential Adverse Effects and Related Topics. Hauppauge, NY: Nova Science Publishers Inc.; 2014. p. 323.
21. Chinnadurai S, Sathe NA, Surawicz T. Laser treatment of infantile hemangioma: A systematic review. Lasers Surg Med. 2016;48(3):221-33.
22. Wang JY, Ighani A, Ayala AP, Akita S, Lara-Corrales I, Alavi A. Medical, surgical, and wound care management of ulcerated infantile hemangiomas: A systematic review. J Cutan Med Surg. 2018;22(5):495-504.
23. George C, Deroide F, Rustin M. Pyoderma gangrenosum: A guide to diagnosis and management. Clin Med (Lond). 2019;19(3):224-8.

SECTION 2

Therapeutics

9. Immunosuppressants in Dermatology
10. FAQs on Biologics and JAKis
11. Antihistamines
12. Antibiotics in Dermatology

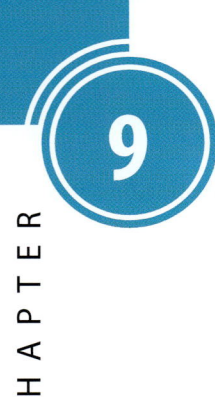

CHAPTER 9: Immunosuppressants in Dermatology

INTRODUCTION

This chapter is designed to provide a broad overview of immunosuppressant therapies which are commonly used for various dermatoses. When choosing therapy for an individual patient, certain general principles must be known. First, the physician should be aware of all the therapeutic modalities available and become familiar with the drugs that are frequently used and are likely to yield optimal results.

The use of each drug during pregnancy and lactation is reviewed. In general, one should be careful in prescribing systemic medications to women of childbearing potential. It is not adequate merely to ask the patient if she is using birth control measures before prescribing most of the medications discussed in the chapter; the patient must be aware of the risks associated with using the medication and the risks of continuing therapy if pregnancy occurs.

Systemic drugs used in dermatology may be subdivided into broad categories, such as immunosuppressive, cytotoxic, and antiproliferative **(Table 1)**.

AZATHIOPRINE

Azathioprine is thiopurine class of drug that is useful in the treatment of a number of inflammatory and autoimmune skin disorders. Its precursor, 6-mercaptopurine (6-MP), and the structurally related compound 6-thioguanine (6-TG) were first developed for their anticancer properties. However, because of their anti-inflammatory and immunosuppressive qualities, thiopurines are now used more frequently.

Mechanism of Action

The body transforms azathioprine nonenzymatically into 6-MP, which is subsequently broken down via one of three routes. In two of these, thiopurine methyltransferase (TPMT) or xanthine

TABLE 1: Systemic drugs in dermatology.

Immunosuppressive/Anti-inflammatory	Cytotoxic	Antiproliferative
Azathioprine	Cyclophosphamide	Methotrexate
Mycophenolate mofetil	Chlorambucil	Hydroxyurea
Cyclosporine	Bleomycin	
Tacrolimus		
Thalidomide		

oxidase (XO) breaks it down into inactive metabolites. Hypoxanthine-guanine phosphoribosyltransferase (HGPRT) is involved in the third metabolic pathway, converting 6-MP into 6-thioguanine nucleotides. By disrupting the regular synthesis of deoxyribonucleic acid (DNA) and ribonucleic acid (RNA), these active metabolites have immunosuppressive effects. Furthermore, it is believed that a derivative of imidazole that is produced during metabolism plays a major role in the medication's anti-inflammatory properties.

Licensed Indications

Autoimmune Bullous Disorders

Despite azathioprine's official approval for the treatment of pemphigus vulgaris, there is still little evidence to support its application in this condition. Despite the generally poor quality of the included studies, azathioprine showed a steroid-sparing effect that seemed more noticeable than that of cyclophosphamide or mycophenolate mofetil, according to a recent systematic review assessing treatments for both pemphigus vulgaris and pemphigus foliaceus.[1,2] Nevertheless, there is currently insufficient evidence to conclusively demonstrate that azathioprine, or any other second-line medication such as cyclophosphamide and mycophenolate, is superior to glucocorticoids alone in terms of inducing remission.

Lupus Erythematosus

Evidence indicates that azathioprine is more effective than cyclophosphamide for maintenance therapy after induction in patients with lupus nephritis, and it is approved for the treatment of systemic lupus erythematosus (SLE).[3] Although there are not any randomized controlled trials (RCTs) that explicitly support its use in cutaneous lupus, a number of case series have suggested that azathioprine might be a useful therapeutic option in these situations.

Dermatomyositis and Polymyositis

In patients with dermatomyositis (DM) and polymyositis (PM), azathioprine has demonstrated efficacy as a second-line treatment; multiple case series have reported clinical improvement in 57–75% of cases.[4] It has shown a steroid-sparing effect in juvenile DM and could be a useful treatment option for patients who have failed other immunosuppressive therapies.

Recommendations: Off-label Indications for Azathioprine

There is evidence to support the use of azathioprine outside its product license for the following indications:
- Atopic eczema (strength of recommendation A; level of evidence 1+).
- Maintenance therapy for Wegener's granulomatosis (strength of recommendation B; level of evidence 1+).
- Behçet's disease (strength of recommendation B; level of evidence 1+).
- AI-VBDs (strength of recommendation B; level of evidence 1).

Inflammatory Skin Diseases

Atopic Dermatitis

Two RCTs have provided compelling evidence of azathioprine's efficacy in treating atopic eczema, despite the medication's lack of official approval. When azathioprine was administered orally as a monotherapy to patients with moderate-to-severe, treatment-resistant disease, both studies showed a statistically significant and clinically meaningful improvement.[5,6]

Psoriasis

Nowadays, azathioprine is rarely used in standard clinical practice for moderate-to-severe psoriasis because there is little evidence to support its use as monotherapy.[7] However, a recent retrospective review suggests azathioprine may be combined with biologics such as infliximab as an alternative to methotrexate (MTX) for long-term maintenance.[8]

Checklist for Use Prior to Prescribing Azathioprine

- Patients should be informed that they should not anticipate an instant alleviation of their symptoms, and its effect may not be apparent for 2–3 months.
- Because of the possibility of hematological toxicity, regular monitoring of complete blood count (CBC), liver function tests (LFTs), and renal function tests (RFTs) is necessary. Azathioprine should not be prescribed to patients who are incapable or unwilling to adhere to monitoring requirements.
- Inform the patient that although the medication is not officially approved for the condition, it is frequently used due to clinical evidence and experience in cases of unlicensed use. Make sure to clearly record this conversation.
- Due to the possibility of azathioprine hypersensitivity, bone marrow suppression, or liver impairment, patients who experience any of the following symptoms are advised to contact a doctor right away:
  - Extreme flu-like illness or a high fever
  - Unexpected bleeding or bruises
  - Recent onset of jaundice
- Ensure that the usage of azathioprine is not contraindicated.
- *Review the baseline investigations*:
  - CBC
  - Electrolytes and urea
  - LFTs
  - Serology for hepatitis B and C
  - Human immunodeficiency virus (HIV) serology, particularly in populations at high risk.
  - Activity of TPMT (rarely also genotype—when available)
  - Serology for the varicella-zoster virus (VZV) (if no history of varicella).
- *Precautions must be taken into consideration in the following groups*:
  - Young and the elderly age group
  - Liver or kidney impairment
  - Premalignant diseases such as actinic keratoses and cervical intraepithelial neoplasia (CIN).
  - *VZV nonimmune*: Immunization is required.
  - *Hepatitis B virus (HBV) nonimmune*: In at-risk groups, immunization is necessary.
  - HIV infected individuals.
- Pneumococcal vaccination should be advised prior to beginning treatment, along with yearly immunization against influenza.
- Educate regarding the possibility of elevated risk of malignancy associated with prolonged use.
- Give advice on sun protection, encourage the use of broad-spectrum sunscreens.

- Given that azathioprine may be hazardous during pregnancy, provide advice on effective contraception with its use.
- Rule out potential drug interactions, if any.
- Plan for a gradual withdrawal and, if possible, describe the anticipated length of treatment.
- If it has not been given already, provide a patient information leaflet and note its availability in the case notes.

Adverse Effects

It can be divided into short-term, medium-term, and long-term toxicity.

Short-term Toxicity

Nausea

The most frequently observed adverse effect of azathioprine is isolated, dose-dependent nausea. Patients with true azathioprine hypersensitivity also exhibit nausea as part of a wider symptom complex, but management of these patients is different and is described separately.

Recommendations

Managing nausea (strength of recommendation D; level of evidence 4)
- Increasing the dosage gradually could help reduce the initial nausea.
- *You can control moderate nausea by*:
  - With divided daily dosages
  - Intake of azathioprine after meals
  - Short-term dosage reduction
  - Antiemetics
- When nausea is accompanied by other symptoms such as fever, myalgia, and arthralgia, it indicates hypersensitivity and needs to be managed differently.

Hypersensitivity

Azathioprine hypersensitivity is an uncommon, idiosyncratic, and immunologically mediated reaction that usually manifests a few weeks after starting treatment. Despite being severe, it is rarely lethal. Symptoms of hypersensitivity can be organ-specific or generalized and commonly include nausea, fever, myalgia, and arthralgia; infrequently, hepatitis, interstitial nephritis, or renal failure may also occur. In fatal cases, hypotension and shock may develop.[9] There are reports of occasional maculopapular rash. Instead of hypersensitivity, the underlying illness may be the cause of eruptions like erythema nodosum.

Using the smallest dose of azathioprine possible is advised when considering rechallenging to confirm hypersensitivity because rechallenge with conventional azathioprine dose can lead to severe, unwarranted symptoms. It is recommended to rechallenge in a hospital setting with access to resuscitation facilities if the hypersensitivity symptoms are severe. 6-MP may be a safe substitute in as many as 60% of azathioprine-hypersensitive patients, indicating that in these patients, immunological sensitivity is focused on the imidazole rather than the thiopurine component of the azathioprine molecule.

Medium-term Toxicity

Myelotoxicity
A potentially dangerous and rather frequent dose-dependent side effect of azathioprine is bone marrow suppression, which most frequently manifests as neutropenia.[10]

Susceptibility to Infection
Although there is currently little evidence to support this, azathioprine may raise the risk of infection even in the absence of neutropenia. This increased susceptibility may be attributed to mild lymphopenia, which is a fairly common finding in patients receiving thiopurine treatment.

Recommendations
Managing VZV in patients receiving azathioprine[11] (strength of recommendation D; level of evidence 4).
- Consider temporary withdrawal of azathioprine
- Prompt use of oral antivirals (aciclovir, valaciclovir, or famciclovir) in all patients
- Intravenous antiviral therapy is desirable for disseminated or ophthalmic VZV.

Hepatotoxicity
Patients on azathioprine frequently experience mild liver enzyme abnormalities, which typically do not have any serious clinical repercussions. On the other hand, severe hepatotoxicity is uncommon but crucial to identify. There are two patterns in which liver injury presents: (1) Acute idiosyncratic drug-induced liver injury (DILI) and (2) Nodular regenerative hyperplasia. The former could be a cholestatic disproportionate to rise in bilirubin and alkaline phosphatase, or hepatocellular (disproportionately elevated transaminases).

Recommendations
Managing hepatotoxicity (strength of recommendation B; level of evidence 2++).
    Mild LFT abnormalities are common and might not necessitate changing treatment.
    Rarely, at any point during azathioprine therapy, different patterns of severe liver damage can be observed.
    Any abnormal LFT results should be carefully evaluated, and more frequent monitoring should be performed; medication withdrawal or dose reduction may be necessary.

Long-term Toxicity

Carcinogenesis
Azathioprine has also been linked to carcinogenicity.

Ultraviolet Radiation and Skin Cancer
It is commonly known that recipients of solid organ transplants who take azathioprine for an extended period of time have a much higher chance of developing non-melanoma skin cancer (NMSC).
    The concurrent use of several immunosuppressive medications probably exacerbates this increased risk,[12,13] with some studies indicating a risk increase of >200 times.[14]

Lymphoma Risk

Long-term azathioprine use is linked to a higher risk of developing a number of malignancies, particularly in solid-organ transplant recipients who also receive other immunosuppressive medications. After NMSC, non-Hodgkin lymphoma is the second most common type of cancer.[15]

Drug Interactions (Table 2)

Caution is advised when considering concomitant use with drugs such as cotrimoxazole, trimethoprim, and clonazipine.

Toxicity Monitoring

Frequency

The British National Formulary (BNF) states that patients beginning azathioprine should be monitored weekly for the first month and then monthly thereafter. On the other hand, a more cautious approach is suggested by the azathioprine manufacturer's datasheet, which calls for weekly monitoring for the first 8 weeks. The frequency of monitoring can be decreased once the patient is stable on a fixed dosage, but it should always be done at least once every 3 months.

Monitoring for Myelosuppression

During long-term azathioprine therapy, routine CBC monitoring is essential. A common and usually harmless side effect, macrocytosis can also be used as a proxy for medication compliance. Leukopenia is the most frequent hematological side effect, though anemia, thrombocytopenia, and in rare instances, pancytopenia, can also happen. In addition to macrocytosis, the appearance of any hematological abnormalities should trigger careful observation and suitable azathioprine dosage modification.

METHOTREXATE

- In 1948, aminopterin, a folate antagonist, was introduced, followed by amethopterin (methotrexate).
- In 1951, Gubner and colleagues recognized its efficacy for the treatment of psoriasis.
- In 1971, the United States Food and Drug Administration (US FDA) approved its use in psoriasis.

TABLE 2: Drug risks/interactions—drugs that can cause hematological adverse drug reactions (ADRs).

• Allopurinol and febuxostat	• Risk of severe, life-threatening myelotoxicity
• Immunosuppressant drugs	• Immunosuppressant drugs. Combination with other drugs such as cyclophosphamide, methotrexate, and cyclosporine increases the risk of myelotoxicity
Warfarin	Warfarin resistance is reported, and the warfarin dose may need to be increased. Close monitoring of anticoagulation parameters is advised
Ribavirin	Severe pancytopenia has been reported. This drug inhibits inosine monophosphate dehydrogenase (IMPD), an enzyme in the purine salvage pathway
Live vaccines	Should not be prescribed to immunocompromised individuals
Aminosalicylates	Inhibit thiopurine methyltransferase (TPMT) in vitro, but the clinical importance of this is unknown. The drugs are often coprescribed for inflammatory bowel disease (IBD), and increased monitoring of full blood count (FBC) is advised

Pharmacology

- *Structure:* A synthetic analog of folic acid, 4-amino-N10-methyl-pteroylglutamic acid.
- *Pharmacokinetics:*
    - Can be administered orally, intravenously, or intramuscularly.
    - Methotrexate is readily absorbed from the gastrointestinal (GIT) at doses < 25 mg/m^2.
    - Absorption is influenced by food and milk in children, but not in adults.
    - Bioavailability in adults—67%; reaches peak plasma level in 1–3 hours.
    - Distributed widely in all tissues except the brain.
    - 50–60% bound to plasma proteins
    - Minimally metabolized in the liver. Methotrexate is converted to methotrexate polyglutamates, which have prolonged intracellular storage. After high doses, however, metabolites do accumulate; these include 7-OH methotrexate, which is potentially nephrotoxic.
    - Clearance is via the kidneys, both glomerular filtration and tubular secretion—about 60–95% of the single dose appears unchanged in urine.
    - Biliary excretion is <10%.
    - Lower dose (dermatological use)—biphasic elimination, mean half-life 6–7 hours.

Mechanism of Action (Flowchart 1)

- Inhibition of cell division–specific for the S phase of the normal cell cycle
- Toxicity is limited to proliferating cells (in contrast to alkylating agents) and has less potential for mutagenicity.

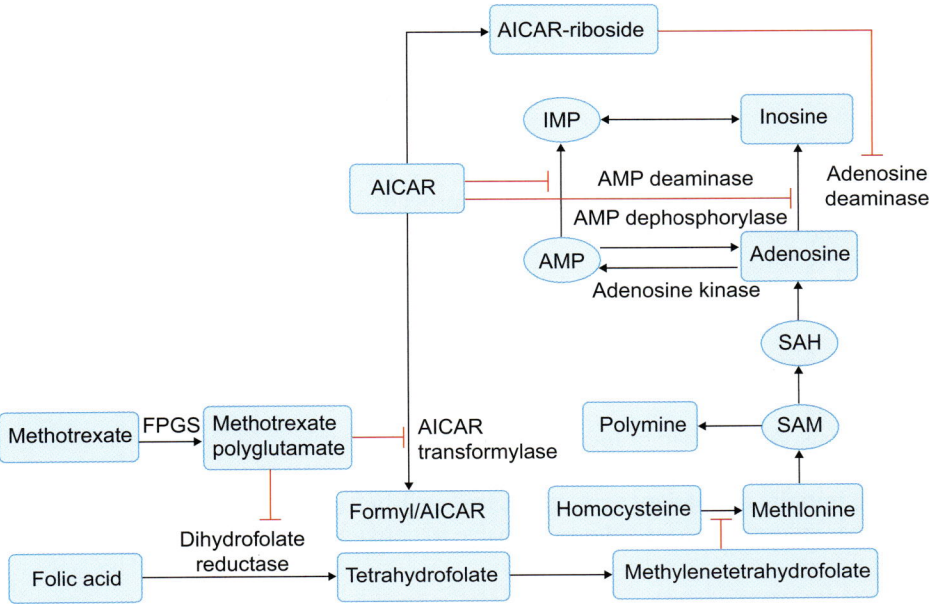

FLOWCHART 1: Mechanism of action of methotrexate.
(AICAR: 5-aminoimidazole-4-carboxamide-1-β-D-ribofuranoside; AMP: adenosine monophosphate; FPGS: folylpolyglutamate synthase; IMP: inosine monophosphate; SAH: S-adenosylhomocysteine; SAM: S-adenosyl methionine)

- Inside the cells, additional glutamyl residues are added—polyglutamylated forms
  - Binds more tightly to dihydrofolate reductase (DHFR).
  - Persists longer in the cells.
  - Spectrum of inhibition increased.

Anti-inflammatory Properties

- Methotrexate polyglutaminate → inhibits 5-aminoimidazole-4-carboxamide ribonucleotide (AICAR) which, increases local tissue adenosine.
- *Release of adenosine by fibroblasts and endothelial cells occurs by three distinct mechanisms*: The inhibition of superoxide anion generation in neutrophils, the inhibition of the adherence of neutrophils to endothelium, and the reduction of tumor necrosis factor (TNF) synthesis is activated in neutrophils.[16]
- Suppression of inflammatory cell chemotaxis decreases Langerhans cell activity and LTB_4 synthesis, inhibiting inflammation caused by C5a.
- Inhibits the histamine release from basophils.

Immunosuppressant Action

- Shown by an in vitro experiment the effect of methotrexate on lymphoid cells is 1,000 times more than its effect on human keratinocytes.
- Methotrexate acts via an immunosuppressant mechanism rather than an antiproliferative agent directed against the keratinocytes.
- The effect probably occurs because of the inhibition of DNA synthesis in immunologically competent cells.
- Methotrexate suppresses primary and secondary antibody responses but does not affect delayed-type hypersensitivity.
- However, in the case of acute methotrexate toxicity, inhibition of epidermal proliferation is likely pertinent.

Clinical Uses

- *Psoriasis:* Most widely accepted and US-FDA approved.
- *Dose:* 0.2–0.4 mg/kg/week
- Available as a 2.5, 5,10,15 mg tablet
- 2 mL vials with 2.5, 15, 20 and 25 mg/mL.

Indications of Methotrexate Therapy in Psoriasis

- Psoriatic arthritis
- Pustular psoriasis, generalized or localized variant
- Erythrodermic psoriasis
- Psoriasis that impairs the patient's psychological well-being.
- Extensive severe plaque psoriasis not responsive to conventional therapy (>10% BSA).

Two Types of Intermittent Weekly Regimens

- *Triple dose regimen (Weinstein FROST)*: 2.5–5 mg at 12-hourly intervals–aimed at providing a therapeutic level for 36 hours, which is the duration of the psoriatic cell cycle.

- It is now acknowledged that the previously put forth justification for giving methotrexate in three divided doses once weekly[17] is not valid,[18] and this regimen may carry a higher risk of hepatic fibrosis.[19]

Single Dose Weekly Regimen (Oral, Intramuscular, Intravenous, or Subcutaneous)
- To identify patients who might be hypersensitive to methotrexate, a small test dose (typically 2.5–5 mg) is advised at first.
- Depending on the clinical response and any toxicity, subsequent doses should be progressively increased (usually in 2.5–5 mg increments) if the CBC at 7 days after the test dose does not reveal leukopenia.[20]
- The majority of patients can be effectively managed with 7.5–15 mg/week; in older patients, even lower dosages might be sufficient.
- The goal of treatment is to attain optimal control (75–80%) clearance.
- Although a maximal response may take 4–8 weeks, a clinical response is typically observed within 7–14 days.
- Within 48 hours, acute generalized pustular psoriasis may improve.
- *Clinical improvement sequence*:
    - *Clearing of scale*: 1 month later.
    - Decrease in erythema following the second month.
    - By the end of the third month, plaques will have broken up with islands of normal skin.
- Quality-of-life (QOL) data and desired retreatment scores from a number of clinical trials and concluded that a 50% reduction in the Psoriasis Area and Severity Index score (PASI 50) represents a meaningful change in a person's life and a better endpoint.
- After adequate clearing, methotrexate is decreased by 2.5–5 mg every month to determine the lowest effective minimum dose or to extend the interval between doses.
- After complete remission patient may be maintained on a weekly or biweekly dose of methotrexate. The lesion-free period after complete remission ranges from 1 month (no maintenance therapy) to 1 year (with maintenance therapy), and it is not well-established whether methotrexate discontinuation will result in a rebound phenomenon.

How Long can or should a Patient be Maintained on Methotrexate?
- If a patient takes low-dose methotrexate continuously for >3 years, the approximate cumulative dose they could receive is 1.5 g.
- Methotrexate therapy rest periods, which typically last a few months each year (summer is usually a good time), may help lower cumulative toxicity.
- Weekly intramuscular (IM) doses of methotrexate can be given in the following situations:
    - When taking oral medication, the patient is unreliable.
    - Oral methotrexate's efficacy has decreased.
    - Treatment is being limited by GIT side effects.
    - Because methotrexate has a shorter plasma half-life when given parenterally, doses are typically higher than weekly oral doses.

Combination Therapy in Psoriasis
Combining different therapies at low doses improves overall treatment efficacy while lowering toxicity.

Methotrexate and Phototherapy (Flowchart 2)

- *Combination of methotrexate and psoralen plus ultraviolet A (PUVA)*:
    - Controversial
    - Higher risk of squamous cell carcinoma (SCC)
- *With UVB*: Will halve the number of UVB treatments and above one-third to one-half the total dose required to clear psoriasis.
- Throughout the course of treatment, the total dosage of methotrexate given using this method usually stays below 200 mg.
- Usually, this combination is well tolerated.
- Radiation recall phenomenon—rarely seen with methotrexate and UVB.
- Narrow band UVB and methotrexate—good results
- Recently in a placebo-controlled randomized study ($n = 24$) has concluded that methotrexate pretreatment allows physicians to clear psoriasis in fewer phototherapy (UVB—narrow band) sessions than when phototherapy is administered alone.

Methotrexate and Retinoids (Acitretin)

- Both are hepatotoxic.
- So LFT could be monitored at baseline, 1 week, and monthly thereafter.

Methotrexate and Cyclosporine

- Cyclosporine (CsA)—causes renal abnormality → decrease the excretion of methotrexate.
- Methotrexate—hepatotoxicity → CsA is not adequately metabolized.
- Both are immunosuppressive—increased incidence of opportunistic infections.
- But used in severe psoriatic arthritis and recalcitrant plaque psoriasis.
- Maximal tolerated dosages of methotrexate + CsA 5 mg/kg can be tapered rapidly.
  No flare-up even if CsA is discontinued abruptly.
  A recent prospective study by Aydir F, et al. ($n = 20$), median duration of combination therapy was 9.5 weeks, short-term side effects were minimal, concluded that maximal improvement at the start of combination therapy, healing rate was decreased after tapering and cessation of one drug. Long-term follow-up of the patient is needed.

Methotrexate and Biological Agents

A chest X-ray and baseline purified protein derivative (PPD) testing should be done in addition to routine methodology. Treatment with alefacept may also necessitate routine lymphocyte count monitoring.

Methotrexate and Etanercept

- Both in severe psoriasis and psoriatic arthritis
- Add 25 mg subcutaneous twice per week to the methotrexate regimen.
- No additional monitoring required, and good remission.

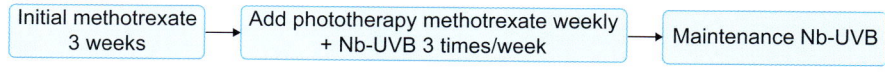

FLOWCHART 2: Methotrexate and phototherapy.

Methotrexate and Infliximab—in Severe Recalcitrant Psoriasis
- Slow IV infusion of infliximab (5 mg/kg), repeat at 2 and 6 weeks.
- Methotrexate can be tapered rapidly—good remission.

Methotrexate and Alefacept
- Recent randomized, placebo-controlled, double blind study by Mease PJ, et al. in severe psoriatic arthritis (*n* = 185), Alefacept 15 mg IM once weekly for 12 weeks + methotrexate > 54% patients responded well.
- Most adverse events were mild-to-moderate in severity.

Rotational Therapy
- Concept by Weinstein and white.
- Each form of therapy for 1–2 years and switching to the next form.
- Cumulative toxicity, such as hepatic fibrosis, can be reduced.

Other Proliferative Disorders Responding to Methotrexate
- *Pityriasis subra pilaris (PRP)*:
  - Responds less well to methotrexate than does psoriasis.
  - Doses are 1.5–2 times greater, and reports suggest daily low-dose regimen responds better than weekly regimens.
- *Pityriasis lichenoides et varioliformis acuta (PLEVA)*: Small doses of methotrexate (weekly) can be used to control the disease process
- *Reiter's disease*:
  - Doses required are slightly higher than for psoriasis.
  - Beneficial for both rheumatologic and cutaneous aspects.

Other Indications of Methotrexate and Its Efficacy
Dermatomyositis
- Methotrexate is increasingly advocated for cutaneous lesions of DM.
- Oral methotrexate 2.5–30 mg weekly (*n* = 13), whose cutaneous lesions have not been completely responsive to corticosteroid, oral antimalarial, or oral prednisone.[21]
  Oral methotrexate is effective (75% of patients have complete clearing) and frequently enables a reduction or discontinuation of corticosteroid therapy.[7]

Childhood Dermatomyositis
Early introduction of methotrexate in children in doses of 15 mg/m²/week, along with oral corticosteroids is more effective therapy than traditional long-term steroid therapy for children.[8]

Systemic Lupus Erythematosus
- *Methotrexate*: Effective in patients with subacute cutaneous lupus erythematosus (LE) unresponsive to standard therapy.

- Wenzel et al. studied 43 patients of cutaneous LE (recalcitrant to topical treatments and first-line systemic drugs, antimalarials), a highly significant ($p < 0.01$) decline in disease activity, 98% patients recorded improvement, and side effects that led to discontinuation of methotrexate in only 16%.[9]
- Intravenous (IV) was tolerated better than oral administration.
- Also, an increase in circulating lymphocyte numbers in patients with lymphopenia.

Atopic Dermatitis
- Open retrospective study by Goujan et al. ($n = 20$) of adult patients.
- >75% had improvement in the fourth to eight weeks after methotrexate doses.
- Placebo-controlled trials are needed to confirm observations.

Systemic Sclerosis and Morphea
- Role controversial—cutaneous scores improved in all studies.
- Methotrexate (0.3–0.6 mg/kg/week) along with IV methyl prednisolone (pulse) (30 mg/kg for 3 days monthly for initial 3 months)—effective (median time to response—3 months) and well tolerated in the treatment of pediatric localized scleroderma.

Cutaneous Sarcoidosis
- Effective for the treatment of patients with chronic cutaneous sarcoidosis where topical corticosteroids and antimalarials failed.[22]
- But the improvement in skin lesions may be slow.
- Less successful in treating pulmonary sarcoidosis; only one-third of patients showed an improvement in lung function.

Bullous Pemphigoid
- Treatment of BP with low-dose methotrexate is an effective alternative with a favorable benefit/side effect ratio.
- In elderly patients with generalized BP, not responding to potent topical steroid—methotrexate in low dose weekly worked as an effective monotherapy and was well tolerated.
- Pemphigus and epidermolysis bullosa acquisita (EBA) → Also respond (as an adjuvant to corticosteroids).

Other Dermatoses
Individual Case Reports or Small Series
- Cutaneous small vessel vasculitis
- Polyarteritis nodosa
- Behçet's disease
- Pyoderma gangrenosum (PG)
- Multisystem Langerhans histiocytosis
- Multicentric reticulohistiocytosis
- Lymphomatoid papulosis
- Scleromyxedema
- Keratoacanthoma
- Sézary syndrome

Methotrexate in Human Immunodeficiency Virus Infected Patients
- Methotrexate in low doses—tolerated by HIV individuals.
- Careful laboratory monitoring for methotrexate toxicity and avoidance of concomitant medications that alter methotrexate metabolism.
- Possibility of added immunosuppression by methotrexate in HIV patients → first-line systemic treatment for psoriasis in PLHIV is acitretin.

Methotrexate in Children
- Indicated for unresponsive psoriasis, exfoliative erythroderma, pustular psoriasis, and psoriatic arthritis.
- Test dose 2.5 mg → gradually increase up to 20 mg/week.
- Screening tests and side effect profile are similar to adults.
- Liver biopsy is unnecessary as hepatotoxicity is rare.
- Live vaccines are contraindicated when taking methotrexate (killed vaccines can be substituted)
- Long-term oncogenic risk–great concern; not clearly delineated.

Adverse Effects
Gastrointestinal
- Nausea, vomiting—common.
- Dose related and seen in 10–30%.
- Gastric ulcerations, diarrhea—infrequently.
- *Treatment*—H_2 blockers, metoclopramide, prochlorperazine, or even ondansetron.
- Large parenteral doses are frequently followed by bursting headaches, which usually last for a day or so.
- Following full doses, psoriatic plaques frequently experience a burning sensation that lasts for several days.

Hematopoietic
- Most important adverse effect to look for.
- Maximum myelosuppression 7–10 days after an oral dose.

Risk Factors for Methotrexate-induced Pancytopenia
- *Drug interactions*: Trimethoprim (TMP)/sulfamethoxazole (SMX)/nonsteroidal anti-inflammatory drugs (NSAIDs).
- Renal disease
- Elderly patients
- No folate supplementation
- First 4–6 weeks of therapy
- Albumin < 3.0 g/dL
- Major illnesses
- Patients should have a weekly CBC before the pulse methotrexate up to 1 month of therapy.
- If serum hemoglobin <10 g%/total leukocyte count (TLC) < 3,500/PC <1 lakh → drug should be temporarily stopped.

- If the TLC falls further to 500 cells/mL and does not show improvement → start treatment for drug-induced neutropenia.
- Marrow recovery usually occurs in 3 weeks.
- Drug may be restarted at a lower dose after 2–3 weeks rest period, if laboratory abnormality is resolved.

Acute Toxicity and Overdose

Acute toxicity from an absolute or relative overdose of methotrexate can manifest as mucosal ulceration, myelosuppression, and, in rare instances, cutaneous necrolysis. Early treatment may be life-saving. The metabolic effects of methotrexate can be bypassed by the administration of folinic acid. As soon as overdose is suspected, serum should be collected for measurement of methotrexate levels, and folinic acid should be administered intravenously. The dose of folinic acid should be at least as high as the total dose of methotrexate thought to be responsible for the overdose and should, in any event, not be <20 mg. Until the serum methotrexate level drops below 0.01 μmol/L, subsequent doses (which can be taken orally if they do not exceed 20 mg) should be given every 6 hours. The serum methotrexate concentration determines the necessary folinic acid dosage. When the concentration of methotrexate is 0.5 μmol/L or less, a dose of 20 mg is sufficient; for higher concentrations, the folinic acid dose can be computed as 100 mg/1 μmol/L of serum methotrexate.[21]

Hepatic Toxicity

- Most common long-term adverse drug reaction (ADR) of methotrexate.
- 8–67% have hepatotoxicity.
- Patients with psoriasis have been shown to have an increased incidence (2.5–5 fold) of hepatic fibrosis than those with rheumatoid arthritis.
- Negligible incidence in doses < 1.5 g of cumulative dose—high incidence > 4 g.
- Nonaggressive course—some patients are able to continue taking methotrexate without worsening of liver biopsy findings.

Risk Factors for Methotrexate-induced Hepatic Fibrosis

- *Age:* Increased risk > 60 years
- *Dose:*
  - Increase dose
  - Dose frequency
  - Duration of therapy
  - Total dose
- *Alcohol:* Increased risk with daily levels of >15 g (one to two drinks).
- *Obesity:* Increased risk and diabetes mellitus.
- Preexisting liver disease
- Impaired renal function
- *Other drugs:* NSAIDs, vitamin A, arsenic, and other hepatotoxic drugs.
- LFT may be transiently raised after each dose to ensure normalization of the level before the next dose.
- Methotrexate should normally be stopped if liver enzyme levels suddenly rise above three times the upper limit of normal.

- *Current dermatology guideline:* Liver biopsy is no more recommended.
- Liver elastography is better to evaluate changes in liver.[23,24]
- Nonetheless, a number of studies show that patients receiving closely monitored, once-weekly low-dose methotrexate have a low risk of suffering serious liver damage.[25-30] Therefore, considering the low frequency of identifying significant liver pathology, the routine use of repeated liver biopsies may be difficult to justify due to their expense and associated risks.
  - Blinded percutaneous
  - Ultrasound-guided
- Liver biopsy should be done 2 weeks after the last methotrexate dose in order to minimize the possibility of acute toxicity changes noted in liver histology.
- The risk of bleeding is 1 in 1,000.
- Death in 1/10,000.

Other Noninvasive Tests
- Liver ultrasound screening
- *Dynamic hepatic scintigraphy*:
  - Measures reduction in the portal venous contribution to total hepatic blood flow
  - Sensitivity 83.5% and specificity 81.5%.
- Magnetic resonance imaging (MRI), static radionucleotide scanning.
- Serum levels of aminoterminal propeptide of type III procollagen (P-III-NP).

Limitations of p3NP
- Lack of site specificity regarding identifying which organ is undergoing fibrosis.
- Not reliable in patients with significant psoriatic arthritis.
  - Serial testing at 3-month intervals to detect active fibrogenesis
  - Khan et al. conducted an audit to assess the practice of P3NP monitoring. It concluded that a median P_3NP value of 5.8 μg/L or higher had a stronger correlation with histological severity.
  - Combining these tests may eventually lead to a decreased number of liver biopsies.

Pulmonary Toxicity
- Acute pneumonitis/more insidious pulmonary fibrosis.
- Idiosyncratic reaction and not dose-related.
- Smoking is a risk factor for pulmonary toxicity.
- Renal impairment and concomitant use of NSAIDs increase pulmonary toxicity
- If suspected → PFT should be advised.
- Methotrexate should be stopped immediately, and the condition responds to corticosteroids.

Methotrexate Osteopathy
- A complication of long-term low dosage
- *Consists of a triad of*:
  - Intense pain in the distal tibia.
  - Presence of osteoporosis.
  - Compression fracture of the distal tibia.
- *Treatment*: Withdrawal of methotrexate.

Teratogenicity
- Methotrexate is a teratogen and abortificient.
- During treatment, sperm count decreases but recovers within 2-3 months.
- No reports of abnormal children fathered by men receiving methotrexate therapy.

However, men on the medication should wait 3 months after stopping treatment, and women of childbearing potential must use effective contraception during methotrexate treatment and for at least three menstrual cycles after discontinuation. Additionally, methotrexate should not be taken while nursing.

Mucocutaneous Side Effects
- Alopecia (6%)—generally telogen effluvium; sometimes anagen alopecia.
- Intermittent high dosage—horizontal pigmented banding of hair (flag sign).
- Photosensitivity (5%)—reactivation of sunburn.
- Urticaria (4%) and urticarial vasculitis.
- Local epidermal necrosis.
- Anaphylactic reactions.
- Macular erythema (capillaritis), vasculitis, toxic epidermal necrolysis (TEN)—rarely reported.
- Mucocutaneous ulceration and ulcerative stomatitis—warning signs of bone marrow suppression or overdosage usually develop within 2-7 days of therapy.

Renal Effects

Fatal consequences include acute renal failure: Secondary to precipitation of methotrexate in renal tubules, especially with high-dose therapy (50-250 mg/m^2).

Secondary Malignancy
- Methotrexate can cause mutations in laboratory animals
- Development of lymphoma after long-term methotrexate-reported in a patient with psoriasis
- Metastasizing SCC of skin—documented in patients exposed to high doses over an extended period of time (>3 mg over 4 years).

Potential Drug Interactions with Methotrexate

Folate Supplementation
- Folic acid enters cells by active transport without competing with methotrexate, but methotrexate does compete with folinic acid.
- Folic acid supplementation decreases side effects such as GIT side effects, chiefly nausea, mild myelosuppression, and elevated liver transaminase—without reducing efficacy.
- No effect on liver fibrosis, cirrhosis, pneumonitis, and moderate myelosuppression
- Dose 1-5 mg/day appears to be adequate.
- Folic acid—5 mg/day, including day of methotrexate dosing, folinic acid—not on methotrexate days.[29-31]

- Folate also decreases the associated increase in homocysteine levels due to methotrexate treatment, thus reducing the risk of cardiovascular disease.
- Drawback of folate supplementation—mask vitamin B12 deficiency macrocytosis in red blood cells (RBCs) deleterious side effect seen in patients with decreased renal function, daily ingestion of methotrexate, or concomitant use of another folate antagonist.
- Leucovorin (folinic acid)—antidote to methotrexate overdose.
- Any dose that exceeds 10^6 mole/L plasma methotrexate level—needs leucovorin treatment.
- Should preferably be started within 4 hours and continued for 24–48 hours.
- Rescue doses of 10 mg/m² (~20 mg) are administered IV, followed by fumonisim B (f/b) 20 mg orally (a 20 mg dose is sufficient when methotrexate concentration is <0.5 µmol/L).
- Blood levels of methotrexate are assessed every 12–24 hours; leucovorin should be given every 6 hours till drug levels fall below 10^{-8} M on the methotrexate assay.

Contraindications to Methotrexate Therapy

Absolute Contraindications
- Pregnancy
- Lactation

Relative
- Unreliable patients, including excessive alcohol intake.
- Decreased renal function (creatinine clearance < 50 mL/min).
- *Metabolic*: Diabetes mellitus and obesity.
- *Hepatic diseases*: Abnormal LFT, active hepatitis.
- Man/woman contemplating conception.
- Active infectious disease or history of potentially serious infection.
- *Immunodeficiency syndrome*: Hereditary or acquired.

Monitoring

Baseline (Premethotrexate Evaluation)
- Careful history and physical examination
- Identification of patients at risk
- Recording concomitant medications, if any.

Laboratory
- CBC and platelet count, peripheral smear.
- LFT (especially transaminases).
- Serological tests for hepatitis A, B, and C antibodies.
- *Renal function tests*: Blood urea nitrogen, creatinine clearance.
- HIV testing, if at risk.
- Pregnancy testing.
- Chest radiography.

Follow-up
- Blood CBC, platelet count, and LFT.
  - Weekly for 1 month
  - 7 days after dose escalations
  - Gradually, decrease the frequency of tests to once in 4 weeks and finally to once in 3–4 months.
- *RFT*: Once in 6 months
- *Chest X-ray*: Once in 6 months or when the patient is symptomatic.

Topical Methotrexate
- *Much reduced efficacy due to*:
  - Decreased local penetration
  - Different target sites might be involved
  - No suppression of the immune system
  - No suppression of systemic production of psoriatic factors.
- Controlled trials suggested—topical methotrexate is ineffective
- Kumar B, et al. tried topical 0.25% methotrexate gel in a hydrogel base for palmoplantar psoriasis (*n* = 14).
- Well tolerated, not very effective in controlling lesions.
- A higher concentration in a different base with better penetration could possibly provide better results.
- In vitro percutaneous penetration of methotrexate is enhanced with 1-dodecylazacychloheptan 2-one, laurocapram (Azone).
- Two center double blind pilot study (*n* = 42) in chronic plaque psoriasis—0.1, 0.5, and 1% methotrexate in a laurocapram formulation.
- Overall, improvement around—50%.
- The same formulation is also useful for treatment of early-stage mycosis fungoides.
- In India, topical methotrexate 1% gel is available.

Electroporation
- To increase transdermal transport of methotrexate within a short application time.
- Pilot study by Wong TW, et al. concluded that electroporation of methotrexate with an anion lipid enhancer under a mild hyperthermic environment provided an effective means of drug delivery, and avoided potential systemic toxicity.

CYCLOPHOSPHAMIDE

It is a derivative of nitrogen mustard. It is an alkylating agent.

Pharmacology
- High bioavailability (~75%) is demonstrated by oral cyclophosphamide, which reaches peak plasma concentrations 1–2 hours after administration. It has a half-life of roughly 5–9 hours and is metabolized by the cytochrome P450 (CYP450) enzyme system.[32]

- As a prodrug in the body, cyclophosphamide is converted by the liver to 4-hydroxycyclophosphamide, which exists in equilibrium with aldophosphamide. These metabolites are not directly cytotoxic, but they readily permeate cells.
- Aldophosphamide, in turn, is cleaved intracellularly to phosphoramide mustard, an active metabolite that is directly cytotoxic, and acrolein.[33,34]
- Acrolein itself is highly reactive and may enhance cellular damage by depleting glutathione stores.
- While 30–60% of cyclophosphamide's active metabolites are eliminated in the urine, mostly as carboxyphosphoramide, <20% of the drug's unmetabolized form is removed by the kidneys.

Mechanism of Action

- As a "cell-cycle nonspecific" agent, cyclophosphamide's cytotoxic effects are independent of the cell cycle phase.
- The primary metabolites of the parent compound alkylate DNA by establishing covalent bonds with nucleophilic sites, despite the parent compound's pharmacological inactivity.
- DNA cross-linking, abnormal base pairing, cleavage of the imidazole ring with loss of purine bases, and strand breaks are all caused by this alkylation.
- Cell death, carcinogenesis, or mutagenesis may result from such extensive damage that exceeds the cell's ability to repair itself.
- Cyclophosphamide preferentially affects suppressor T-cells over helper T-cells and exhibits higher cytotoxicity toward B-lymphocytes than T-lymphocytes. Reduced cellular uptake, competition from other nucleophiles, improved DNA repair mechanisms,[35] or increased drug metabolism can all lead to the development of resistance.

FDA Approved Indications in Dermatology

Mycosis Fungoides

The FDA has approved cyclophosphamide for the treatment of mycosis fungoides. It has also been used to treat advanced stages of cutaneous T-cell lymphoma in combination with other therapeutic agents and modalities, like total skin electron beam therapy.[36]

Off-label Dermatologic Uses

Vasculitis

Various types of vasculitides, including Churg–Strauss syndrome, leukocytoclastic vasculitis[37] (like, Henoch–Schönlein purpura, microscopic polyangiitis, polyarteritis nodosa, Wegener's granulomatosis,[38] and many other forms of necrotizing vasculitis not otherwise specified, have been found to respond well to cyclophosphamide, either by itself or in conjunction with corticosteroids.

Mucous Membrane Pemphigoid (Cicatricial Pemphigoid)

Mucous membrane pemphigoid, also called cicatricial pemphigoid, is commonly treated with cyclophosphamide, particularly when there is moderate to severe involvement of the ocular mucosa.[39]

Pemphigus

All forms of pemphigus,[40] even paraneoplastic pemphigus, may be treated with cyclophosphamide. Combination therapy using dexamethasone and cyclophosphamide is effective in limiting disease activity in pemphigus and serves to lower the doses and consequences of systemic glucocorticosteroids.

Neutrophilic Dermatoses
- Behçet disease[41]
- Erythema elevatum diutinum[42]
- Pyoderma gangrenosum (PG)[43,44]

Autoimmune Connective Tissue Diseases
- DM[45,46]
- Relapsing polychondritis[47,48]
- Scleroderma[49,50]
- Severe cutaneous LE

Other
- Bullous drug eruptions (Stevens–Johnson and erythema multiforme major)
- Subcutaneous panniculitic T-cell lymphoma
- Cytophagic histiocytic panniculitis
- Ichthyosis linearis circumflexa
- Lichen myxedematosus/scleromyxedema
- Langerhans' cell histiocytosis
- Xanthoma disseminatum
- Multicentric reticulohistiocytosis

Contraindications

Absolute
- Drug allergy[51-54] (conflicting reports about cross-reactivity with chlorambucil)
- Lactation and pregnancy[55,56]
- Prior history of bladder cancer
- Depressed bone marrow function

Relative
- Active infection
- Impaired renal function
- Impaired hepatic metabolism
- Pregnancy prescribing status—category D

Adverse Effects

Hemorrhagic Cystitis and Bladder Cancer[57]
- One of the most well-known side effects of using cyclophosphamide is genitourinary toxicity. About 5–41% of patients who receive treatment with cyclophosphamide develop hemorrhagic cystitis.

- The main cause of this adverse effect is acrolein, a hazardous byproduct of cyclophosphamide. A thiol compound called mesna (sodium 2-mercaptoethane sulfonate) binds acrolein in the bladder and reduces irritation.
- For prophylaxis, mesna can be given intravenously or orally.
- Although mesna successfully lowers the risk of hemorrhagic cystitis, some patients may experience cutaneous side effects like maculopapular rash or fixed drug eruption.
- In oncology settings, mesna is typically recommended for patients undergoing prolonged or high-dose cyclophosphamide therapy. Increasing fluid intake also helps to reduce the risk of bladder toxicity. Cyclophosphamide-induced bladder damage can dramatically increase the risk of transitional cell carcinoma if left unchecked when used for prolonged duration of therapy. Therefore, for all patients who have previously been exposed to this drug, continuous monitoring of the lower urinary tract is necessary.

Carcinogenesis
- Cyclophosphamide exposure is associated with non-Hodgkin's lymphoma, leukemia,[58] and SCC in addition to the risk of bladder cancer.
- While patients treated with lower doses and shorter courses, which are typical for most skin conditions,[59] are likely to face a lower risk, this risk is primarily observed in transplant and oncology patients receiving high doses over extended periods of time.

Gastrointestinal
About 70–90% of patients experience nausea and vomiting, the most common GIT side effects of cyclophosphamide. Hemorrhagic colitis, stomatitis, liver toxicity (particularly from high dosages), and appetite loss can also occur as side effects.

Hematologic
One of the frequent and dose-limiting side effects linked to cyclophosphamide use is suppression of bone marrow function, which can present as leukopenia and/or thrombocytopenia.

Reproductive
- About 27–60% of women receiving cyclophosphamide experience amenorrhea, and up to 80% of those who experience it may present with premature ovarian failure.
- The medication has the potential to cause azoospermia in men. Testosterone administration might reduce its risk.
- Cyclophosphamide should typically not be advised as a first-line therapy in men and women planning to conceive following therapy.[57]

Dermatologic[60,61]
- Alopecia (anagen effluvium, seen in 5–30%, usually reversible)
- Urticaria or bullous eruptions (Stevens–Johnson syndrome)
- Pigmentation of nails and skin
- Pigmented band on teeth (irreversible).

Drug Interactions

Drugs that may Lower Cyclophosphamide Levels
Rifampin, prednisolone, nevirapine, ondansetron, phenobarbital, phenytoin, and dexamethasone.

Drugs that may Raise Cyclophosphamide Levels
Allopurinol, chlorpromazine, ciprofloxacin, cimetidine, fluconazole, thiotepa, busulfan, and chloramphenicol.

Immunosuppressive Agents
Azathioprine, CsA.

Cytotoxic Agents
Chlorambucil.

Therapeutic Guidelines

Cyclophosphamide is available in 25 and 50 mg tablets, as well as an intravenous form. The usual oral dosage is 1–3 mg/kg/day, given either divided or as a single morning dose. At doses of 0.5–1 g/m², it can also be given parenterally via pulse therapy. Cyclophosphamide alone or in combination with dexamethasone can be administered as monthly infusions. Parenteral pulse dosing may have fewer side effects than daily oral administration. Vigorous hydration should be started 24 hours before therapy and continue during the dosing period to reduce bladder toxicity.

CYCLOSPORINE

Pharmacology

Structure
- 11 amino acids make up the neutral, cyclic peptide known as CsA.
- It is available in original formulation (Sandimmune) or in a more consistently bioavailable microemulsion formulation (Neoral). Neoral is the only formulation of CsA that is approved for the treatment of psoriasis. Neoral is available as an oral solution or in capsules.
- The CsA oral solution contains a 100 mg/mL concentration and should be diluted right before use, ideally with apple or orange juice to enhance flavor. Avoiding grapefruit juice is advised because it may disrupt the metabolism of CsA.
- Soft gelatin capsules provide a more convenient option and are available in strengths of 25, 50, and 100 mg.

Metabolism and Excretion
- The cytochrome P450 3A4 (CYP3A4) enzyme system in the liver extensively metabolizes CsA. Only around 6% of the administered dose (including the parent drug and its metabolites) is eliminated in the urine.

- The half-life of CsA may be extended in hepatic impairment cases, requiring dose modification. Dialysis and renal failure, however, have little effect on the drug's clearance.
- Breastfeeding is not advised during treatment because CsA is also excreted in breast milk.

Mechanism of Action

- CsA primarily works to treat psoriasis by inhibiting T-lymphocyte activity. This is accomplished by inhibiting the calcineurin enzyme, which is activated by the CsA-cyclophilin complex.[62]
- Nuclear factors of activated T-cells (NFAT-1), a transcription factor, are less active when calcineurin is inhibited. This, in turn, lowers the expression of multiple cytokine genes, most notably interleukin-2 (IL-2). Reduced IL-2 production leads to fewer activated T-cells in the epidermis because IL-2 is essential for the activation and proliferation of $CD4^+$ helper T-cells and $CD8^+$ cytotoxic T-cells.
- Additionally, CsA may directly affect mast cells, keratinocytes, and antigen-presenting cells (like Langerhans' cells).
- Furthermore, intercellular adhesion molecule 1 (ICAM-1) is downregulated as a result of CsA's inhibition of interferon-gamma (IFN-γ) production. Dermal capillary endothelial cells and keratinocytes both express ICAM-1, which leads to the "trafficking" of various inflammatory cells.
- The inflammatory cascade is thus hindered by CsA, which helps limit leukocyte trafficking into the epidermis by blocking IFN-γ and lowering ICAM-1 expression.

Clinical Use

Food and Drug Administration-approved Indications
Psoriasis
There are at least three types of psoriasis that can come under consideration for CsA therapy:
1. First, patients who present with a sudden, severe flare-up or with widespread, intensely inflammatory psoriasis are likely to benefit the most from CsA.
2. Patients with moderate to severe psoriasis or disabling psoriasis who are either (i) unable to tolerate, (ii) contraindicated for, or (iii) have not responded to other systemic therapies that make up the second group of patients. CsA may occasionally enable a patient to attain enough clearing that a previously ineffective treatment may prove more beneficial in sustaining the remission.
3. The third patient group consists of people going through significant life events, like a wedding, where it is necessary to have significant psoriasis clearance for a brief period of time. In addition, to its effectiveness against all types of psoriasis, CsA can be strongly considered for erythrodermic and pustular psoriasis.[63]

Off-label Dermatologic Uses

The most common "off-label" indications for CsA are likely pyoderma gangrenosum and severe atopic dermatitis, which are "on-label" in the majority of developed countries outside the United States.
- *Atopic dermatitis:* In Europe, it is approved for this indication. CsA doses of 2.5–5 mg/kg daily are typically used at the outset.
- *PG:* 7 PG patients who were unresponsive to conventional therapies were reported by Elgart and colleagues. Overall, six of seven patients treated with CsA showed improvement. In this study, three

patients remained in remission after 3–7 months of treatment with CsA at 5–7 mg/kg daily, without subsequent relapse after CsA was discontinued.
- *Chronic idiopathic urticaria:* When conventional therapies are ineffective for chronic idiopathic urticaria (CIU), CsA may be a viable alternative.
- *Papulosquamous dermatoses*: Lichen planus
- *Bullous dermatoses:*
    - Pemphigus
    - Pemphigoid
    - Linear immunoglobulin A (IgA) bullous dermatosis
    - Epidermolysis bullosa acquisita
- *Autoimmune connective tissue diseases:*
    - DM
    - LE
    - Scleroderma
- *Neutrophilic dermatoses:*
    - Pyoderma gangrenosum
    - Behçet's disease
- *Dermatitis*: Atopic dermatitis
- *Alopecia:*
    - Lichen planopilaris
    - Alopecia areata
- *Granulomatous dermatoses:*
    - Granuloma annulare
    - Sarcoidosis
- *Disorder of keratinization*: Pityriasis rubra pilaris
- *Photosensitivity dermatoses*: Chronic actinic dermatitis
- *Other dermatoses:*
    - Eosinophilic cellulitis
    - Kimura's disease
    - Morphea
    - Prurigo nodularis
    - Papuloerythroderma of Ofuji
    - Purpura pigmentosa chronica
    - Persistent papular acantholytic dermatosis
    - Reiter's syndrome
    - Scleromyxedema

Contraindications

Absolute
- Significantly impaired renal function
- Uncontrolled hypertension
- Known hypersensitivity to CsA or any of its ingredients
- Clinically cured or persistent malignancy (except NMSC)
- Cutaneous T-cell lymphoma.

Relative

- *Age group*: Under 18 to over 64 years.
- Controlled hypertension.
- Planning to receive live-attenuated vaccinations.
- On medications that increase renal toxicity or disrupt CsA metabolism.
- Evidence of immunodeficiency or any active infections.
- Concurrent administration of immunosuppressants such as methotrexate or receiving photo-therapy.
- Pregnancy or on lactation.
- Unreliable patients.

Adverse Effects

Renal Effects

Risk for nephrotoxicity rises with therapy duration and dose. If serum creatinine rises by 25% or more from baseline, the FDA recommends modifying the CsA dosage. Nonetheless, a slightly more lenient threshold of a 30% increase is frequently employed in dermatological practice to initiate dose modification or additional assessment.

Steps to follow with rising creatinine are given in **Flowchart 3**.

Hypertension

One known side effect of CsA therapy is hypertension, which is usually defined as a mean systolic blood pressure of >140 mm Hg or a mean diastolic blood pressure of >90 mm Hg. Although it could also

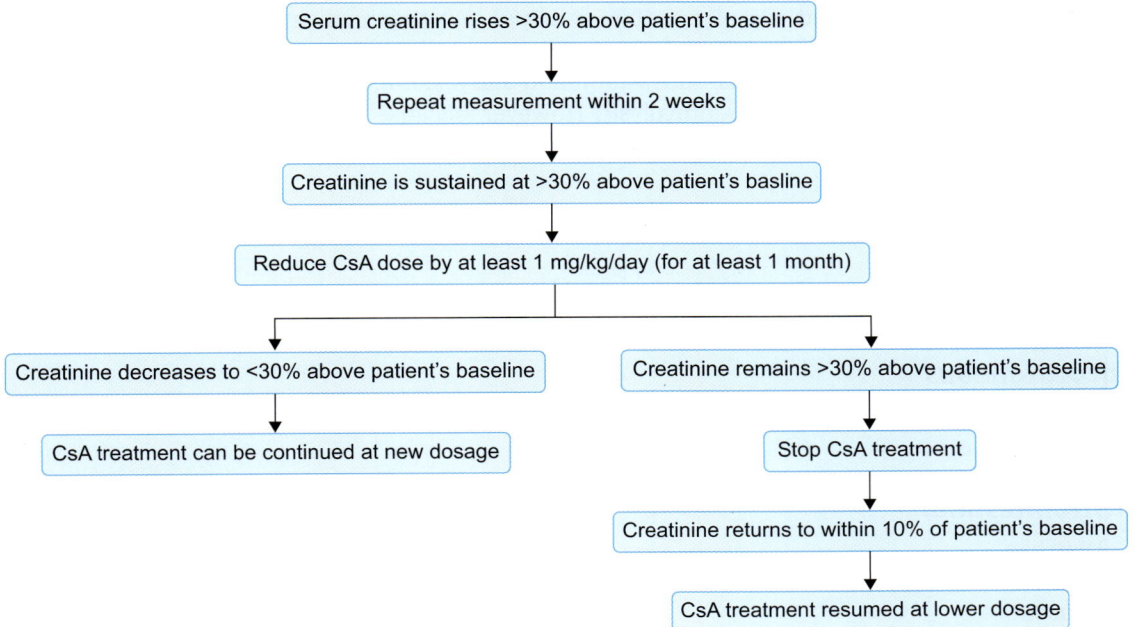

FLOWCHART 3: Steps to follow with rising creatinine.

be secondary to CsA-induced renal impairment, this increase in blood pressure is thought to be caused by CsA's direct vasoconstrictive action on renal vascular smooth muscle. Usually mild, hypertension can be resolved by lowering the dosage or stopping the medication. If blood pressure remains above 140/90 mm Hg for longer than 2 weeks:
   Add an antihypertensive drug (preferably calcium channel blockers- amlodipine) or decrease the CsA dose 25–50%.

Malignancy Risk

Patients with psoriasis receiving long-term CsA treatment are likely to have a higher risk of developing NMSC. Psoriasis patients treated with CsA had a sixfold higher incidence of skin cancer than the general population, with SCC accounting for the majority of these cases. Following CsA treatment for psoriasis, at least three B-cell lymphomas and two cutaneous T-cell lymphomas have been documented. The treatment duration with CsA before diagnosis ranged from 1.5 months to 6 years. When CsA was stopped after less than a year of treatment, the lymphoma spontaneously went into remission. The following usage of CsA has not yet been proven to increase the risk of internal malignancy:
- The maximum "dermatologic" dosage is 5 mg/kg/day.
- Duration of continuous therapy for <2 years.
- In patients with psoriasis who do not take any additional systemic immunosuppressants at the same time.
- In patients with psoriasis who are otherwise healthy.

Hyperlipidemia

One of the more frequent side effects of CsA is hyperlipidemia. Dietary adjustments and increased physical activity should form the basis for initial intervention. If these approaches prove ineffective, the dose of CsA may be decreased, if at all possible, or a lipid-lowering medication may be added to treat hyperlipidemia. It is crucial to be mindful of a significant possible drug interaction between CsA and lovastatin, as well as other statins like simvastatin and atorvastatin. Concurrent CsA raises lovastatin levels, which raises the risk of rhabdomyolysis. However, because they are not CYP3A4 substrates, fluvastatin, rosuvastatin, and pravastatin do not interact with CsA.

Neurologic

- Headache
- Tremor
- Paresthesia and hyperesthesia

Mucocutaneous

- Gingival hyperplasia
- Hypertrichosis

Gastrointestinal

- Diarrhea
- Abdominal discomfort
- Nausea

Musculoskeletal
- Arthralgia
- Myalgia and lethargy

Laboratory Abnormalities
- Hyperkalemia
- Hyperuricemia (occasionally precipitates gout)
- Hyperlipidemia
- Hypomagnesemia

Drug Interactions

Drugs that inhibit CYP3A4 and raise CsA *levels:*
- *Antibiotics* include cephalosporins, doxycycline, norfloxacin, azithromycin, clarithromycin, and erythromycin.
- *Antifungals*: Fluconazole, itraconazole, and ketoconazole.
- Ritonavir, indinavir, saquinavir, and nelfinavir are antivirals (HIV protease inhibitors).
- *Calcium channel blockers*: Nicardipine, verapamil, and diltiazem > all others.
- Cimetidine, ranitidine, and famotidine are H2 receptor antagonists.
- Additional medications include furosemide, thiazides, methylprednisolone, and azacitidine.
- *Other*: Warfarin, metoclopramide, amphotericin B, bromocriptine, allopurinol, and oral contraceptives.

Drugs that decrease CsA *drug levels—CYP3A4 induction:*
- Carbamazepine, phenobarbital, phenytoin, and valproic acid
- Rifampin, rifabutin, and nafcillin
- Octreotide and ticlopidine

The following medications may increase renal toxicity when taken with CsA:
- *Aminoglycosides*: Gentamicin and tobramycin.
- *Additional antibiotics*: Vancomycin and trimethoprim/sulfamethoxazole.
- *Antifungal*: Amphotericin B (ketoconazole, probably through CYP3A4)
- *NSAIDs*: Diclofenac, naproxen, and indomethacin
- *H2 blockers*: Ranitidine and cimetidine
- *Other*: Melphalan and tacrolimus

REFERENCES

1. Martin LK, Werth V, Villanueva E, Segall J, Murrell DF. Interventions for pemphigus vulgaris and pemphigus foliaceus. Cochrane Database Syst Rev. 2009;21(1):CD006263.
2. Chams-Davatchi C, Esmaili N, Daneshpazhooh M, Valikhani M, Balighi K, Hallaji Z, et al. Randomized controlled open-label trial of four treatment regimens for pemphigus vulgaris. J Am Acad Dermatol. 2007;57(1):622-8.
3. Pisoni CN, Karim Y, Cuadrado MJ. Mycophenolate mofetil and systemic lupus erythematosus: an overview. Lupus. 2005;14 (Suppl 1):s9-11.
4. Iorizzo LJ III, Jorizzo JL. The treatment and prognosis of dermatomyositis: an updated review. J Am Acad Dermatol. 2008;59(1):99-112.

5. Berth-Jones J, Takwale A, Tan E, Barclay G, Agarwal S, Ahmed I, et al. Azathioprine in severe adult atopic dermatitis: a double-blind, placebo-controlled, crossover trial. Br J Dermatol. 2002;147(2):324-30.
6. Meggitt SJ, Gray JC, Reynolds NJ. Azathioprine dosed by thiopurine methyltransferase activity for moderate-to-severe atopic eczema: a double-blind, randomized controlled trial. Lancet. 2006;367(9513):839-46.
7. Du Vivier A, Munro DD, Verbov J. Treatment of psoriasis with azathioprine. Br Med J. 1974;1(5897):49-51.
8. Dalaker M, Bonesronning JH. Long-term maintenance treatment of moderate-to-severe plaque psoriasis with infliximab in combination with methotrexate or azathioprine in a retrospective cohort. J Eur Acad Dermatol Venereol. 2009;23(3):277-82.
9. Sinico RA, Sabadini E, Borlandelli S, Cosci P, Di Toma L, Imbasciati E. Azathioprine hypersensitivity: report of two cases and review of the literature. J Nephrol. 2003;16(2):272-6.
10. Anstey A, Lennard L, Mayou SC, Kirby D. Pancytopenia related to azathioprine--an enzyme deficiency caused by a common genetic polymorphism: a review. J R Soc Med. 1992;85(12):752-6.
11. Ahmed AM, Brantley JS, Madkan V, Mendoza N, Tyring SK. Managing herpes zoster in immunocompromised patients. Herpes. 2007;14(2):32-6.
12. Taylor AE, Shuster S. Skin cancer after renal transplantation: the causal role of azathioprine. Acta Derm Venereol. 1992;72(2):115-19.
13. McLelland J, Rees A, Williams G, Chu T. The incidence of immunosuppression-related skin disease in long-term transplant patients. Transplantation. 1988;46(6):871-4.
14. Euvrard S, Kanitakis J, Pouteil-Noble C, Claudy A, Touraine JL. Skin cancers in organ transplant recipients. Ann Transplant. 1997;2(4):28-32.
15. Karran P, Attard N. Thiopurines in current medical practice: molecular mechanisms and contributions to therapy-related cancer. Nat Rev Cancer. 2008;8(1):24-36.
16. Crostein BN, Levin RI, Belanoff J, Weissmann G, Hirschhorn R. Adenosine: an endogenous inhibitor of neutrophil-mediated injury to endothelial cells. J Clin Invest. 1986;78(3):760-70.
17. Weinstein GD, Frost P. Methotrexate for psoriasis. A new therapeutic schedule. Arch Dermatol. 1971;103(1):33-8.
18. Zanolli MD, Sherertz EF, Hedberg AE. Methotrexate: anti-inflammatory or antiproliferative? J Am Acad Dermatol. 1990;22:523-4.
19. Roenigk HH, Auerbach R, Bergfeld WF. A cooperative prospective study of the effects of psoriasis on liver biopsies. In: Farber EM, Cox AJ (Eds). Psoriasis: Proceedings of the Second International Symposium. New York: Yorke Medical; 1977. pp. 243-8.
20. Jih DM, Werth VP. Thrombocytopenia after a single test dose of methotrexate. J Am Acad Dermatol. 1998;39(2 Pt 2):349-51.
21. Kasteler JS, Callen JP. Low-dose methotrexate administered weekly in an effective corticosteroid-sparing agent for the treatment of the cutaneous manifestations of dermatomyositis. J Am Acad Dermatol. 1997;36(1):67-71.
22. Veien NK, Brodthagen H. Cutaneous sarcoidosis treated with methotrexate. British Journal of Dermatology. 1977;97(2):213-6.
23. Ramanan AV, Campbell-Webster N, Ota S, Parker S, Tran D, Tyrrell PN, et al. The effectiveness of treating juvenile dermatomyositis with methotrexate and aggressively tapered corticosteroids. Arthritis and Rheumatism. 2005;52(11):3570-8.
24. Aithal GP, Haugk B, Das S, Card T, Burt AD, Record CO. Monitoring methotrexate-induced hepatic fibrosis in patients with psoriasis: are serial biopsies justified? Aliment Pharmacol Ther. 2004;19(4):391-9.
25. Wenzel J, Brähler S, Bauer R, Bieber T, Tüting T. Efficacy and safety of methotrexate in recalcitrant cutaneous lupus erythematosus: results of a retrospective study in 43 patients. Br J Dermatol. 2005;153(1):157-62.
26. Gary A, Modeste AB, Richard C, Jubert C, Majour F, Nouvet G, et al. Methotrexate for the treatment of patients with chronic cutaneous sarcoidosis: 4 cases. Ann Dermatol Venereol. 2005;132(8-9 pt 1):659-62.
27. Boffa MJ, Smith A, Chalmers RJ. Comment on: Liver fibrosis in patients with psoriasis and psoriatic arthritis on long-term, high cumulative dose methotrexate therapy. Rheumatology (Oxford, England), 2009;48(11):1464-5.
28. Khan S, Subedi D, Chowdhury MMU. Use of Amino Terminal Type III Procollagen Peptide (P3NP) Assay in Methotrexate Therapy for Psoriasis. Postgrad Med J. 2006;82(967):353-4.
29. Boffa MJ, Chalmers RJ, Haboubi NY, Shomaf M, Mitchell DM. Sequential liver biopsies during long-term methotrexate treatment for psoriasis: a reappraisal. Br J Dermatol. 1995;133(5):774-8.

30. Lanse SB, Arnold GL, Gowans JD, Kaplan MM. Low incidence of hepatotoxicity associated with long-term, low-dose oral methotrexate in treatment of refractory psoriasis, psoriatic arthritis, and rheumatoid arthritis. An acceptable risk-benefit ratio. Dig Dis Sci. 1985;30(2):104-9.
31. Strober BE, Menon, K. Folate supplementation during methotrexate therapy for patients with psoriasis. J Am Acad Dermatol. 2005;53(4):652-9.
32. Arnold H, Bourseaux F. Synthese und Abbau cytostatisch wirkeamer cyclisher N-phosphamidester des bis (β-chloroethyl)-amins. Angew Chem. 1958;70:539-44.
33. de Jonge ME, Huitena ADR, Rodenhuis S, Beijnen JH. Clinical pharmacokinetics of cyclophosphamide. Clin Pharmacokinet 2005;44(11):1135-64.
34. Blomgren H, Hallstrom M. Possible role of acrolein in 4-hydroxyperoxycyclophosphamide-induced cell damage in vitro. Methods Find Exper Clin Pharmacol. 1991;13(1):11-4.
35. Hall AG, Tilby MJ. Mechanisms of action of, and modes of resistance to, alkylating agents used in the treatment of haematological malignancies. Blood Rev. 1992;6(3):163-73.
36. Bunn PA Jr, Hoffman SJ, Norris D, Golitz LE, Aeling JL. Systemic therapy of cutaneous T-cell lymphomas (mycosis fungoides and the Sézary syndrome). Ann Intern Med. 1994;121(8):592-602.
37. Holle JU, Gross WL, Latza U, Nölle B, Ambrosch P, Heller M, et al. Improved outcome in 445 patients with Wegener's granulomatosis in a German vasculitis center over four decades. Arthritis Rheum. 2011;63(1):257-66.
38. Stone JH, Merkel PA, Spiera R, et al. Rituximab versus cyclophosphamide for ANCA-associated vasculitis. N Engl J Med. 2010;363(3):221-32.
39. Thorne JE, Woreta FA, Jabs DA, Seo P, Langford CA, Hoffman GS, et al. Treatment of ocular mucous membrane pemphigoid with immunosuppressive drug therapy. Ophthalmology. 2008;115(12):2146-52.
40. Mimouni D, Nousari CH, Cummins DL, Kouba DJ, David M, Anhalt GJ. Differences and similarities among expert opinions on the diagnosis and treatment of pemphigus vulgaris. J Am Acad Dermatol. 2003;49(6):1059-62.
41. Alpsoy E, Akman A. Behçet's disease: an algorithmic approach to its treatment. Arch Dermatol Res. 2009;301(10):693-702.
42. Chow RK, Benny WB, Coupe RL, Dodd WA, Ongley RC. Erythema elevatum diutinum associated with IgA paraproteinemia successfully controlled with intermittent plasma exchange. Arch Dermatol. 1996;132(11):1360-4.
43. Wollina U. Clinical management of pyoderma gangrenosum. Am J Clin Dermatol. 2002;3(3):149-58.
44. Kaminska R, Ikäheimo R, Hollmen A. Plasmapheresis and cyclophosphamide as successful treatments for pyoderma gangrenosum. Clin Exp Dermatol. 1999;24(2):81-5.
45. Stringer E, Bohnsack J, Bowyer SL, Griffin TA, Huber AM, Lang B, et al. Treatment approaches to juvenile dermatomyositis (JDM) across North America: The Childhood Arthritis and Rheumatology Research Alliance (CARRA) JDM Treatment Survey. J Rheumatol. 2010;37(9):1953-61.
46. Tsujimura S, Saito K, Tanaka Y. Complete resolution of dermatomyositis with refractory cutaneous vasculitis by intravenous cyclophosphamide pulse therapy. Intern Med. 2008;47(21):1935-40.
47. Ruhlen JL, Huston KA, Wood WG. Relapsing polychondritis with glomerulonephritis. Improvement with prednisone and cyclophosphamide. JAMA. 1981;245(8):847-8.
48. Rapini RP, Warner NB. Relapsing polychondritis. Clin Dermatol. 2006;24(6):482-5.
49. Valentini G, Paone C, La Montagna G, Chiarolanza I, Menegozzo M, Colutta E, et al. Low-dose intravenous cyclophosphamide in systemic sclerosis: an open prospective efficacy study in patients with early diffuse disease. Scand J Rheumatol. 2006;35(1):35-8.
50. Quillinan NP, Denton CP. Disease-modifying treatment in systemic sclerosis: current status. Curr Opin Rheumatol. 2009;21(6):636-41.
51. Weiss RB, Bruon S. Hypersensitivity reactions to cancer chemotherapy agents. Ann Intern Med. 1981;94(1):66-72.
52. Kritharides L, Lawrie K, Varigos GA. Cyclophosphamide hypersensitivity and cross reaction with chlorambucil (letter). Cancer Treat Rep. 1987;71:1323-4.
53. Levin M, Libster D. Allergic reaction to chlorambucil in chronic lymphocytic leukemia presenting with fever and lymphadenopathy. Leuk Lymphoma. 2005;46(8):1195-7.
54. Cornwell GG 3rd, Pajak TF, McIntyre OR. Hypersensitivity reactions to iv melphalan during treatment of multiple myeloma: Cancer and Leukemia Group B experience. Cancer Treat Rep. 1979;63(3):399-403.
55. Wiernik PH, Duncan JH. Cyclophosphamide in human milk. Lancet. 1971;1:912.

56. Amato D, Niblett JS. Neutropenia from cyclophosphamide in breast milk. Med J Aust. 1977;1(11):383-4.
57. Clowse ME, Magder L, Petri M. Cyclophosphamide for lupus during pregnancy. Lupus. 2005;14(8):593-7.
58. Baltus JA, Boersma JW, Hartman AP, Vandenbroucke JP. The occurrence of malignancies in patients with rheumatoid arthritis treated with cyclophosphamide: a controlled retrospective follow-up. Ann Rheum Dis. 1983;42(4):368-73.
59. Baker GL, Kahl LE, Zee BC, Stolzer BL, Agarwal AK, Medsger TA Jr. Malignancy following treatment of rheumatoid arthritis with cyclophosphamide. Long-term case-control follow-up study. Am J Med. 1987;83(1):1-9.
60. Despain JD. Dermatologic toxicity of chemotherapy. Semin Oncol. 1992;19(5):501-7.
61. Bronner AK, Hood AF. Cutaneous complications of chemotherapeutic agents. J Am Acad Dermatol. 1983;9(5):645-63.
62. Schreiber SL, Crabtree GR. The mechanism of action of cyclosporin A and FK506. Immunol Today. 1992;13(4):136-42.
63. Rosenbach M, Hsu S, Korman NJ, Lebwohl MG, Young M, Bebo BF Jr, et al. Treatment of erythrodermic psoriasis: from the medical board of the National Psoriasis Foundation. J Am Acad Dermatol. 2010;62(4):655-62.

CHAPTER 10

FAQs on Biologics and JAKis

INTRODUCTION

Biological therapy (BT) includes all substances derived from living material (human, plant, animal, or microorganism) used for the treatment, prevention, or cure of disease in humans.

Biologic therapies are specifically designed to resemble identical molecular targets, which are key factors for the pathogenesis of particular diseases, and these comprises of various licensed molecules for the management of patients with severe diseases or in specific need when traditional therapies may be contraindicated.

Questions and Answers

Rituximab

Q.1. What is the mechanism of action of rituximab?

Ans. It is a chimeric *(xi)* murine-human monoclonal immunoglobulin G1 (IgG$_1$) κ antibody *(mab)* against the specific CD20 cell surface antigen of the B cell. The expression of CD20 is almost exclusive on B cells from the pre-B cell lineage to the mature, activated, and memory B cells. CD20 is not expressed on the hematopoietic stem cells, common lymphocyte precursor, pro-B cells, long and short-lived plasmablasts; hence, these cell lines are not affected by rituximab. However, indirect depletion of short-lived plasmablasts is possible due to depletion of CD20+ precursors. And as long-lived plasma cells are responsible for the immunity acquired through natural infection or vaccination. The rest of the innate immunity acquired by the individual is not suppressed by rituximab. CD20: Hematopoietic stem cells, common lymphocyte precursor, and pro-B cells are spared, allowing gradual recovery of the immune response postrituximab.

Short-lived plasmablasts are responsible for the production of antidesmoglein antibodies.
There are three known mechanisms by which rituximab causes B-cell destruction:
1. *Antibody-dependent cell-mediated cytotoxicity*: Natural killer cells target the rituximab-coated CD20+ B cells by releasing perforins and granzymes, leading to death of B cells via cytolysis.
2. *Complement-mediated cytolysis*: The classical complement pathway gets activated, resulting in insertion of the membrane attack complex into the plasma membrane of the rituximab-coated B cells.
3. *Signaling-induced cell death*: Binding of rituximab disrupts growth/survival signals [nuclear factor kappa B (NF-κB), mitogen-activated protein kinase (MAPK), extracellular signal-regulated kinase (ERK), and anti-tubercular therapy (ATT) pathways] and induces apoptosis in B cells.

Q.2. For which conditions is the use of rituximab Food and Drug Administration (FDA)-approved?

Ans. In 1997 FDA approved the first monoclonal antibody, rituximab, for the treatment of CD20+ non-Hodgkin B cell lymphoma. In 2018, it gained approval for use in pemphigus vulgaris.[1]

Licensed indications (by FDA):
- CD20 +ve non-Hodgkin B-cell lymphoma.
- CD20 +ve chronic lymphocytic leukemia.
- Rheumatoid arthritis (RA)
- Pemphigus vulgaris[1]
- Granulomatosis with polyangitis
- Microscopic polyangitis

Q.3. What are the protocols for rituximab infusion?

Ans.
- *RA protocol*: Two doses, 1 g intravenous (IV) infusion 15 days apart.
- *Lymphoma protocol*: 375 mg/m² dose given 4 weekly.
- RA protocol has shown higher response and lower mortality rates.
- One should note that to achieve remission and prevent flare postinfusion, the use of low-dose corticosteroids should be continued. However, concurrent use with other immunosuppressants is not supported by data.
- Lymphoproliferative diseases have a higher burden of the B-cell and hence may require repeated and higher doses than to be used for autoimmune diseases.
- Even doses as low as 1 mg/m² in comparison with 375 mg/m² used in lymphoma protocol can deplete about 97% B-cell population. 100 mg of rituximab infusion will lead to depletion of B cells for about 3 months. Some researchers have even tried ultralow doses of 30–40 mg.

Q.4. What pretreatment workup should be done before giving injection of rituximab?

Ans.

Baseline investigations:
- Detailed history and examination
- Complete blood count (CBC) with peripheral smear (PS), liver function test (LFT), renal function test (RFT), and urine analysis.
- Urine pregnancy test (UPT)
- Fasting blood sugar (FBS) and postprandial 2-hour blood sugar (PP2BS)
- Electrocardiogram (ECG)
- Chest X-ray
- Abdominal ultrasonography (USG) and two-dimensional (2D) Echo
- Mantoux test interferon-gamma release assay (IGRA)
- Human immunodeficiency virus (HIV), Hepatitis B surface antigen (HBsAg), and hepatitis C virus (HCV).

Special investigations:
- Anti-desmoglein 1 (anti-Dsg1) and Dsg3
- Baseline immunoglobulin levels
- CD19 B-cell counts

Q.5. What are the contraindications of rituximab?
Ans.
- *Absolute*:
  - Patients having known anaphylaxis to components of rituximab or murine proteins, Chinese hamster ovary (CHO) cells.
  - Progressive multifocal leukoencephalopathy
  - Active, severe infection.
- *Relative*:
  - History of hepatitis B infection
  - Severe infusion reaction during first infusion then do not administer subsequent infusion or be very cautious for development of bronchospasm, hypotension, or angioedema.
  Pregnancy prescribing status-C.

Q.6. How to infuse injection rituximab?
Ans.
First infusion:
- 1 g (100 mL) (two vials, 500 mg each) + 150 mL normal saline
- Therefore, concentration = 1,000 mg/250 mL (4 mg/mL)

Infusion rate **(Table 1)**—start at 50 mg/h, increase by 50 mg/h every 30 minutes till maximum—400 mg/h.
In terms of dial flow.
Hence, total time—4 hours 15 minutes for 250 mL infusion
Subsequent infusion—(if tolerated first dose well)
Start at 100 mg/h, increase by 100 mg/h till a maximum of 400 mg/h.
Use dial flow **(Table 2)**.
Total time—3 hours 15 minutes for 250 mL infusion.

TABLE 1: Infusion rate chart for rituximab at the induction dose.		
Hour	mL/h	mL infusion at end-finished
0 (at 50 mg/h)	12.5	
0.5	25	
		1 hour: 18.75 mL infused
1	37.5	
1.5	50	
		2 hours: 62.5 mL infused
2	62.5	
2.5	75	
		3 hours: 131.25 mL infused
3		
3.5 (at 400 mg/h)		
		4 hours: 225 mL infused
4	100	
4.5	100	

TABLE 2: Infusion rate chart for rituximab maintenance dose.		
Hour	Rate	mL infused at the end
0 (at 100 mg/h)	25	
0.5	50	
		1 hour: 18.75 mL infused
1	75	
1.5 (at 400 mg/h)	100	
		2 hours: 106.25 mL infused
2	100	
2.5	100	
		3 hours: 206.25 mL infused
3	100	
3.5	100	

Q.7. What are the warnings and precautions that should be kept in mind while infusing the injection of rituximab?

Ans.
- Should not be given during active infections.
- Keep at least a gap of 4 weeks between administration of nonlive vaccine and rituximab; if given, defer giving rituximab infusion for about 4 weeks.
- Screen for latent viral infection, namely (hepatitis B, herpes simplex, and varicella zoster virus).
- *Special populations*:
  - Pregnancy—category C, can cause first-trimester miscarriage and preterm deliveries.
  - *Lactating mothers*: Human IgG can pass through breastmilk; hence rituximab should be avoided during lactation
  - Pediatric safety and efficacy of rituximab have not been established.
  - Geriatric safety and efficacy are the same as in the younger population.

Q.8. What are the adverse effects reported with rituximab?

Ans.
- *Infusion reactions*: Most common, usually mild, typically 30–120 minutes after infusion.
- *Tumor lysis syndrome*: Rapid decline in renal function, occurs 12–24 hours after rituximab administration.
- *Infections*: Increase in fungal, bacterial, and viral infections during and up to 12 months postrituximab infusion.
- *Neutropenia*: Late onset and self-limiting
- Increased risk of malignancy.
- Chances of developing human antichimeric antibodies (HACA) to the drug specifically in patients with autoimmune disease.
- Hypogammaglobulinemia-risk is greater in patients who received maintenance rituximab.
- Baseline and periodic monitoring of serum IgGs is necessary; symptomatic hypogammaglobulinemia treat with—intravenous immunoglobulin (IVIg).

Q.9. How will you monitor the patient after giving an injection of rituximab?
Ans.
- CBC every 2 weeks during rituximab treatment and 1–3 months thereafter.
- CD20+ B cell counts may be done periodically or in cases with the occurrence of severe infection.

Biologics in Psoriasis

Q.1. Name the biologics used for psoriasis treatment.[2]
Ans. Biologics used for the treatment for psoriasis are discussed in **Table 3**.

TABLE 3: Biological therapies for psoriasis.

Approved TNF Inhibitor	Target	Molecular structure
Adalimumab	TNF	Fully human monoclonal antibody
Etanercept	TNF	Receptor fusion protein
Infliximab	TNF	Chimeric monoclonal antibody
Certolizumab pegol	TNF	Humanized monoclonal antibody
IL-12/23 inhibitor		
Ustekinumab	p40 subunit	Fully human monoclonal antibody
IL-17A inhibitor		
Secukinumab	Il-17A	Fully human monoclonal antibody
Ixekizumab	IL-17A	Humanized monoclonal antibody
Brodalumab (IL-17 RA inhibitor)	IL17RA	Fully human monoclonal antibody
IL-23 inhibitor		
Guselkumab	p19 subunit	Fully human monoclonal antibody
Risankizumab	p19 subunit	Humanized monoclonal antibody
Tildrakizumab	p19 subunit	Humanized monoclonal antibody

(IL: interleukin; RA: rheumatoid arthritis; TNF: tumor necrosis factor)

Q.2. When will you consider a patient with psoriasis for biologic therapy?
Ans.
- Extensive disease in terms of body surface area (BSA) involvement > 10% or Psoriasis Area and Severity Index (PASI) score > 10.
- Inadequate response to previously used immunosuppressives.
- Development of cumulative toxicity or significant adverse effects limiting the use of alternative immunosuppressive drugs (namely, methotrexate and cyclosporine).
- Significant impairment in quality of life as indicated by a Dermatology Life Quality Index (DLQI) or Children's DLQI score > 10, or the presence of clinically significant depressive or anxiety symptoms.
- Psoriasis may be limited but occurs in high-impact areas such as the face and genitals, resulting in considerable functional limitations and/or high levels of emotional distress.
- Associated psoriasis arthritis needing BT.

Q.3. What are the contraindications for the use of tumor necrosis factor alpha (TNF-α) inhibitor agents?

Ans.
- Active tuberculosis.
- *Active cutaneous or systemic foci of infection*: High risk includes chronic leg ulcers, persistent or recurrent chest infections, and an indwelling urinary catheter
- *Severe congestive heart failure*: New York Heart Association (NYHA) grade III or IV.
- Past history of PUVA phototherapy exceeding > 200 treatment sessions.
- History of demyelinating disease or optic neuritis.
- Latent hepatitis B and C infection.
- Immunosuppressive states, such as HIV and acquired immunodeficiency syndrome (AIDS).
- Pregnancy and breastfeeding.

Q.4. What are the pretreatment investigations that should be done before giving biologics?

Ans.
- CBC
- LFT and RFT
- *Urine*: Routine and microscopy
- ± Antinuclear antibodies (ANA)
- Hepatitis B and C serologies
- HIV serology
- Mantoux test/IGRA
- UPT

Q.5. What are the monitoring guidelines for patients on biologics?

Ans. The monitoring guidelines for patients on biologics are discussed in **Table 4**.

TABLE 4: Laboratory monitoring for patients on biologics.

Investigations	Monitoring
Full blood counts	TNF blockers—3 months, then every 6 months
LFT and RFT	At 3 months, then every 6 months
• Urine analysis • Screening for HIV, hepatitis B and C, autoantibodies (ANA, anti-dsDNA), and chest X-ray	Only baseline pre-treatment
Disease severity assessment	
PASI and DLQI	At 3 months, then every 6 months
General health symptom enquiry and clinical examination to rule out infection, demyelination, heart failure, and malignancy	At 3–6 monthly intervals

(ANA: antinuclear antibody; DLQI: dermatology life quality index; HIV: human immunodeficiency virus; LFT: liver function test; PASI: psoriasis area and severity index; RFT: renal function test)

Q.6. In what dosage and at what intervals are biologics given in psoriasis?

Ans. The type of dosage and at what intervals the biologics are given in psoriasis are discussed in **Table 5**.

TABLE 5: Dosing schedule for biologics in psoriasis.

	Secukinumab	Adalimumab	Itolizumab	Etanercept	Infliximab
Dosage schedule	300 mg at weeks 0, 1, 2, 3, and 4 f/b 300 mg every 4 weeks	80 mg initial dose, followed by 40 mg every other week starting 1 week after the initial dose	• 1.6 mg/kg once every 2 weeks for 12 weeks, then 1.6 mg/kg once in 4 weeks up to 24 weeks • Total: 10 (7 + 3)/ year	• *Induction dose*: 50 mg twice weekly for 3 months • *Maintenance dose*: 50 mg once weekly	• *Induction dose*: 5 mg/kg IV at 0, 2, and 6 weeks • *Maintenance dose*: 5 mg/kg every 8 weeks
Route	*Subcutaneous:* • 150 mg in 1 vial • Diluted in 1 mL DW	*Subcutaneous:* • Prefilled syringe 40 mg • 80 mg	IV infusion in 250 mL NS. 50 mL in the 1 hour and the remaining 200 mL in the next hour	*Subcutaneous:* • 25 mg • 50 mg	IV infusion in 250 mL NS over a period of not <2 hours

Q.7. How are newer biologics, i.e., IL-23 inhibitors, administered?

Ans. Table 6 discusses the administration of new biologics, i.e., IL-23 inhibitors.

All IL-23 inhibitors are administered subcutaneously, and they are available as prefilled syringes.

TABLE 6: IL-23 inhibitors: Dosage and frequency of administration.

Guselkumab	Tildrakizumab	Risankizumab
100 mg at week 0, 4, then every 8 weeks	100 mg at weeks 0, 4, then every 12 weeks	150 mg at weeks 0, 4, then every 12 weeks

Q.8. How will you choose biologics in psoriasis?

Ans. With multiple biologic agents now approved for psoriasis, the clinician has to decide which biologic would suite the need of the individual patient and it depend on the disease factors like presence or absence of psoriatic arthropathy, prior use of medication, risk of development of tuberculosis or past history of tuberculoid, economic factors and availability and ease of administration at the place of therapy. Usually, the starting drug is either a TNF-α inhibitor or an IL-17 inhibitor.

Etanercept may be considered for use in patients who require a TNF-α inhibitor and have not responded to other biologics or cannot use them.

Patients with a history of treatment with biologics from one class of drugs (TNF inhibitors) would respond better after switching to other class of drug, like IL-17 inhibitors.

Q.9. What is the definition of minimal response criteria for patients with psoriasis on biologics?

Ans.
- It is defined as a 50% reduction in baseline disease severity, measured by a PASI 50 response, or a decrease in the percentage of BSA affected from baseline.
- Clinically relevant improvement in physical, psychological, or social functioning (e.g., more than four points).

Note: According to National Institute for Health and Care Excellence (NICE) guidelines, minimal response criteria include:
- PASI 75% reduction from baseline, *or*
- PASI 50% reduction from baseline and a five-point reduction in DLQI from the start of treatment.

Q.10. When will you consider a patient on biologics for dose escalation?

Ans.
- If there is an insufficient primary response, as defined above, or if patient-related factors such as obesity or severe disease led to relapse during the treatment cycle, or if drug levels are considered subtherapeutic.
- This could increase the risk of infection and, depending on the specific medication (e.g., ustekinumab or infliximab), may involve off-label use.
- *Suggested dose escalation*:
    - Adalimumab can be escalated by giving 40 mg every week in place of prescribing it every other week.
    - Etanercept 50 mg given twice weekly rather than once.
    - Reducing the dosage interval between subsequent Infliximab 5 mg/kg infusion from every 8 weeks to every 6 weeks.
    - Doubling the dose of ustekinumab [from 45 mg every 12 weeks (<100 kg) to 90 mg every 12 weeks] and from [90 mg every 12 weeks (>100 kg) to 90 mg every 8 weeks].
    - Certolizumab pegol 200 mg every 2 weeks to 400 mg every 2 weeks.
    - Tildrakizumab 100 mg every 12 weeks to 200 mg every 12 weeks (high disease burden or ≥90 kg).

Q.11. When will you change a patient on a biologic therapy to another biologic?

Ans.
- Consider switching to an alternative treatment, including a different biologic therapy, if any of the following conditions apply in a biologic-naïve patient.
    - *In case of primary failure*: Not achieving the minimum response criteria.
    - *In case of secondary failure*: When the disease responds initially but subsequently loses this response.
    - If the current biologic is not tolerated by the patient or develops a serious adverse event.
- Advice on how to change biologics in a biologic-experienced patient:
    - Improve adherence.
    - Encourage weight loss in an obese person.
    - Determine if the dose and frequency of the drug are adequate.
    - Introduce adjunctive therapy [e.g., transitioning from oral to subcutaneous (SC) methotrexate].
    - Switch to a biologic from a different class.
    - Consider alternative or complementary nonbiologic treatment options (e.g., topical therapies, phototherapy, or systemic treatments).

Q.12. When will you stop biologic therapy in a patient with psoriasis?

Ans.
- The remission rates vary with each biologic. As of now, there is no endpoint defined for patients who have reached PASI 99 clearance with a biologic.
- In scenarios where therapy is not successful, failure to achieve an adequate response (according to minimal response criteria) following treatment initiation or when treatment response is not maintained.
- *Also indicated due to the following*:
    - Serious adverse events—which may justify withdrawal include malignancy, severe drug-related toxicity, severe intercurrent infection (temporary withdrawal).

- Pregnancy (temporary withdrawal).
- Elective surgical procedures.

Q.13. How will you transition a patient from one biologic to another?
Ans. While contemplating changing one biologic to another, one should consider either a 1-month washout period or the duration equivalent to the gap between two cycles of ongoing biologic, whichever is longer of the two is preferred, following which a new biologic can be started.

Q.14. Can biologics be given in special populations?
Ans.
Pediatric population:
- Fulfilling the criteria to initiate biologic therapy
- Offer adalimumab (age ≥ 4 years)
- Etanercept (≥ 4 years)
- Ixekizumab (age ≥ 6 years) or ustekinumab (≥6 years)

Pregnant and lactating women:
- Successful outcomes have been reported in most pregnancies incidentally occurring while on biologic therapy.
- Most pregnancies reported in women taking biologic therapy at conception and during pregnancy have successful outcomes.
- Most available data on the effect of biologic therapy on conception and pregnancy originates from the usage of TNF antagonists in rheumatological and inflammatory bowel disease, suggesting potential risk with exposure to these agents.
- Maternal IgG, including biologic drugs approved for psoriasis, is actively transferred to the developing fetus during the second and third trimesters. However, the effects of this transfer on fetal and neonatal development, as well as the risk of infection, have not been thoroughly studied.
- Live vaccines should be avoided in infants born to mothers who have received biologic therapy beyond 16 weeks' gestation. The use of live vaccines should be postponed until the infant reaches 6 months of age.
- Advise on the appropriate use of contraception and supervision of the same on each visit.
- If a female becomes incidentally pregnant while on biologic therapy, such a woman should be counseled about the risk of continuing pregnancy and/or flare-up of disease upon stoppage of biologic, e.g., flare-up of pustular psoriasis along with discussion on alternative nonbiologic therapy.

If the decision to use biologic therapy when planning conception or during pregnancy has been made:
- Use of *certolizumab pegol should be considered as a first-line option* when starting biologic therapy *in women planning conception or during the second or third trimester*.
- Aim to minimize fetal exposure by discontinuing biologic therapy during the second and third trimesters.
- Good knowledge of which biologics transfer across the placenta also helps to limit risk in the neonate.

Q.15. What adverse effects are encountered with biologics?
Ans. The adverse effects are discussed in **Table 7**.

TABLE 7: Side effects of biologics.	
Biologic agent	Toxicities
Etanercept	Mildly pruritic injection site reaction, rarely serious infections such as (i.e., TB) and malignancies, lupus without renal and CNS complications, cytopenia, MS, and exacerbation and new onset of CHF
Infliximab	Infusion reactions and serum sickness, rarely serious infections (i.e., TB), lupus without renal or CNS complications, malignancies including hepatosplenic T-cell lymphoma (in children), cytopenia, MS, and exacerbation and new onset of CHF
Itolizumab	Infusion reactions, precipitation of erythrodermic psoriasis, serious infections, and rarely exfoliative dermatitis, adjustment disorder with anxiety, and bacterial arthritis
Secukinumab	Nasopharyngitis, diarrhea, and upper respiratory tract infections. Infection, inflammatory bowel disease, increased risk of candidal infection
Guselkumab	Nasopharyngitis, URTI, myocardial infarction (more with risankizumab), malignancies, and nonmelanoma skin cancers
Adalimumab	Injection site reactions and antidrug antibodies

(CHF: congestive heart failure; CNS: central nervous system; MS: multiple sclerosis; TB: tuberculosis; URTI: upper respiratory tract infection)

Q.16. Which oral phosphodiesterase 4 (PDE-4) inhibitor has been approved for psoriasis?

Ans. *Apremilast* was the first FDA-approved small molecule inhibitor, belonging to the group of oral PDE-4 inhibitors for psoriasis in 2014[3] based on the significant efficacy demonstrated in various randomized controlled trials (RCTs) of moderate-to-severe plaque psoriasis, demonstrating an acceptable safety profile and a low rate of discontinuation.

Q.17. Which oral tyrosine kinase 2 (TYK-2) inhibitor is under study for psoriasis?

Ans. *Deucravacitinib*: It demonstrated PASI-75 response in 69.0% of patients at week 24. With nasopharyngitis, upper respiratory infections (URIs), and low incidences of headaches, diarrhea, and nausea are commonly reported as adverse events.

Q.18. Which are the newer topicals, small-molecule inhibitors for psoriasis?

Ans.
- *Tapinarof*: An aryl hydrocarbon receptor-modulating agent.
- *Roflumilast*: Topical PDE-4 inhibitor.

Q.19. Which biologic agent is FDA-approved for the treatment of hidradenitis suppurativa?[4,5]

Ans. Adalimumab is an FDA-approved for Hidradenitis suppurativa in adults > 12 years of age.
- Route—SC
- 40 mg/0.8 mL—prefilled syringe
- *Dosage regimen*:
    - *At week 0*: 160 mg
    - *At week 2*: 80 mg
    - *At week 4*: 40 mg

Followed by weekly 40 mg till clinical resolution
- *Secukinumab*: Now approved for HS

Omalizumab

Q.1. What kind of biologic is omalizumab?
Ans.
- A humanized monoclonal anti-immunoglobulin E (anti-IgE) antibody featuring a human IgG framework, with complementarity-determining regions derived from a murine anti-IgE antibody.
- 95% IgG1 kappa human framework.
- 5% mouse sequence, which is hidden from the immune system when omalizumab binds to IgE.

Q.2. What is the mechanism of action of omalizumab?
Ans.
- It binds to free IgE in the bloodstream and interstitial space, creating biologically inactive IgE complexes that cannot bind to FcεRI receptors on the surface of mast cells and basophils. This reduces the activation of mast cells and basophil degranulation, thereby decreasing the subsequent inflammatory response.
- Downregulates IgE receptors.
- Reduces mast cell releasability.
- Reverses basopenia and improves basophil IgE receptor function.
- Gene expression in lesional skin was altered to levels seen in nonlesional skin.

Q.3. What preinjection investigations should be done before giving omalizumab?
Ans.
- CBC
- Random blood glucose
- Renal function test
- Liver function test
- Urine routine and microbiology
- Chest X-ray
- ECG

Q.4. What dosage of omalizumab should be given?
Ans. Omalizumab 300 mg by SC injection every 4 weeks—dosage not dependent on serum IgE or body weight.

Q.5. How is omalizumab reconstituted and administered?
Ans.
- Before starting, calculate how many vials need to be reconstituted based on the total dosage required. Each vial contains 150 mg of omalizumab in 1.2 mL.
- Using a 3 mL syringe and a 1", 18-G needle, draw 1.2 mL of Sterile Water for Injection (SWFI).
- With the vial held upright, injected the SWFI into the vial containing the omalizumab powder. Gently swirl the vial for about 1 minute to ensure the powder is evenly moistened.

- After the initial 1-minute swirl, gently swirl the vial for 5–10 seconds every 5 minutes to aid in dissolving any remaining powder. If the contents do not dissolve fully within 40 minutes, discard the vial.
- Once reconstituted, the omalizumab solution would be somewhat viscous and would appear clear or slightly opalescent.
- Using a new 3 mL syringe with a 1", 18-G needle, insert the needle into the inverted vial. Place the needle tip at the very bottom of the vial to withdraw the solution. After drawing the solution, replace the 18-G needle with a 25-G needle for the SC injection.
    - Administer the injection slowly, as the solution is slightly viscous, taking 5–10 seconds to inject.
    - Do not inject > 150 mg (the amount in one vial) into a single injection site.
    - The reconstituted solution should be used within 8 hours if stored at 2–8ºC, or within 4 hours if kept at room temperature.
    - Protect the reconstituted vials from sunlight.

Q.6. What are the indications of omalizumab?
Ans.
- *Chronic idiopathic urticaria (CIU)*:[6] FDA-approved.
- Omalizumab is indicated for the treatment of chronic idiopathic urticaria in adults and adolescents aged 12 years and older who continue to experience symptoms despite the use of H1 antihistamines. It is not recommended for the treatment of other types of urticaria.

Pregnancy category B:
- *Off label indications*: Atopic dermatitis, systemic mastocytosis, and bullous urticaria.
- *Contraindications*: Hypersensitivity to omalizumab or any ingredient.

Q.7. What are the warnings and precautions that should be considered while giving the injection of omalizumab?
Ans.
- Anaphylaxis
- *Malignancy*: Breast, nonmelanoma skin, prostate, melanoma, and parotid.
- Acute asthma, i.e., acute bronchospasm or status asthmaticus.
- *Corticosteroid reduction*: Do not abruptly discontinue corticosteroids upon initiation of omalizumab therapy.
- Worsening pulmonary symptoms—flu-like symptoms.
- Chest tightness and tachycardia.

Q.8. What are the adverse effects encountered with injection omalizumab?
Ans.
- Anaphylaxis
- Nausea
- Nasopharyngitis and sinusitis
- Headache and fatigue
- Fever and arthralgia
- *Local site reactions*: Swelling, bruising, itching, pain, and urticaria.

Q.9. Name new biologics for the treatment of urticaria.[6]
Ans.
- *Mepolizumab*: IL-5 inhibitor- humanized IgG1 kappa monoclonal antibody—200 mg SC at week 0, 2, 4, 6, and 8 (phase 1 clinical trial).
- *Ligelizumab*: High-affinity humanized monoclonal IgG1 kappa anti-IgE-single dose (0.1–10 mg/kg) IV or two to four doses (0.2–4 mg/kg) SC at 2-week intervals (under clinical trial).
- *Ibrutinib*: Bruton kinase inhibitor, in clinical trials for chronic spontaneous urticaria.

Tofacitinib
Q.1. What is the mechanism of action of tofacitinib?
Ans.
- Tofacitinib is a first-generation Janus kinase (JAK) inhibitor and inhibits JAK 1, 2, and 3.
- JAK are a family of non-receptor tyrosine kinases that, in response to several cytokines, initiate a variety of downstream intracellular effects.
- Based on their selective response to extracellular signals, there are four members in the JAK family: JAK1, JAK2, JAK3, and Tyk2.
- Signal transducer and activator of transcription (STAT) are latent cytoplasmic transcription factors that increase the expression of proinflammatory cytokines and cause the maturation of dendritic cells.
- *7 STAT proteins*: 1, 2, 3, 4, 5a, 5b, and 6.
- Many dermatologically relevant cytokines rely on the JAK-STAT pathway.
- These include—IFN-α/β, IFN-γ, IL-2 receptor common γ-chain interleukins (IL-2, IL-4, IL-7, IL-9, IL-15, and IL-21), and IL-5, IL-6, IL-12, IL-13, and IL-23.
- Although other cytokines, such as TNF-α, IL-1, and IL-17 do not signal via the JAK-STAT pathway.
- In some instances, JAK inhibitors can indirectly suppress these cytokines (i.e., IL-17) by inhibition of other STAT-dependent cytokines (i.e., IL-23) that act upstream.

Q.2. What are the indications of tofacitinib?[7]
Ans.
Food and Drug Administration approved:
- Psoriatic arthritis
- RA
- Ulcerative colitis

Off-label:
- *Autoimmune dermatoses*:
  - *Psoriasis*:
    - Alopecia areata
    - Vitiligo
    - Dermatomyositis
- *Dermatitis*: Atopic dermatitis
- *Photodermatoses*: Chronic actinic dermatitis
- *Others*:
  - Erythema multiforme
  - Hypereosinophilic syndrome

Anecdotal reports:
- Cutaneous lupus erythematosus
- Dermatomyositis
- Chronic actinic dermatitis
- Erythema multiforme
- Hyper eosinophilic syndrome
- Cutaneous graft-versus-host disease
- Pyoderma gangrenosum (PG)
- Lichen planus
- Sjögren's syndrome

Q.3. What oral tofacitinib formulations are available in the market?
Ans.
- *Tofacitinib tablets*: 5 and 10 mg.
- *Tofacitinib XR tablets*: 11 and 22 mg
- *Tofacitinib oral solution*: 1 mg/mL tofacitinib.
- Topical tofacitinib 2% ointment.

Q.4. In what dosages is oral tofacitinib prescribed, and what is its method of administration?
Ans.
- *RA (2012) standard*: 5 mg BD, XR: 11 mg OD.
- *Psoriatic arthritis (2017) standard*: 5 mg BD, XR: 11 mg OD.
- *Ulcerative colitis (2018) standard*: 10 mg BD.
- Usual dose for any inflammatory disorder is 5 mg BD and can be uptitrated to 10 mg BD.

Method of administration:
- Oral use, orally with or without food.
- For patients who have difficulties swallowing, tofacitinib tablets may be crushed and taken with water.

Q.5. What are the warnings and precautions to be considered while prescribing oral tofacitinib?
Ans.
- *Hematologic*: Lymphocytopenia, neutropenia, and anemia have been observed. Avoid if lymphocytes < 500 cells/mm^3, absolute neutrophil count < 500 cells/mm^3, Hb < 9 g/dL.
- *Hepatic*: Baseline LFT recommended. Alteration of liver enzymes is seen mostly in patients on concomitant disease-modifying anti-rheumatic drugs (DMARD) therapy, especially methotrexate.
- *Metabolic*: Maximum lipid abnormalities noted at 6–8 weeks. To be used with caution in diabetic patients, as they are predisposed to recurrent infections.
- *Renal*: Dose reduction required in patients with moderate-severe fall in glomerular filtration rate (GFR).
- *Infections*: Avoid use of tofacitinib during an active serious infection, including localized infections. Screen for latent TB infection, HIV, and viral hepatitis. Monitor for opportunistic infections.

- *Immunizations*: Live vaccines—avoid concurrent use with tofacitinib to be given 2 weeks (preferably 4 weeks) before drug initiation.
- *Thrombosis (including pulmonary, deep venous, and arterial, some fatal)*: Has been reported more commonly in patients treated with tofacitinib 10 mg twice daily compared to 5 mg twice daily. Avoid tofacitinib in patients at risk. Promptly evaluate patients with symptoms of thrombosis and discontinue tofacitinib.
- *Cardiovascular*: Decreased HR and prolonged PR interval have been seen in clinical trials.
- *Pulmonary*: Caution to be taken in patients with interstitial lung disease and in patients on concomitant methotrexate therapy.
- *Gastrointestinal*: Bowel perforations have been reported, especially in patients with diverticulitis, those on nonsteroidal anti-inflammatory drugs (NSAIDs), or steroids.
- *Pregnancy*: As a precautionary measure, the use of Tofacitinib during pregnancy is contraindicated. Breastfeeding is not recommended during treatment and for at least 18 hours after the last dose of tofacitinib (approximately six elimination half-lives).
- *Pediatric population*: The safety and efficacy of tofacitinib in children aged 0 to <18 years have not been established, but a few clinical studies in children are available in alopecia areata.
- *Malignancy*: Lymphoma is the most commonly reported. Caution to be exercised in patients on concomitant immunosuppressive medications, biologics.

Q.6. How will you monitor a patient on oral tofacitinib?

Ans.
- *Baseline*:
  - CBC and differential leukocyte count (DLC)
  - Liver enzyme panel
  - Lipid profile
  - Renal function test
  - Hepatitis B
  - Hepatitis C
  - HIV
  - Tuberculin skin test (TST)/IGRA
  - UPT (child-bearing age)

Follow-up: 4–8 weeks after therapy initiation and then every 3 months thereafter.
- CBC with DLC
- Liver enzyme panel
- Lipid profile

Dupilumab

Q.1. What is the mechanism of action of dupilumab?

Ans.
- It is a fully human monoclonal antibody
- Binds IL-4 receptor alpha subunit and blocks downstream signaling of 2 cytokines- IL-4 and IL-13

Q.2. What are the indications of dupilumab?

Ans. FDA-approved—moderate-to-severe atopic dermatitis in adults and adolescents at least 12 years old, refractory to topical treatments or when those therapies are not advisable.

Off-label dermatologic uses:
- Alopecia areata
- Idiopathic chronic eczematous eruption of pregnancy
- Prurigo nodularis

Q.3. How is dupilumab supplied and administered?

Ans. It is available as:
- 300 mg/2 mL
- 200 mg/1.14 mL
- Single-dose syringe

Route: SC
Dosing:
- Adult and adolescents > 60 kg—initial dose—600 mg
    - Followed by: 300 mg every 2 weeks
- Adolescents (<60 kg)—initial dose—400 mg
    - Followed by 200 mg every 2 weeks

Q.4. What are the contraindications and adverse effects of dupilumab?

Ans.
Contraindications:
- Type I hypersensitivity to dupilumab or its components.
- *Pregnancy and lactation*: Safety and efficacy not established.

Adverse effects:
- Herpes simplex infections
- Headache
- Arthralgia
- Nasopharyngitis, conjunctivitis, and keratitis
- Development of antidrug neutralizing antibodies
- Urticaria and serum sickness-like reactions

Tralokinumab and Lebrikizumab

FDA-approved anti-IL-13 monoclonal antibody for the treatment of moderate-to-severe atopic dermatitis in adults (18 years and older).

Q.1. What are the reported adverse effects of tralokinumab?

Ans. The side effects profile is similar to dupilumab. It is linked to a higher incidence of conjunctivitis.

Q.2. What are the reported adverse effects of lebrikizumab?

Ans. They are generally mild forms of conjunctivitis (4.6%) and headaches (4.6%) not requiring discontinutation.[4]

Table 8 enlists all the newer biological molecules for atopic dermatitis.[8]

TABLE 8: Biologics available for atopic dermatitis.			
Biological	**Target**	**Current phase of clinical trials**	**Main findings in clinical trials**
Tralokinumab	IL-13	Approved for clinical use by EMA	EASI-75 improvement and IGA 0 or 1 after 16 weeks of trial compared to placebo (phase III)
Lebrikizumab	IL-13	3, still recruiting	Up to 72.1% improvement in EASI (250 mg dose) after 16 weeks of trial compared to placebo (phase IIb)
Nemolizumab	IL-31	3, still recruiting	Up to 63.1% change in the pruritus VAS score after 12 weeks compared to placebo (Phase IIb)
Tezepelumab	TSLP	2b, still recruiting	Numerical EASI50 improvement after 12 weeks of trial compared to placebo (Phase IIa)
Etokimab	IL-31	2b, still recruiting	83% improvement of EASI50 and 33% EASI75 after 29 days of a single dose (Phase IIa)
Fezakinumab	IL-22	2a, completed	SCORAD improvement was greater compared to placebo at 12 weeks of trial (Phase IIa)

Q.3. Which are the newer small-molecule inhibitors for atopic dermatitis?

Ans. Newer small-molecule inhibitors for atopic dermatitis **(Table 9)**.

TABLE 9: Small molecules for atopic dermatitis.			
Drug	**Target**	**Route of administration**	**Status for AD**
Crisaborole 2% ointment	PDE-4	Topical	Approved (ages > 3 months) for mild-to-moderate AD
Upadacitinib	JAK1	Oral	Approved (ages 12 years)
Abrocitinib	JAK1	Oral	Approved (ages 18)
Baricitinib	JAK1 and JAK2	Oral	Phase III trials completed
Ruxolitinib 1.5% cream	JAK1 and JAK2	Topical	Approved (ages > 12 years)
Tofacitinib	JAK1 and JAK3	Topical	Phase II trials are complete. No active trials
Delgocitinib	JAK1, JAK2, and JAK3	Topical	Phase III trials completed and active
Serlopitant	NK-1	Oral	Phase II trial terminated
Tradipitant	NK-1	Oral	Phase III trials completed

(AD: atopic dermatitis; JAK: Janus kinase; NK-1: neurokinin-1; PDE-4: phosphodiesterase-4)

Q.4. Which are the topical phosphodiesterase-4 inhibitors for atopic dermatitis?

Ans. Crisaborole is approved for use in patients aged 3 months and older. Clinical studies showed that 40% of participants experienced clear or almost clear skin after just 8 days of treatment.[4]

Q.5. Which are the newer systemic JAK-pathway inhibitors for atopic dermatitis?

Ans. *Approved molecules*: Upadacitinib and abrocitinib.
- *Upadacitinib*, an oral JAK-1 inhibitor, was approved in January 2022 for the treatment of atopic dermatitis in patients aged 12 years and older. It is also indicated for RA, psoriatic arthritis, and ankylosing spondylitis. A common side effect associated with its use is acne.

- *Abrocitinib*, an oral JAK-1 inhibitor, was approved in January 2022 for the treatment of atopic dermatitis in adults aged 18 years and older. Its safety profile includes warnings similar to other JAK inhibitors, such as the risk of serious infections, increased mortality, malignancy, cardiovascular events, and thrombosis.[4]

Q.6. Which are the newer topical JAK-pathway inhibitors for atopic dermatitis?[9]

Ans. *Ruxolitinib*:[4] It selectively inhibits JAK-1/2 and was approved in September 2021 for the treatment of mild-to-moderate atopic dermatitis in patients aged 12 years and older. In July 2022, ruxolitinib 1.5% cream also received approval for the treatment of nonsegmental vitiligo.

Delgocitinib is a topical inhibitor of JAK-1/2/3 and Tyk2, approved in Japan for atopic dermatitis. Common side effects include folliculitis (2.4%) and acne (2.2%).

Q.7. Which are the newer neurokinin-1 (NK-1) inhibitors for atopic dermatitis?[10]

Ans. Newer NK-1 inhibitors for atopic dermatitis are serlopitant and tradipitant.

REFERENCES

1. Kanwar AJ, Vinay K. Rituximab in pemphigus. Indian J Dermatol Venereol Leprol. 2012;78(6):671-6.
2. Sivamani RK, Correa G, Ono Y, Bowen MP, Raychaudhuri SP, Maverakis E. Biological therapy of psoriasis. Indian J Dermatol. 2010;55(2):161-70.
3. Moyle M, Cevikbas F, Harden JL, Guttman-Yassky E. Understanding the immune landscape in atopic dermatitis: The era of biologics and emerging therapeutic approaches. Exp Dermatol. 2019;28(7):756-68.
4. Dodson J, Lio PA. Biologics and small molecule inhibitors: an update in therapies for allergic and immunologic skin diseases. Curr Allerg Asthma Rep. 2022;22(12):183-93.
5. Santillan RM, Morss PC, Porter ML, Kimball AB. Biologic therapies for the treatment of hidradenitis suppurativa. Expert Opin Biol Ther. 2020;20(6):621-33.
6. Mustari AP, Bishnoi A, Kumaran MS. Biologicals in Treatment of Chronic Urticaria: A Narrative Review. Indian Dermatol Online J. 2023;14(1):9-20.
7. Sonthalia S, Aggarwal P. Oral tofacitinib: Contemporary appraisal of its role in dermatology. Indian Dermatol Online J. 2019;10(5):503-18.
8. Schneider S, Li L, Zink A. The new era of biologics in atopic dermatitis: a review. Dermatol Pract Concept. 2021;11(4):e2021144.
9. Szalus K, Trzeciak M, Nowicki RJ. JAK-STAT inhibitors in atopic dermatitis from pathogenesis to clinical trials results. Microorganisms. 2020;8(11):1743.
10. Alam M, Buddenkotte J, Ahmad F, Steinhoff M. Neurokinin 1 receptor antagonists for pruritus. Drugs. 2021;81(6):621-34.

Antihistamines

INTRODUCTION

Antihistamines are a heterogeneous group of drugs that act as inverse agonists of histamine, the primary mediator of inflammation in most dermatoses.

There are four classes according to the receptors on which they act:
1. H_1-receptor antagonists
2. H_2-receptor antagonists
3. H_3-receptor antagonists (not relevant in dermatology)
4. H_4-receptor antagonists (not relevant in dermatology)

H_1 ANTIHISTAMINES

Mechanism of Action

Antihistamines are now perceived as inverse agonists, as they work by downregulating the constitutively activated state of the corresponding receptor **(Table 1)**.[1] Systemic adverse effects of first-generation antihistamines:
- *Central nervous system (CNS):* Sedation and hyperexcitability, impaired cognitive function, and increased appetite
- *Gastrointestinal tract (GIT):* Dry mouth and constipation
- *Genitourinary tract (GUT):* Dysuria and erectile dysfunction
- *Cardiac:* Tachycardia and arrhythmia
- *Others:* Glaucoma and blurred vision

Indications

Indications are as follows:
- Allergic skin disorders, e.g., urticaria, angioedema and drug hypersensitivity
- Severe pruritus associated with skin lesions, e.g., scabies, lichen planus, atopic dermatitis, contact dermatitis, dermatitis herpetiformis, etc.
- Pruritus without skin lesions, especially, if interfering with sleep

TABLE 1: Classification of antihistamines.

	Dosage	Peak plasma concentration (hours)	Pregnancy category
First-generation antihistamines			
Ethanolamines			
Diphenhydramine	20–50 mg TID	0.6–2.8	B
Clemastine	2 mg BID	–	B
Alkylamines			
Chlorpheniramine	4–8 mg BID	2.0–3.6	B
Piperidines			
Cyproheptadine	4–8 mg BID	2–3	B
Azatadine	1–2 mg TID	–	B
Phenothiazines			
Promethazine	12.5–25 mg TID	2–3	C
Piperazines			
Hydroxyzine	12.5–25 mg TID	1.7–2.5	C
Second-generation antihistamines			
Piperazines			
Cetirizine	10 mg OD/BID	0.5–1.5	B
Levocetirizine	5 mg OD	–	B
Piperidines			
Loratadine	10 mg OD	1–2.5	B
Fexofenadine	180 mg	1–3	C
Desloratadine	5 mg OD	3	C
Mizolastine	10 mg OD	1.5	No adequate data
Ebastine	10–20 mg OD	2.6	No adequate data
Astemizole	10 mg OD	Days	C

Contraindications

Contraindications include:
- Drivers/Pilots
- Machine operators during work hours
- Elderly individuals with benign prostatic hyperplasia (BPH)
- Glaucoma (precipitates glaucoma)

Special Points

- Alcohol, opioid analgesics such as morphine and codeine, and benzodiazepines use is contraindicated in patients taking first-generation antihistamines as it causes more CNS depression.

- In pregnancy, H_1 antihistamines are considered unsafe, especially during 4 weeks of pregnancy. After assessing risk–benefit ratio, in a case of urticaria, chlorpheniramine and diphenhydramine can be given.
- Tachyphylaxis and/or reduced sensitivity toward the specific molecule of antihistamine, which is characterized by diminished response after administration of repeated doses of a drug is frequently observed problem with H_1 antihistamines.[2]
- Hydroxyzine showed highest while chlorpheniramine shows the lowest risk of developing tachyphylaxis.

Second-generation Antihistamines

Fexofenadine

Fexofenadine is the pharmacologically active metabolite of the prodrug terfenadine. There is no evidence for cardiotoxicity with fexofenadine.

Fexofenadine is a selective H_1 receptor inverse agonist that has few or no sedative or anticholinergic adverse effects.

There is no evidence of tolerance after repeated administration.

The currently recommended dosage of fexofenadine is 60–180 mg twice daily. Present evidence also suggests that there is no need for dosage adjustment in the elderly or in patients with mild renal or hepatic impairment.

Loratadine

- It is a long-acting.
- It has minimal sedating potential.
- It is not contraindicated in patients with chronic liver or renal disease; however, cautious administration of reduced dosage is advisable.
- It is not cardiotoxic.
- It has no significant adverse drug reactions (ADRs)

Cetirizine

Cetirizine is a long-acting, low-sedation H_1 antihistamine. It also has an inhibitory action on eosinophil accumulation in tissues, including the skin. Reduction in dose is recommended in patients with chronic hepatic or renal disease. It does not have significant cardiotoxicity.

Desloratadine

- Dosage for chronic urticaria is 5 mg daily.
- As compared to desloratadine in suppression of histamine wheal response, its potency is 5 times higher.
- It has minimal anticholinergic activity, minimal sedation, and no cardiac toxicity.

Levocetirizine

Levocetirizine, the *R*-enantiomer of cetirizine and its major active metabolite, is second-generation H_1 antihistamine. It has higher potency than loratadine in suppression of histamine wheal in healthy volunteers. The incidence of sedation and anticholinergic-like adverse effects is low.

TABLE 2: Differences between first- and second-generation antihistamines.	
First-generation antihistamines	**Second-generation antihistamines**
Competitively blocks H_1 receptors	Noncompetitively blocks H_1 receptors
Highly sedating	Low sedating
Has anticholinergic and antiemetic effects	No anticholinergic and antiemetic effects
Short-acting and frequent dosing required	Long-acting and frequent dosing not required
Early tachyphylaxis	No tachyphylaxis
Example: Promethazine	*Example:* Cetirizine

Key point: Sedating potential of second-generation antihistamines is in the following order: Cetirizine > levocetirizine > desloratadine > fexofenadine.

Mizolastine

Mizolastine, a benzimidazole derivative is a new, nonsedating second-generation oral antihistamine with additional anti-inflammatory properties. This new H_1-receptor antagonist is highly selective for peripheral histamine H_1 receptors.

Mizolastine is associated with less sedation, psychomotor impairment, and anticholinergic activity than the first-generation agents, and tolerance does not appear to develop with long-term use.

Olopatadine

Olopatadine hydrochloride is one of the second-generation nonsedating antihistamines that is used for treating allergic disorders, such as urticaria, rhinitis, and atopic dermatitis.

Olopatadine is a selective histamine H_1-receptor antagonist possessing inhibitory effects on the release of inflammatory lipid mediators, such as leukotriene and thromboxane, from human polymorphonuclear leukocytes and eosinophils.

Olopatadine is useful for the treatment of allergic rhinitis and chronic urticaria.

Dosage is 5 mg once to twice daily after meals.

Differences between first-generation and second-generation antihistamine are depicted in **Table 2**.

H_2 ANTIHISTAMINES

The H_2 antihistamines have the following characteristics:
- Inhibit H_2 receptor in cutaneous vasculature
- *Drugs include:* Famotidine and ranitidine
- *Indications:* Refractory chronic idiopathic urticaria, physical urticaria, and mastocytosis
- *Side effects:* Susceptibility to arrhythmia (ranitidine)

MAST-CELL STABILIZERS

Mast-cell stabilizers include cromolyn sodium, doxantrazole, and ketotifen.

Ketotifen

Mechanism of Action
Ketotifen prevents release of histamine from mast cells, calcium-channel blocker, and H_1-type antihistamine. It inhibits the Ca^{++} passage through the mastocyte and basophil membrane.

Indications
- Chronic idiopathic urticaria
- Physical urticaria
- Mastocytosis
- Neurofibromatosis-associated pruritus

Dosage
1 mg BD

Adverse Drug Reaction
Sedation and weight gain are ADRs.

Key Point
It may take up to 10 weeks for the complete effect of ketotifen to occur.

REFERENCES

1. Leurs R, Church MK, Taglialatela M. H1-antihistamines: Inverse agonism, anti-inflammatory effects and cardiac effects. Clin Exp Allergy. 2002;32(4):489-98.
2. Long WF, Taylor RJ, Wagner CJ, Leavengood DC, Nelson HS. Skin test suppression by antihistamines and the development of subsensitivity. J Allergy Clin Immunol. 1985;76(1):113-7.

CHAPTER 12
Antibiotics in Dermatology

INTRODUCTION

We must follow antibiotic policy of our own hospital wherever we are working. Usage of antibiotics is frequent in every dermatology ward, in conditions such as:
- Where causative agent is primarily bacteria, e.g., cellulitis, necrotizing fasciitis, etc.
- Where superantigens are thought to play a role in the exacerbation of the disease. For example, staphylococcal scalded skin syndrome, toxic shock syndrome,[1] cutaneous T-cell lymphoma,[2] erythrodermic psoriasis,[3] and atopic dermatitis.[3]
- Primary dermatoses getting secondarily infected, e.g., autoimmune vesiculobullous dermatoses (AI-VBDs)

Skin and skin-structure infections are common and range from minor pyodermas to severe necrotizing infections. Classification schemes for these infections are varied. Distinguishing characteristics include the etiological agent(s), clinical context and findings, depth of tissue involvement, and rate of progression. The most common pathogens are aerobic gram-positive cocci but frequently involve gram-negative bacilli and anaerobic bacteria. Initial antibiotic therapy is usually based on treating physician's experience, and later on modified by the results of culture and sensitivity tests.

Superantigens (SAgs) **(Fig. 1)** are virulent microbial proteins (22–29 kD), formed as an evolved mechanism of immune evasion, that are produced by a variety of infectious organisms like bacteria,

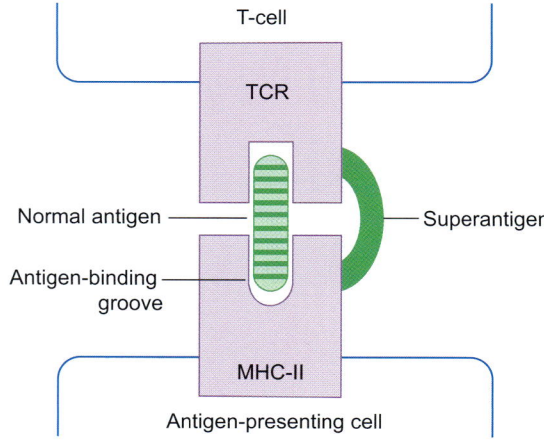

FIG. 1: Super antigen.
(MHC-II: major histocompatibility complex class II; TCR: T-cell receptor)

mycoplasma, viruses, etc. They are capable of causing nonspecific "polyclonal" T-cell activation by circumventing normal antigen processing in the human host, leading to massive cytokine release.[1]

Surgical debridement is important for many complicated infections and is the critical element in managing necrotizing fasciitis and myonecrosis.[4]

The patients in dermatology ward—with large areas of their skin denuded due to a primary dermatoses, and thus, with severely compromised barrier and immune function of the skin—are especially susceptible to develop sepsis. The risk of sepsis is further accentuated by the use of steroids and other immunosuppressive/cytotoxic agents, which are often given in high doses and for prolonged periods.[5] The mortality in dermatology ward can predominantly be ascribed to it directly or indirectly.[6]

CULTURE AND SENSITIVITY PATTERN[7]

A total of 48 positive cultures were obtained from blood, pus, urine, or respiratory tract; the organisms isolated are shown in **Table 1**. The commonly cultured organisms from skin and blood were *Staphylococcus* species (n = 20 isolates); methicillin resistant *Staphylococcus aureus* (MRSA) (n = 16), methicillin sensitive *Staphylococcus aureus* (MSSA) (n = 4), followed by *Acinetobacter* species (9 isolates). *Pseudomonas aeruginosa* and *Klebsiella pneumoniae* were also grown in significant number of cultures (6 isolates each).

In patients with vesiculobullous diseases, *Staphylococcus aureus* was the predominant organism in both blood and skin, while in patients having Stevens–Johnson syndrome (SJS)–toxic epidermal necrolysis (TEN), *Acinetobacter* species was the main organism grown **(Table 2)**. *Pseudomonas aeruginosa* and *Klebsiella pneumoniae* growth did not correlate with a specific dermatosis.

Study by Sharma et al.[7] is an attempt to understand the organisms responsible for sepsis in our dermatology ward and their current sensitivity patterns. Empirical antibiotic guidelines are proposed for adequate coverage of sepsis in admitted patients before culture reports become available:
- Avoid using same class of antibiotics in all ward patients at the same time; otherwise, development of resistance will be faster.
- Affordability and availability factors should also be considered.

TABLE 1: Bacterial isolates in cultures from different sites.					
Isolate	Pus (from skin)	Blood	Urine	Sputum or tracheal aspirate	Total
Methicillin-resistant Staphylococcus aureus	12	1	–	–	16
Methicillin-sensitive Staphylococcus aureus	4	–	–	–	4
Acinetobacter	2	4	2	1	9
Pseudomonas	3	3	–	–	6
Klebsiella	2	3	1	–	6
Escherichia coli, Proteus, Enterobacter, Streptococci	3	1	3	–	7
Total	26	15	6	1	48

TABLE 2: Correlation between positive culture isolates and diagnosis.

Positive culture isolate	Blood			Skin		
Diagnosis	Pemphigus	Erythroderma	TEN	Pemphigus	Erythroderma	TEN
Staphylococcus aureus	1	3	–	10	4	2
Acinetobacter	1	–	2	0	1	1
Pseudomonas	2	1	–	3	–	–
Klebsiella	1	1	1	2	–	–
Others	–	1	–	1	–	2
Total	5	6	3	16	5	5

TABLE 3: Proposed antibiotics drugs in order of preference.[7]

Type of organism to be covered	Choice of antibiotic	Dose and route
Staphylococcus aureus	Vancomycin or teicoplanin	500 mg 6 hourly or 1 g 12 hourly infused IV over 1 hour in adults, 40 mg/kg in 4 divided doses in children: 400 mg × 3 doses 12 hourly—then 400 mg daily IV or IM
	Linezolid	600 mg 12 hourly IV
	Levofloxacin	500 mg OD IV infusion slowly
Gram-negative organisms	Cefoperazone + sulbactam	1–2 g IV 12 hourly
	Imipenem or meropenem	(500 mg IV 6 hourly)/(imipenem + cilastatin) (1 g every 8 hourly)
	Piperacillin + tazobactam	100–150 mg/kg/day or 4.5 g/day in 3 divided doses
	Amikacin	15 mg/kg/day in 2–3 divided doses

(IM: intramuscular; IV: intravenous)

- Empirical coverage in a sepsis patient should include one antibiotic having anti-staphylococcal activity and one sensitive against gram-negative bacteria and one against the anaerobes **(Table 3)**.
- Individualize the treatment on the basis of clinical assessment. Sometimes, it may not be necessary to give multiple antibiotics, especially if a single antibiotic can cover the whole spectrum of suspected infections.

METHICILLIN-RESISTANT *STAPHYLOCOCCUS AUREUS*

The resistance of MRSA to beta-lactam antibiotics is due to the presence of the *mecA* gene sequence, which is carried as a mobile genetic element in a staphylococcal chromosome cassette (SCC). The *mecA* gene produces transpeptidase penicillin-binding peptide-2a (PBP2a) that decreases the bacterial affinity for beta-lactam antibiotics.[8-10] The *mecA* gene with the entire complex known as the *SCC mec* element.
- The most common route of transmission of community-associated (CA)-MRSA is through an open wound, such as a superficial abrasion, or from contact with a CA-MRSA carrier. Other methods of transmission include poor hand washing, poor personal hygiene (e.g., not showering after workouts), sharing personal items (e.g., razors, towels, and clothing), etc.

- Diagnostic microbiology laboratories and reference laboratories are key for identifying outbreaks of MRSA.[11] Faster techniques for identifying and characterizing MRSA have recently been developed. Normally, the bacterium must be cultured from blood, urine, sputum, or other body-fluid samples, and in sufficient quantities to perform confirmatory tests early-on; these include quantitative polymerase chain reaction (PCR) procedures, which are employed in clinical laboratories for quickly detecting and identifying MRSA strains.

Treatment

Systemic therapy with antistaphylococcal antibiotics is indicated in moderate-to-severe disease, especially in the presence of systemic inflammatory response syndrome (SIRS), as defined by two or more of the following:
- Temperature greater than 38°C or lower than 36°C
- Tachypnea (>24 breaths/min)
- Tachycardia (>90 beats/min)
- White blood cell (WBC) count greater than 12,000 cells/µL or less than 4,000 cells/µL.

Oral Antibiotics

Oral antibiotics include:
- *Trimethoprim–sulfamethoxazole (SXT):* 1 or 2 tablets twice daily for 7 days.[12]
- *Clindamycin:* 300–450 mg 3 times a day; resistance to clindamycin is increasing because of the inducible macrolide–lincosamide–streptogramin B (iMLSb) phenotype, which may result in cross-resistance to clindamycin.
- *Doxycycline:* 100 mg twice daily; not recommended for children younger than 8 years.
- *Linezolid:* 600 mg twice daily.

Intravenous Antibiotics

Intravenous (IV) antibiotics that may be used to treat inpatient cases of CA-MRSA include the following:
- *Vancomycin:* 30 mg/kg/day IV in two divided doses; vancomycin is the parenteral drug of choice for treatment of infections caused by MRSA.
- *Linezolid:* 600 mg IV every 12 hours; this agent may increase central nervous system serotonin levels as a result of monoamine oxidase-A (MAO-A) inhibition, thereby increasing the risk of serotonin syndrome.[13]
- *Clindamycin:* 600 mg IV every 8 hours.
- Daptomycin: 4 mg/kg IV every 24 hours; note that this agent can cause myopathy.
- *Ceftaroline:* 600 mg IV twice daily.[14]
- *Dalbavancin:* 1 g IV once weekly; this agent is a second-generation bactericidal glycopeptide that received US Food and Drug Administration (FDA) approval in May 2014 for the treatment of *S. aureus* infections (MRSA and methicillin-sensitive *S. aureus* [MSSA]) after it was proven to be noninferior to vancomycin IV and then linezolid PO in the DISCOVER-1 and DISCOVER-2 trials, respectively.[15]
- *Tedizolid:* 200 mg IV once daily, infused over 1 hour, for 6 days;[16] this agent is an oxazolidinone antibacterial drug designed to enhance activity against gram-positive pathogens; tedizolid received FDA approval in June 2014 for the treatment of MRSA and MSSA skin and soft tissue infections (SSTIs) after it was proven to be statistically noninferior to linezolid in the ESTABLISH-1 and ESTABLISH-2 trials.[17,18]

VANCOMYCIN-RESISTANT *STAPHYLOCOCCUS AUREUS*

- The expected mechanism of vancomycin resistance in *S. aureus* was plasmid-mediated transfer of the *vanA* gene cluster. *Staphylococcus* bacteria are classified as vancomycin-intermediate *S. aureus* (VISA) if the minimum inhibitory concentration (MIC) for vancomycin is 4–8 µg/mL, and classified as vancomycin-resistant *S. aureus* (VRSA) if the vancomycin MIC ≥16 µg/mL.[19]
- *Linezolid, quinupristin/dalfopristin* and *daptomycin*, and *tigecycline* are effective against VISA. *Ceftobiprole*, tested by Rockefeller University, New York/US in 2008, was found effective against MRSA and VRSA. *Ceftaroline and telavancin are other drugs for VRSA.*

Topical Antibiotics

- Topical silver sulfadiazine is an effective and cheap alternative to other available antibiotic ointments.
- Mupirocin and retapamulin, used twice daily for 5 days, are preferred over framycetin and neomycin because of less resistance and over fusidic acid to prevent resistance to oral fusidic acid. However, in patients with multiple lesions or in outbreak settings, oral treatment is preferred to help reduce transmission of infection.

NOSOCOMIAL INFECTIONS IN DERMATOLOGY

- Healthcare-associated infections (HAI) are defined as infections not present and without evidence of incubation at the time of admission to a healthcare setting. These infections arise after 48 hours of being admitted to the hospital.
- Infectious agents causing healthcare-associated infections may come from endogenous or exogenous sources.
- Endogenous sources include body sites normally inhabited by microorganisms, e.g., external nares, nasopharynx, and gastrointestinal (GI) or genitourinary tracts. Exogenous sources include those that are not part of the patient, like visitors, medical personnel, equipments, catheter, intubation, central venous line, ventilator, and the healthcare environment.
- The major sites of infections, among all healthcare-associated infections, are bloodstream infections and urinary tract infections.
- Symptomatic treatment of shock, hypoventilation, and other complications should be provided, along with administration of broad-spectrum antimicrobial therapy.
- Sepsis is an important cause of morbidity and mortality in dermatology inpatients.

Welsh Regimen and Modifications

Mycetoma is a chronic granulomatous infection that can be caused by fungi or aerobic branching actinomycotic bacteria. The disease is endemic in tropical and subtropical regions of the world. Clinically, mycetoma is characterized by painless subcutaneous swelling with nodules that develop and drain through sinus tracts. The organism causing mycetoma aggregate into grains or sclerotia and are found in the discharge. These grains help to identify the causative organism and guide treatment of the disease.

Worldwide 60% of mycetomas are caused by actinomycetes, although the incidence can vary regionally due to geographic variations (climate and rainfall). The most frequent agents of actinomycetoma are grouped in three genera: (1) *Nocardia,* (2) *Streptomyces,* and (3) *Actinomadura.*

Several antimicrobial combinations have been tried in actinomycosis. Until 1970s, best clinical outcome was obtained with sulfamethoxazole + trimethoprim and injection streptomycin.

Oliverio Welsh et al. decided to administer amikacin along with SXT in 1982. Amikacin, a semisynthetic aminoglycoside, acts by irreversibly binding to 30s ribosomal subunit and inhibiting protein synthesis. It has a better safety profile than streptomycin. In the treatment schedule devised by them, injection amikacin 7.5 mg/kg is given intramuscularly (IM) twice daily for 21 days constituting one cycle. 1–3 cycles are given with a gap of 15 days between them. Tablet cotrimoxazole 8/40 mg/kg/day, i.e., double strength in three divided doses is coadministered during, between, and for 2 weeks after the cycles. This treatment was first tried in a 19-year-old male with severe thoracic mycetoma caused by *Nippostrongylus brasiliensis,* which disseminated to lungs. Patient showed complete remission after 5 weeks of therapy with minimal gastrointestinal side effects and has not had a recurrence. This treatment regimen was subsequently tried in a large number of patients and almost all of them attained remission with minimal side effects. Before starting amikacin, one must investigate for complete blood counts, urine analysis, liver function tests, kidney function tests, and audiometry. These investigations need to be repeated before and after each cycle of amikacin, and thereafter monthly.

Side effects of this therapy can be either due to cotrimoxazole, which are gastrointestinal symptoms, skin rash, SJS, and hematologic side effects such as anemia and leukopenia or they can be due to amikacin. It is mainly nephro, oto, and neurotoxic. There is no evidence of any interaction or any increased side effects on coadministration of these two drugs.

Drugs that can interact with amikacin include penicillins, which are inactivated in vitro and therefore should not be mixed or run in the same tubing. Cephalothin can increase the risk of aminoglycoside nephrotoxicity. Amikacin should be used with caution with nondepolarizing muscle relaxants (atracurium, pancuronium, tubocurarine, and gallamine triethiodide) because of possible enhanced action resulting in possible respiratory depression. Loop diuretics (bumetanide, furosemide, ethacrynic acid, and torsemide) should be avoided because of potential cochlear toxicity (especially with ethacrynic acid). Other nephrotoxic agents (e.g., amphotericin B, vancomycin, foscarnet, cidofovir, and IV contrast dyes) should not be coadministered because they can increase nephrotoxicity. Several drug combinations have since been tried on the philosophy that actinomyces need to be targeted with mutidrug therapy on the lines of mycobacteria to prevent resistance and ensure better therapeutic outcome.

Ramam et al.[20] devised a two-step regimen with intensive and maintenance phases. In the intensive phase, patients received a combination of IV crystalline penicillin 1 MU every 6 hours, IV gentamicin 80 mg twice daily and oral cotrimoxazole (sulfamethoxazole 400 mg and trimethoprim 80 mg), as indicated 2 tablets twice a day. This is continued until about 5–7 weeks depending upon clinical response. After this, patients were discharged on tablet amoxicillin 500 mg thrice a day and cotrimoxazole daily. 6 patients were successfully treated with minimal side effects with this regimen and remained disease-free for >6 months follow-up.

This regimen requires administration of IV penicillin 4 times a day and gentamicin twice a day during the intensive phase. Ramam further modified the two-step regimen, the number of daily injections were reduced to two and intensive phase could be given on outpatient or daycare basis. Gentamicin was given for only 4 weeks thus less monitoring was required. The rationale for using gentamicin was the cost effectivity **(Table 4)**.

Damle et al.[21] modified the original Welsh regimen by adding rifampicin to it. 18 patients suffering from actinomycetoma who had unsatisfactory response with previous therapy (15 patients—dapsone/SXT monotherapy; 3 patients—streptomycin + SXT) were administered with 21-day cycles

TABLE 4: Modified two-step treatment for actinomycetomas.		
Antibiotics	Duration	Monitoring
• Intensive phase (step 1) • Gentamicin (80 mg twice daily, intravenously) and cotrimoxazole (2 tablets of 960 mg, twice daily)	4 weeks	Weekly urine examination, renal function tests, clinical evaluation for auditory/vestibular symptoms, and audiometry if required
• Maintenance phase (step 2) • Doxycycline (100 mg orally, twice daily) and cotrimoxazole (as above)	Till 5–6 months after complete healing of all sinuses	Monthly hemogram and urine examination

of amikacin (15 mg/kg/day IV) along with uninterrupted oral SXT and rifampicin (10 mg/kg/day) for until 3 months after last amikacin cycle. All patients who completed the therapy attained remission.

Pulikot et al.[22] have successfully used a combination of rifampicin + dapsone + SXT to treat actinomycetoma of foot in a 10-year-old child.

Netilmicin has been tried in patients not responding or allergic to amikacin-based regimens with successful outcomes. For an adult, a total daily dose of netilmicin (300 mg/day) combined with SXT (8/40 mg/kg/day orally) is given. Other antimicrobials such as imipenem and meropenem have been used in the treatment of severe actinomycetoma in association with amikacin in patients where the bacteria are resistant to SXT. Patients with actinomycetoma unresponsive to SXT can be treated with other antimicrobials such as amoxicillin–clavulanic acid (1.5 g daily) for up to 6 months to evaluate its therapeutic efficacy. Linezolid, an oxazolidinone, which blocks initiation of protein synthesis has shown promising activity against actinomycetes. Most common adverse events with linezolid are diarrhea, headache, nausea, and myelosupression. Complete blood counts should be monitored weekly in patients who receive linezolid. Peripheral neuropathy and optic neuropathy can also develop. A limiting factor in the use of linezolid is its cost and some adverse effects.

In cases of resistance to antimicrobials, it is necessary to evaluate other drugs, both in vitro and in vivo. Moxifloxacin, gatifloxacin, garenoxacin, and an experimental oxazolidinone, DA-7867, have shown in vitro activity against *N. brasiliensis* and *Actinomadura madurae*.

REFERENCES

1. Macias ES, Pereira FA, Rietkerk W, Safai B. Superantigens in dermatology. J Am Acad Dermatol. 2011;64(3):455-72.
2. Talpur R, Bassett R, Duvic M. Prevalence and treatment of *Staphylococcus aureus* colonization in patients with mycosis fungoides and Sézary syndrome. Br J Dermatol. 2008;159(1):105-12.
3. Tomi NS, Kränke B, Aberer E. Staphylococcal toxins in patients with psoriasis, atopic dermatitis, and erythroderma, and in healthy control subjects. J Am Acad Dermatol. 2005;53(1):67-72.
4. DiNubile MJ, Lipsky BA. Complicated infections of skin and skin structures: When the infection is more than skin deep. J Antimicrob Chemother. 2004;53(suppl 2):37-50.
5. Pasricha JS. Pulse Therapy in Pemphigus and Other Diseases, 2nd edition. New Delhi: Pulse Therapy and Pemphigus Foundation; 2000. pp. 19,30,31.
6. Ahmed AR, Moy R. Death in pemphigus. J Am Acad Dermatol. 1982;7(2):221-8.
7. Sharma VK, Asati DP, Khandpur S, Khilnani GC, Kapil A. Study of sepsis in dermatology ward: A preliminary report. Indian J Dermatol Venereol Leprol. 2007;378-82.
8. Feng Y, Chen CJ, Su LH, Hu S, Yu J, Chiu CH. Evolution and pathogenesis of *Staphylococcus aureus*: Lessons learned from genotyping and comparative genomics. FEMS Microbiol Rev. 2008;32(1):23-37.
9. Baba T, Takeuchi F, Kuroda M, Yuzawa H, Aoki K, Oguchi A, et al. Genome and virulence determinants of high virulence community-acquired MRSA. Lancet. 2002;359(9320):1819-27.

10. Kazakova SV, Hageman JC, Matava M, Srinivasan A, Phelan L, Garfinkel B, et al. A clone of methicillin-resistant *Staphylococcus aureus* among professional football players. N Engl J Med. 2005;352(5):468-75.
11. Fontanilla JM, Kirkland KB, Talbot EA, Powell KE, Schwartzman JD, Goering RV, et al. Outbreak of skin infections in college football team members due to an unusual strain of community-acquired methicillin-susceptible *Staphylococcus aureus*. J Clin Microbiol. 2010;48(2):609-11.
12. Stevens DL, Bisno AL, Chambers HF, Dellinger EP, Goldstein EJ, Gorbach SL, et al. Practice guidelines for the diagnosis and management of skin and soft tissue infections: 2014 update by the Infectious Diseases Society of America. Clin Infect Dis. 2014;59(2):e10-52.
13. US Food and Drug Administration. (2011). FDA Drug Safety Communication: Serious CNS reactions possible when linezolid (Zyvox®) is given to patients taking certain psychiatric medications. [online] Available from http://www.fda.gov/Drugs/DrugSafety/ucm265305.htm. [Last accessed July, 2025].
14. Sader HS, Fritsche TR, Jones RN. Antimicrobial activity of ceftaroline and ME1036 tested against clinical strains of community-acquired methicillin-resistant *Staphylococcus aureus* (CA-MRSA). Antimicrob Agents Chemother. 2008; 52(3):153-5.
15. Boucher HW, Wilcox M, Talbot GH, Puttagunta S, Das AF, Dunne MW. Once-weekly dalbavancin versus daily conventional therapy for skin infection. N Engl J Med. 2014:370(23):2169-79.
16. SIVEXTRO (tedizolid phosphate) (for injection, for intravenous use; for oral use) [package insert]. Lexington, MA: Cubist Pharmaceuticals; 2014. [online] Available from https://www.accessdata.fda.gov/drugsatfda_docs/label/2025/205435s016,205436s013lbl.pdf [Last accessed July, 2025].
17. Prokocimer P, De Anda C, Fang E, Mehra P, Das A. Tedizolid phosphate vs linezolid for treatment of acute bacterial skin and skin structure infections: The ESTABLISH-1 randomized trial. JAMA. 2013;309(6):559-69.
18. Moran GJ, Fang E, Corey GR, Das AF, De Anda C, et al. Tedizolid for 6 days versus linezolid for 10 days for acute bacterial skin and skin-structure infections (ESTABLISH-2): A randomized, double-blind, phase 3, non-inferiority trial. Lancet Infect Dis. 2014;14(8):696-705.
19. Soriano A, Marco F, Martínez JA, Pisos E, Almela M, Dimova VP, et al. Influence of vancomycin minimum inhibitory concentration on the treatment of methicillin-resistant *Staphylococcus aureus* bacteremia. Clin Infect Dis. 2008;46(2):193-200.
20. Ramam M, Bhat R, Garg T, Sharma VK, Ray R, Singh MK, et al. A modified two-step treatment for actinomycetoma. Indian J Dermatol Venereol Leprol.2007;73(4):235-9.
21. Damle DK, Mahajan PM, Pradhan SN, Belgaumkar VA, Gosavi AP, Tolat SN, et al. Modified Welsh regimen: a promising therapy for actinomycetoma. J Drugs Dermatol. 2008;7:853-6.
22. Pulikot AM, Bapat SS, Tolat S. Mycetoma of the sole. Ann Trop Paediatr. 2002;22(2):187-90.

SECTION 3

Miscellaneous

13. Bedside Tests in Dermatology
14. Signs in Dermatology
15. Frequently Asked Questions in Dermatology

CHAPTER 13

Bedside Tests in Dermatology

INTRODUCTION

- We do physical examination of patients to formulate initial differential diagnoses.
- In modern dermatology era, we have an access to sophisticated diagnostic techniques such as direct immunofluorescence (DIF) and polymerase chain reaction (PCR) apart from traditional diagnostic tests such as biopsies and culture.
- It is important to know these bedside tests, as they are:
  - Simple and quick to perform
  - Low cost
  - Help us to narrow down the diagnosis to initiate our treatment rapidly.

LIST OF BEDSIDE TESTS

List of bedside tests is as follows:
- Gram's stain
- Potassium hydroxide (KOH) mount
- Tzanck smear
- Thick drop method (modified Tzanck)
- Slit skin smear
- Diascopy
- Dermoscopy
- Nailfold capillaroscopy (NFC)
- Wood's lamp
- Mineral oil preparation
- Hair pull test
- Pathergy test
- Sexually transmitted infections (STIs), disseminated gonococcal infection (DGI)—Gram's stain, crushed smear, wet mount, and whiff test

GRAM-STAIN

Staining materials and chemicals required for Gram-stain are given in **Figure 1**.
- It was first developed by a Danish physician, Hans Christian Gram in 1884.
- It divides the bacteria into gram-positive and gram-negative.

Principle: The cell wall of the organism retains primary stain even after decolorizing and appears as gram positive **(Figs. 2A and B)**.

Cell wall gets decolorized and takes up the counterstain—gram-negative organisms.

Sampling technique:
- In case of intact bulla, the bulla is deroofed and blister fluid is smeared with a sterile swab.
- In case of erosions, the base of the erosion is smeared with a sterile swab.
- The collected material on swab is then smeared on a clean and dry glass slide.

Indications

Indications are as follows:
- Impetigo **(Fig. 3)**
- Staphylococcal scalded skin syndrome
- Actinomycosis

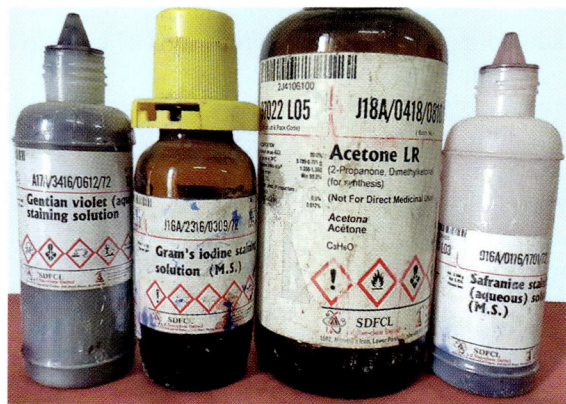

FIG. 1: Staining materials and chemicals required for Gram-stain.

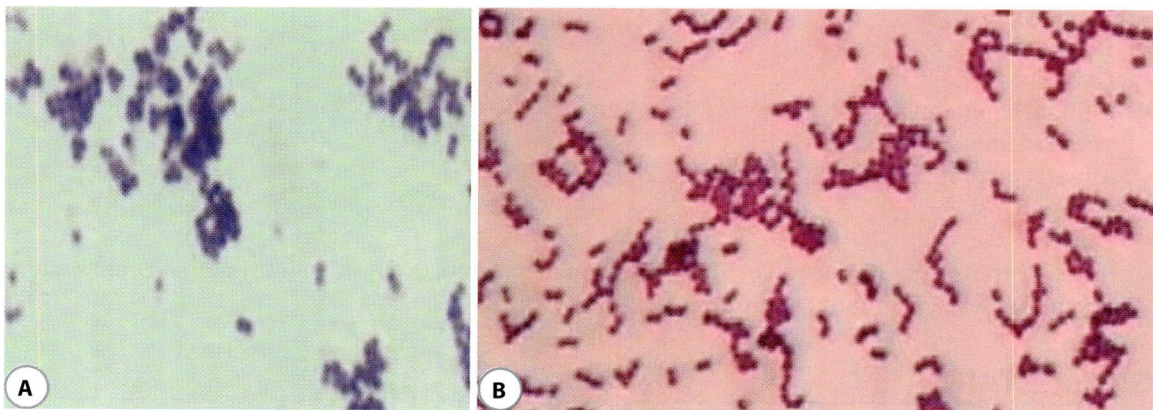

FIGS. 2A AND B: (A) Gram-positive cocci in clusters—*Staphlyococcus* species; and (B) Gram-positive cocci in chains—*Streptococcus* species.

Method[1]

- Cover the fixed smear with *crystal violet* for 1 minute
- Rinse with tap water
- Flood with *Gram's iodine* solution for 1 minute
- Rinse with water
- Decolorize with *acetone* for 10–20 seconds
- Rinse with water
- Counterstain with *safranin* for 1 minute
- Rinse with water
- Air dry the slide, see under the microscope

POTASSIUM HYDROXIDE MOUNT[2]

Potassium hydroxide test is used to demonstrate evidence of fungal infection of skin, hairs, and nails **(Box 1)**.

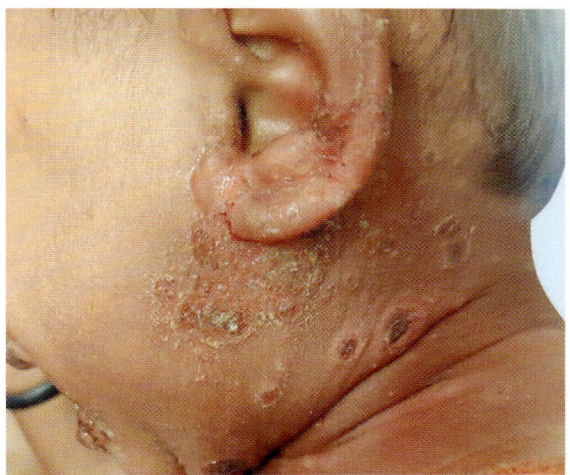

FIG. 3: Clinical image of impetigo-shows gram-positive cocci on Gram-stain.

BOX 1 | Diagnostic steps in fungal microscopy using potassium hydroxide (KOH) mount.

- *Sample collection*:
  - Skin—cleaned with alcohol, scraped with scalpel
  - Hair—plucked with forceps
  - Nail—undersurface of nail plate is scraped
- *KOH mount*: 10% KOH (20% for nails) added and heated, wait for 15–20 minutes for keratin to dissolve nails—24–48 hours
- *Microscopic examination*: Fungal spores or hyphae are seen

Modified KOH mount procedure:
- Cellophane tape can be applied over affected site, pressed firmly, and removed.
- Tape is then stuck on surface of a glass slide.
- Parker's ink can be added to KOH to stain fungal wall blue **(Fig. 4)**.
- Hyphae and spores are visualized **(Figs. 5 to 7)**.

Mechanism of Action

Potassium hydroxide (KOH) dissolves keratin.
- *Dermatophytes*: Long and branched hyphae **(Fig. 5)**
- *Pityriasis versicolor*: Short hyphae and spores **(Figs. 4 to 6)**
- *Candidiasis*: Spores and pseudohyphae **(Fig. 7)**

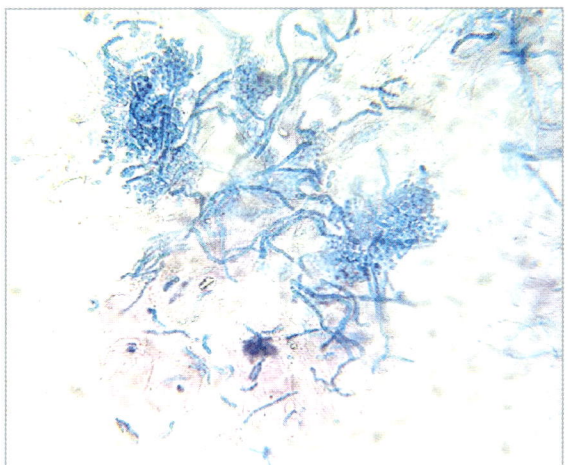

FIG. 4: Parker's ink preparation in case of pityriasis versicolor.

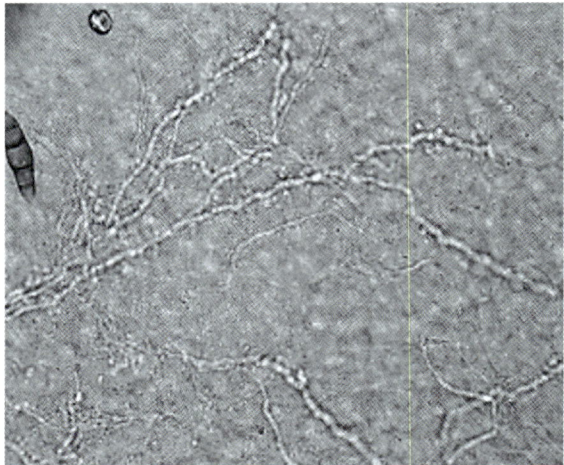

FIG. 5: Refractile, branched septate hyphae.

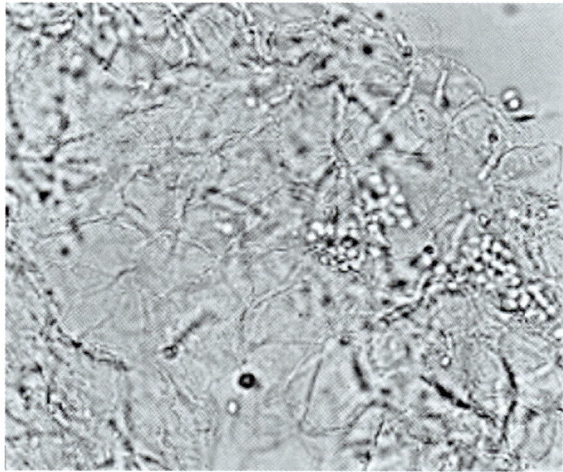

FIG. 6: Yeast-and-mycelia (banana and grapes) appearance on potassium hydroxide (KOH) mount.

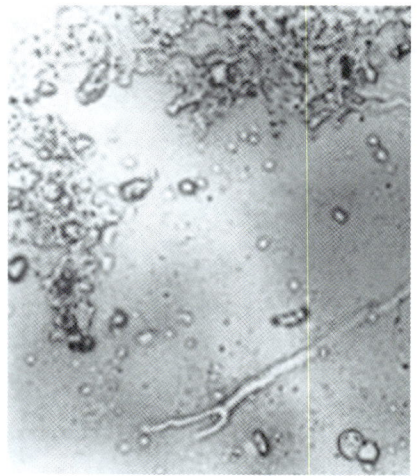

FIG. 7: Budding yeast, pseudohyphae.

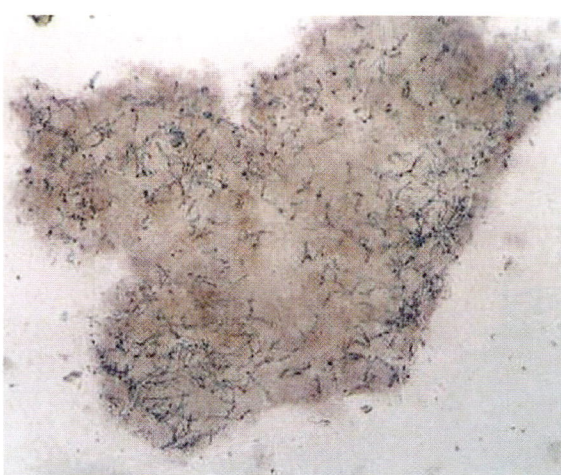

FIG. 8: Chicago sky-blue stain

- *Chicago sky-blue stain* **(Fig. 8)**: Most sensitive method for diagnosis of pityriasis versicolor; easy to perform, rapid, and qualitatively superior.

Pityriasis Versicolor

Other modifications of standard method:
- Parker's ink method
- Eosin 1% method
- Modified Parker's ink and eosin 1% method
- Calcofluor white–fluorochrome stain. When viewed under ultraviolet light, fungal structures display a brilliant apple-green or a ghostly blue–white color.

Whiff Test

Vaginal discharge + drop of 10% KOH = *Fishy smell* (due to presence of amines and trimethylamine)—bacterial vaginosis.

TZANCK SMEAR

The characteristics of Tzanck smear are:
- First used for skin disorder by Tzanck in 1947
- Diagnostic cytology
- Cytology—study of individual cell and their intrinsic characteristic
- Cytology is a Greek word (*kytos* = hollow vessel)

Indications

- Immunobullous disorders: PV, BP, Hailey–Hailey's disease **(Figs. 9 to 13)**
- Infective diseases: Herpes simplex **(Figs. 14 and 15)**
- Genodermatosis

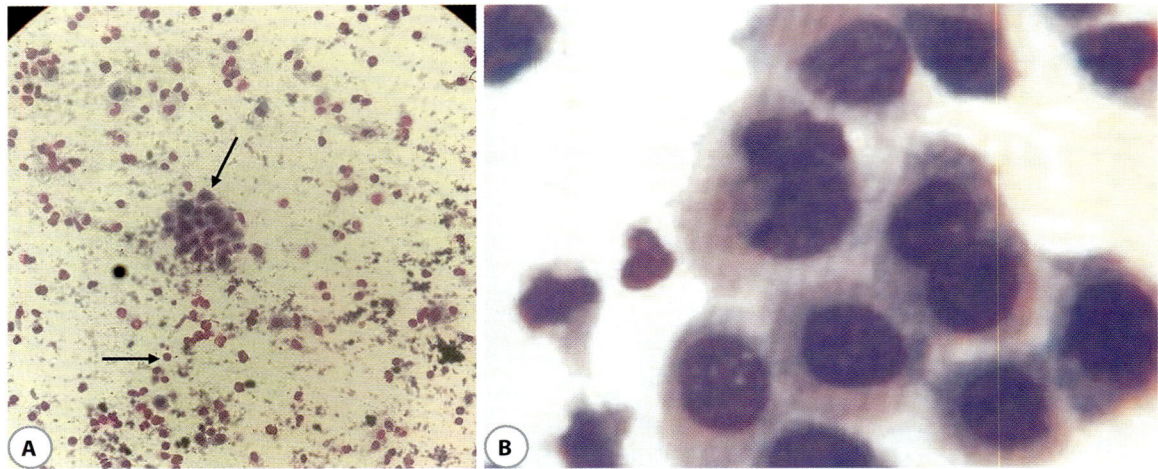

FIGS. 9A AND B: (A) Acantholytic cells as seen in Giemsa stain; and (B) high power view of acantholytic cells.

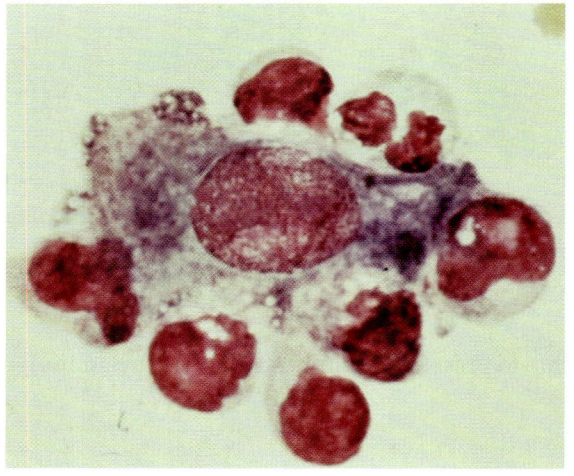

FIG. 10: Isolated epithelial cells surrounded by a ring of leukocytes.

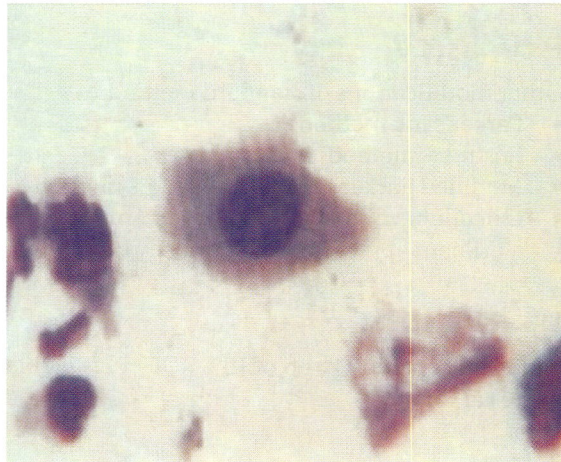

FIG. 11: Hyalinized cytoplasm.

- Neonatal dermatoses **(Fig. 16)**
- Cutaneous tumors

Technique[3]

- Select a fresh blister.
- Remove a blister top with scalpel or sharp scissor.
- Absorb excess fluid with a gauze piece. Avoid bullae fluid and blood.

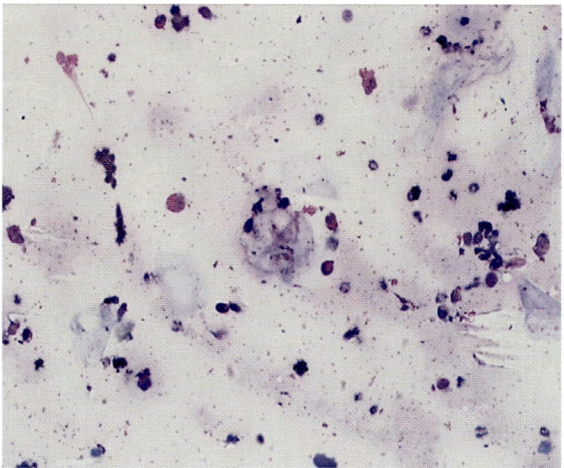

FIG. 12: Abundant eosinophils as seen in Tzanck preparation of bullous pemphigoid.

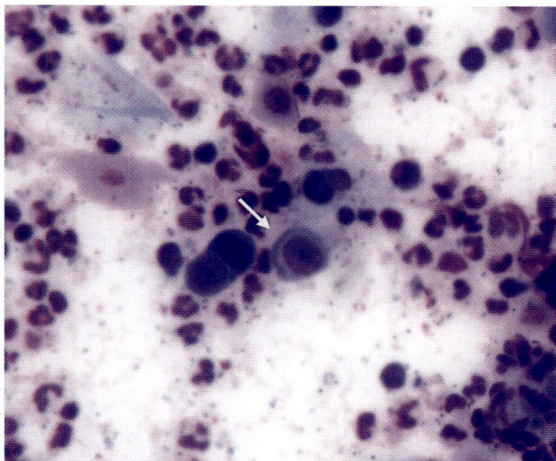

FIG. 13: Hailey–Hailey disease.

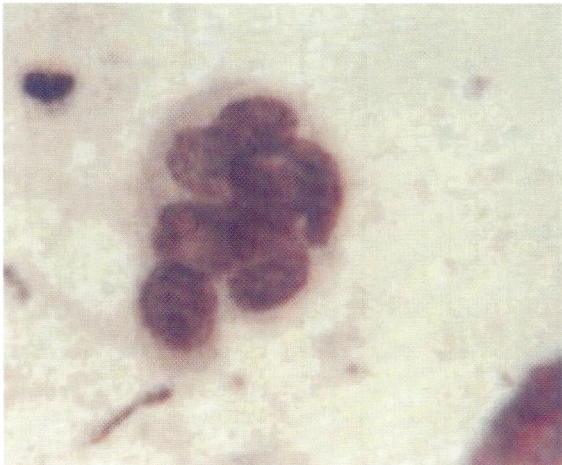

FIG. 14: Multinucleated giant cell formed by fusion of enlarged infected cells.

- Gently scrape the floor and edge of vesicle with no 10 or 15 blade.
- Make a smear on glass slide.
- The slide should be clean, since cells will not adhere to a slide marred by fingerprints.
- Air dry and stain with Giemsa stain **(Figs. 17A and B)**
- Giemsa stain solution is diluted 1:10 with distilled water.
- Diluted solution is poured over smear.
- Kept for 15 minutes.
- Wash with water.
- Examine under the microscope.

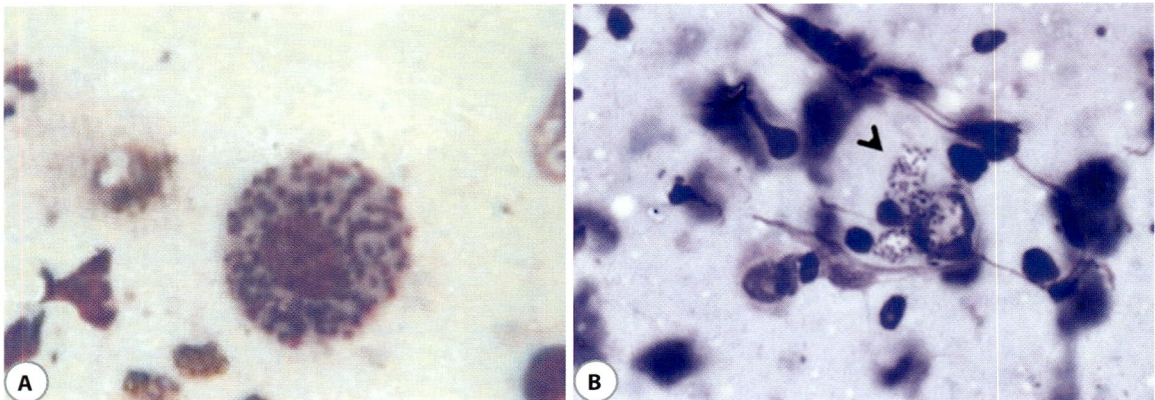

FIGS. 15A AND B: Intracellular LD bodies ("swarm of bees") within large macrophages.

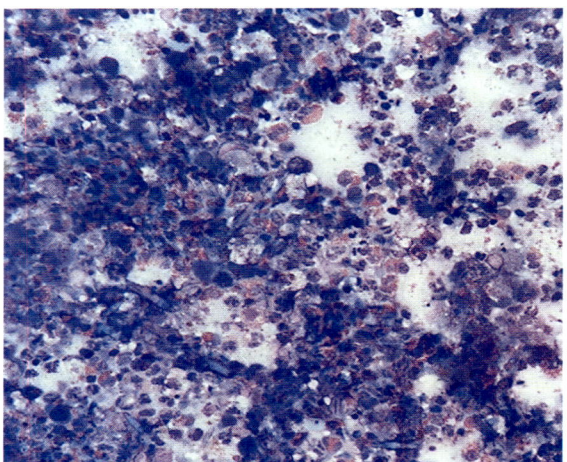

FIG. 16: Numerous neutrophils.

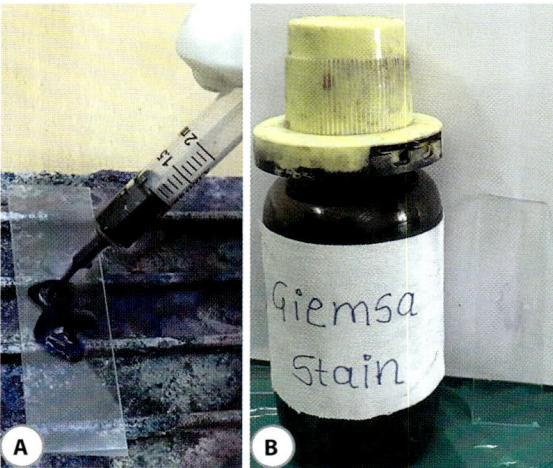

FIGS. 17A AND B: Preparing slide on rack for Tzanck smear with Giemsa stain.

- The stained nuclei may vary in color from reddish blue to purple to pink.
- The cytoplasm stains bluish.

Staining

- Giemsa stain
- Hematoxylin and eosin
- Wright
- Methylene blue
- Papanicolaou

- Toluidine blue
- Azure II-eosin
- Glycerin
- Methanol
- Azure A eosinate
- Azure B eosinate
- Methylene blue chloride
- Methylene blue eosinate

Interpretation

- *Pemphigus vulgaris*:
    - *Acantholytic cells (Tzanck cells)*:
        - Large round keratinocyte
        - Hyperchromatic nucleus
        - Absent or hazy nucleoli
        - Peripherally condensed basophilic cytoplasm, *"mourning edged"* cells
        - Perinuclear halo
        - Due to loss of intercellular bridges, keratinocytes get detached from each other and appear as rounded cells instead of polygonal or hexagonal shaped.
    - *Sertoli rosette*:
        - *Streptocytes*: Chains of white blood cells formed by filamentous, glue-like substances.
- *Pemphigus foliaceous*: Acantholytic cells **(Fig. 11)**
- *Pemphigus vegetans*: Cytological features are identical to pemphigus vulgaris but there are usually more inflammatory cells, particularly *eosinophils*.
- *Bullous pemphigoid*: No acantholytic cells, plenty of eosinophils **(Fig. 12)**
- *Hailey-Hailey disease*: Partial acantholysis **(Fig. 13)**
    - Acantholytic cells do not cluster
    - No streptocytes
    - No Sertoli rosettes
- *Infections:* Herpes simplex, herpes zoster, and varicella
- *Neonatal dermatoses:* Neonatal varicella, transient neonatal pustulosis, and erythema toxicum neonatorum
- *Erythema toxicum neonatorum*: Neutrophils predominance **(Fig. 16)**
- *Cutaneous leishmaniasis:* Intracellular infection of macrophages by protozoal leishmania species

Modified Tzanck Smear: "Thick Drop Method"

- A number 15 scalpel is used to nick the inflamed border of the lesion and drops of the oozing blood are placed onto a glass slide
- The drops of blood are allowed to dry at room temperature without smearing and are then stained using Wright–Giemsa.
- Intracellular amastigotes [Leishman-Donovan (LD) bodies] are readily detected on microscopy as a light blue, round or oval "swarm of bees".[4]

SLIT SKIN SMEAR[5]

Characteristics of slit skin smear are as follows:
- It is the most important laboratory test to detect lepra bacilli **(Figs. 18A and B)** to confirm diagnosis.
- To classify the disease
- Assess progress of disease
- Assess treatment response

Sites
- Right ear lobe
- Forehead
- Chin
- Left buttock in men and left upper thigh in women
- Most active looking part of skin lesion

Method
Method of slit skin smear test is shown in **Figures 19A to G**.

Staining procedure: Modified Ziehl–Neelsen (ZN) stain

DIASCOPY

Indications[6]
- Telangiectasia—central feeder vessel may be distinguished
- Petechiae and purpura
- Port-wine stain or nevus flammeus **(Figs. 20A and B)**
- Granulomatous nodules (sarcoidosis, granuloma annulare, and lupus vulgaris) reveal a brownish-yellow "apple-jelly" translucent quality upon diascopy.

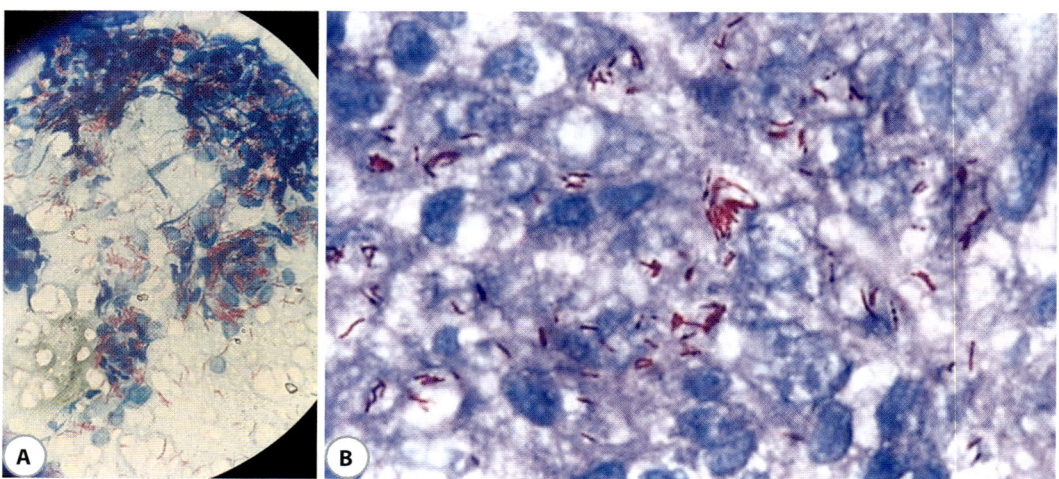

FIGS. 18A AND B: Ziehl–Neelsen stain showing *Mycobacterium leprae*.

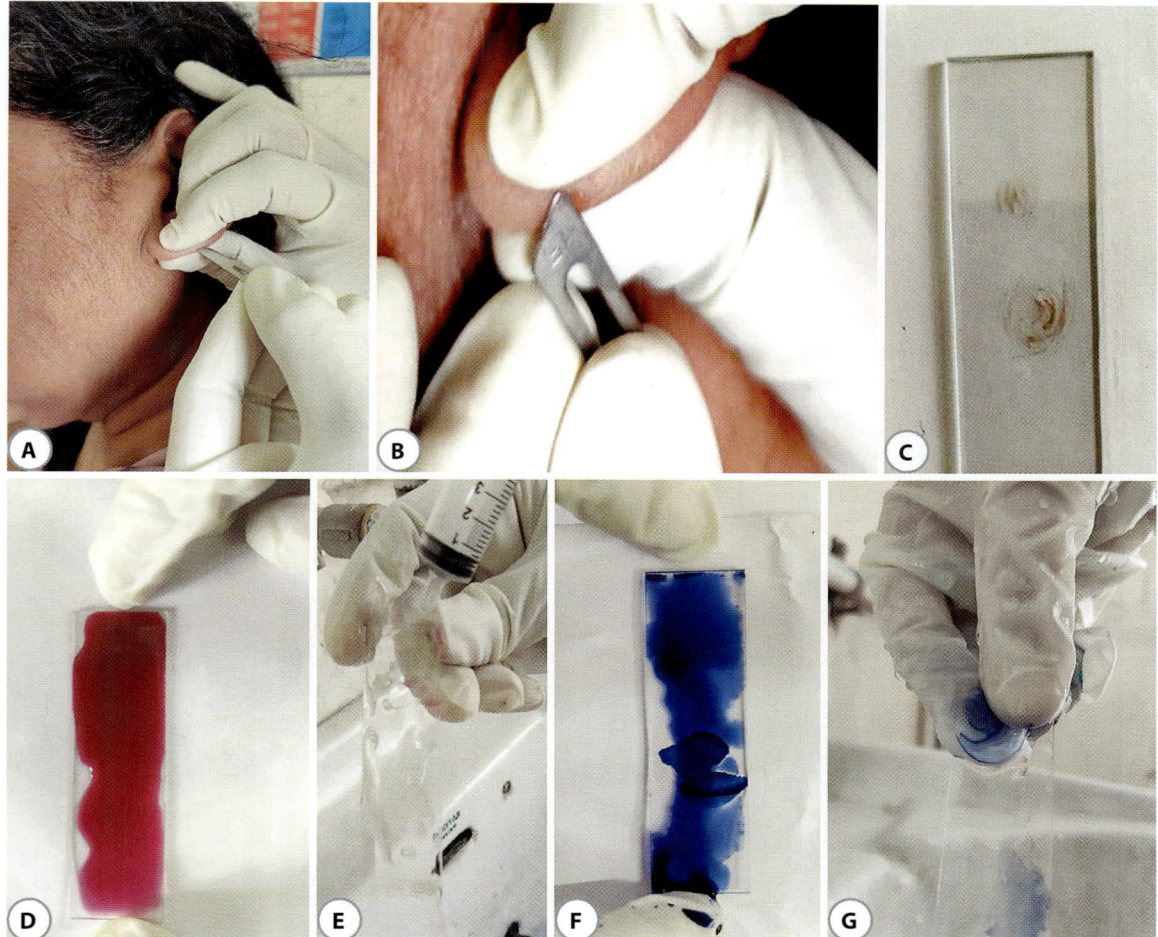

FIGS. 19A TO G: (A) 5 mm long, 2 mm deep cut is made at edge of skin lesion; (B) Sides and bottom of the cut are scraped; (C) Air dried and fix with flaming; (D) Carbol fuchsin for 15–20 minutes; (E) Decolorize with 5% H_2SO_4; (F) Methylene blue 1 minute; and (G) Removing excess counter stain under running water.

Method

Method of diascopy is shown in **Figures 21 and 22**.

DERMOSCOPY

Characteristics of dermoscopy are as follows **(Fig. 23)**:
- Dermoscopy is a noninvasive diagnostic technique that allows recognition of structures, which are not visible by naked eye.
- It is also known as dermatoscopy, epiluminescence microscopy (ELM), incident light microscopy, and skin surface microscopy.

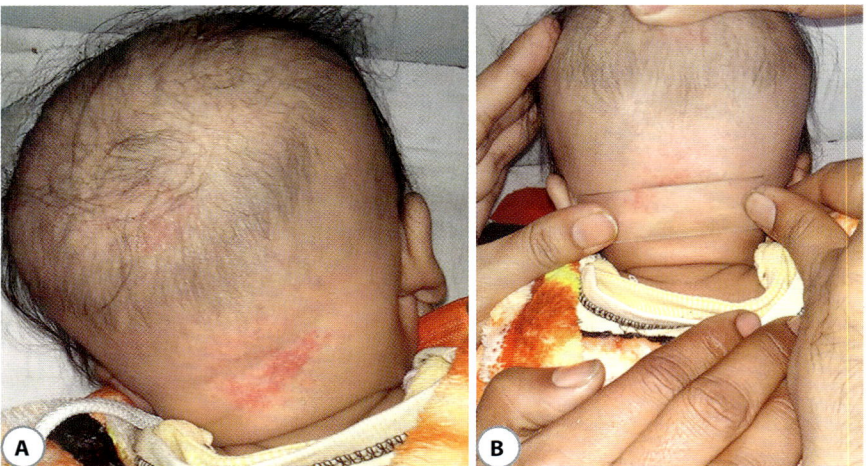

FIGS. 20A AND B: Diascopy test in "Port-wine stain".

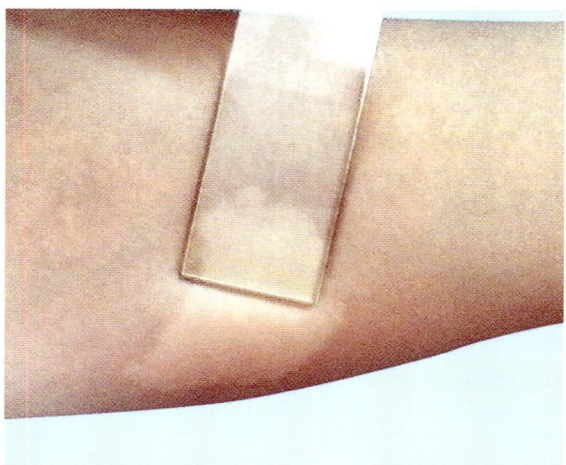

FIG. 21: Performing diascopy test in nevus depigmentosus.

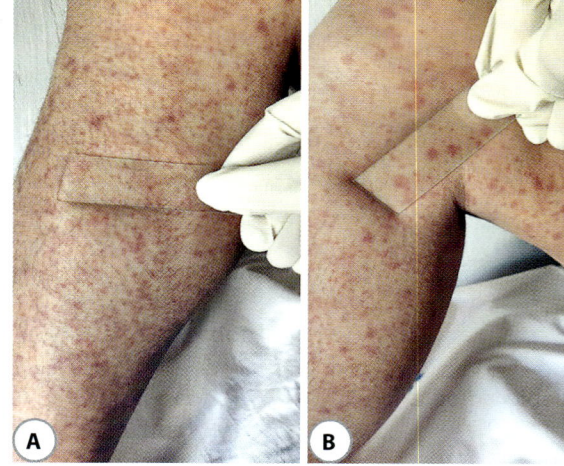

FIGS. 22A AND B: Demonstration of diascopy test to differentiate between "petechiae" and "purpura".

- The term "dermatoscopy" was introduced in 1920 by the German dermatologist Johann Saphier who published a series of communications using a new diagnostic tool resembling a binocular microscope with a built-in light source for the examination of the skin.
- Basically, a dermoscope is functionally similar to a magnifying lens but with the added features of an inbuilt illuminating system, a higher magnification that can be adjusted, the ability to assess structures as deep as in the reticular dermis, and the ability to record images.

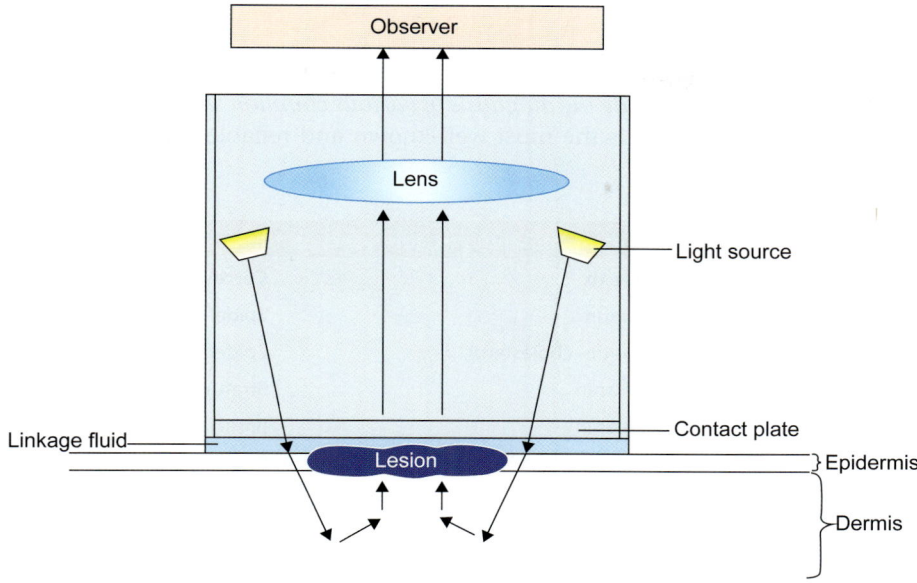

FIG. 23: Principle of dermatoscopy.

Principle

The basic principle of dermoscopy is *transillumination* and *magnification* of a lesion.

Light incident on skin undergoes reflection, refraction, diffraction, and absorption. These phenomena are influenced by physical properties of the skin. Most of the light incident on dry, scaly skin is reflected, but smooth, oily skin allows most of the light to pass through it, reaching the deeper dermis.

Linkage Fluids[7]

- To improve the visibility of subsurface structures, some linkage fluids are used between the skin surface and the dermoscope **(Table 1)**.
- It helps in reducing the reflectivity of the skin and enhances the transparency of the stratum corneum.
- *Various linkage fluids that can be used are*:
    - Liquid paraffin
    - Mineral oil
    - Glycerin
- *Components of a dermoscope include*:
    - Achromatic lens
    - Inbuilt illuminating system
    - Power supply

Patterns of Dermoscopy

Patterns of dermoscopy are given in **Figures 24 to 27**.

Dermoscopic examination can facilitate the diagnosis of various common skin disorders:
- Pattern analysis on dermoscopy is the most well-known and reliable method for differentiating pigmented skin tumors.

TABLE 1: Dermoscopy colors of keratinizing, melanocytic, and vascular tumors.		
Color	**Due to**	**Corresponding layer in skin**
Orange	Keratin	Epidermis
Yellow	Keratin–cholesterol	Epidermis–dermis
Black	Melanin	Stratum corneum
Brown	Melanin	Basal layer
Gray	Melanin	Papillary dermis
White	Fibrosis	Dermis
Blue	Melanin	Papillary and reticular dermis
Red	Hemoglobin	Papillary dermis
Purple	Hemoglobin	Reticular dermis

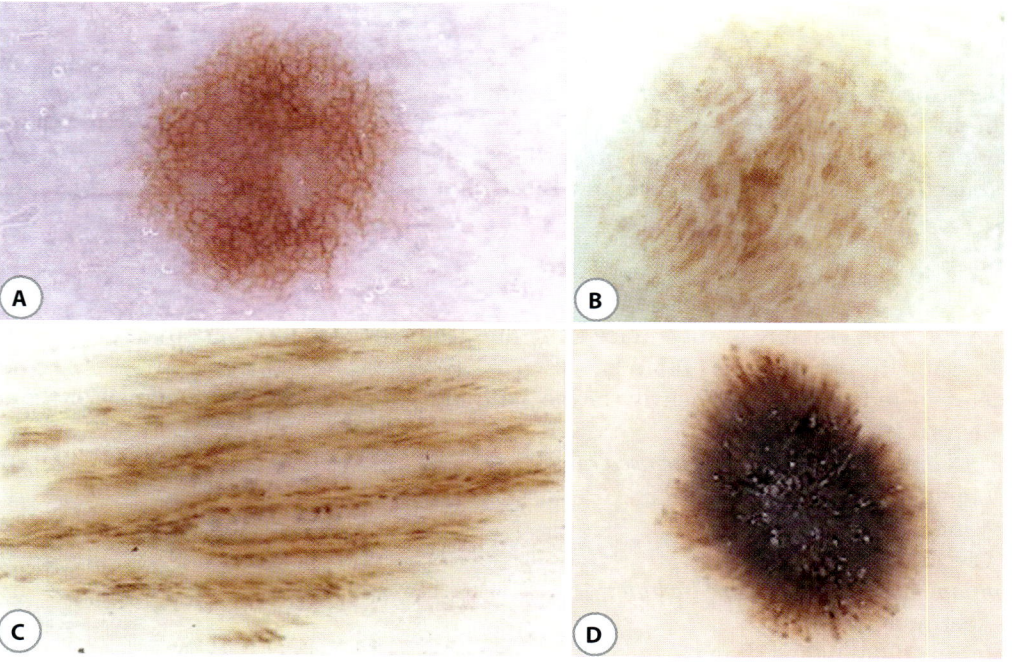

FIGS. 24A TO H: *Continued*

Continued

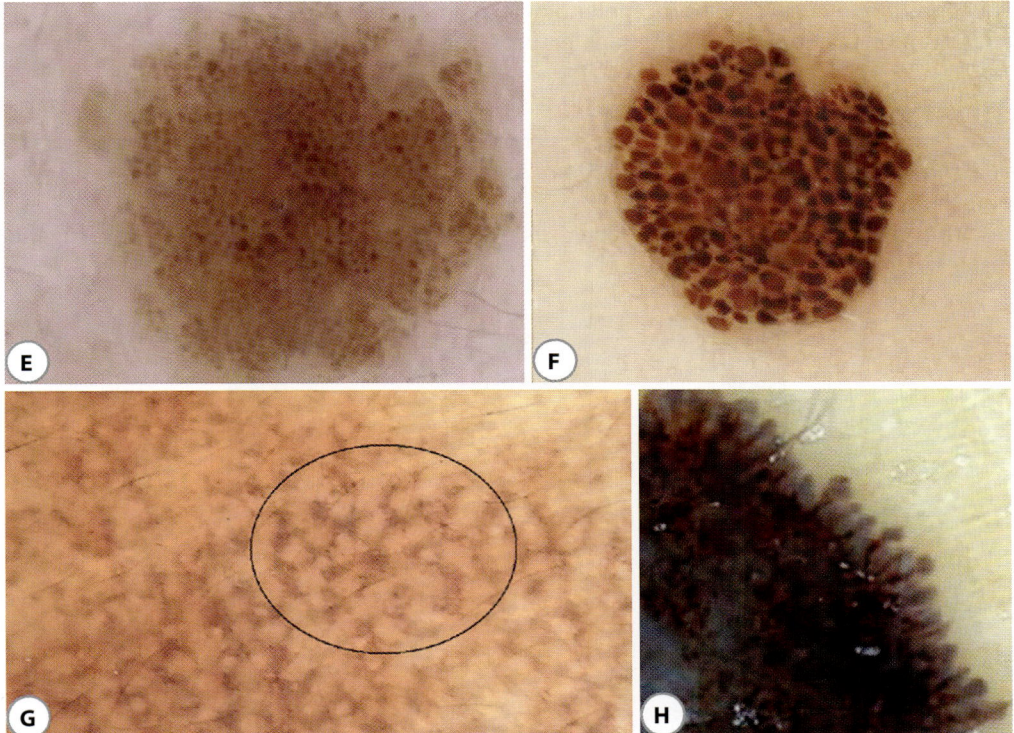

FIGS. 24A TO H: (A) Reticular pattern; (B) Branched; (C) Parallel; (D) Radial arrangement; (E) Pattern of dots; (F) Pattern of clods; (G) Pattern of circles; and (H) Pattern of pseudopods.

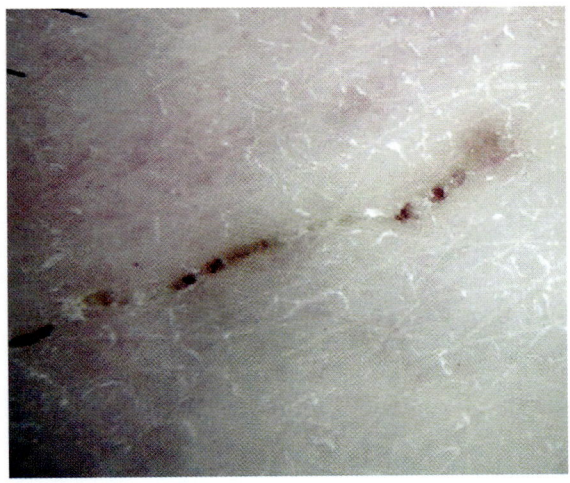

FIG. 25: Scabies—"Jet with contrail" sign.

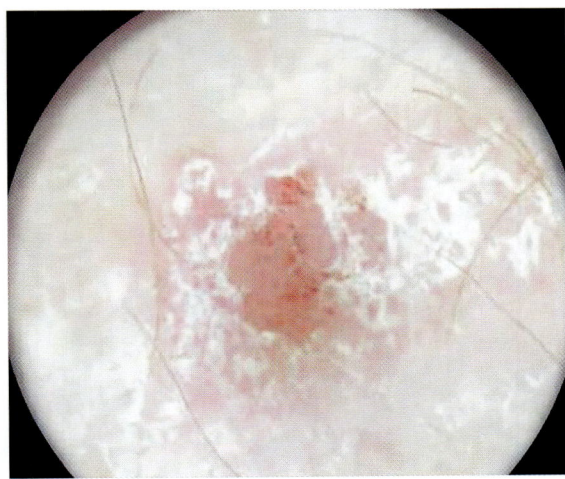

FIG. 26: Psoriasis—red dots and scaling.

- *This is based on a two-step algorithm*:
    1. Recognition of basic criteria for melanocytic and nonmelanocytic tumors.
    2. Recognition of benign and malignant features of melanocytic nevi and melanomas, respectively.

TRICHOSCOPY

*Characteristics of trichoscopy (**Figs. 28 to 36**) are as follows:*
- Dermoscopy of the scalp and hair
- Apart from diagnosing alopecia, it decreases the need for many unnecessary investigations like biopsies to a great extent.

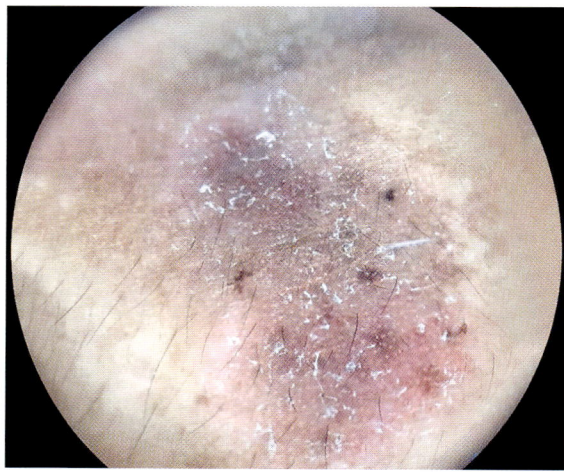

FIG. 27: Lichen planus—Wickham's striae

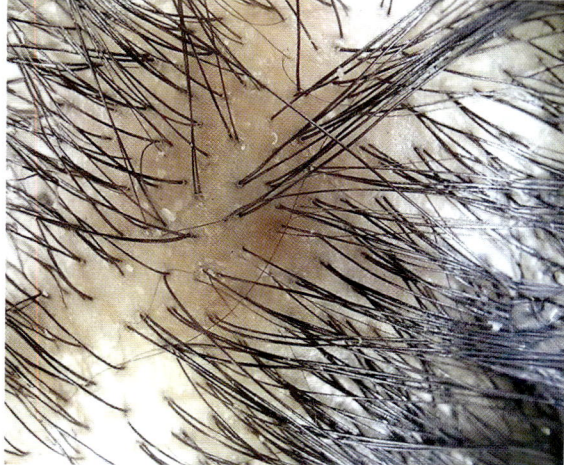

FIG. 28: Normal scalp on trichoscopy.

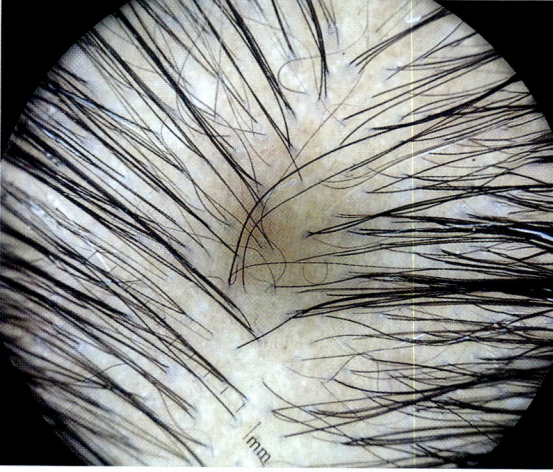

FIG. 29: Female pattern hair loss—hair shaft diameter diversity >20% and increased proportion of vellus hair.

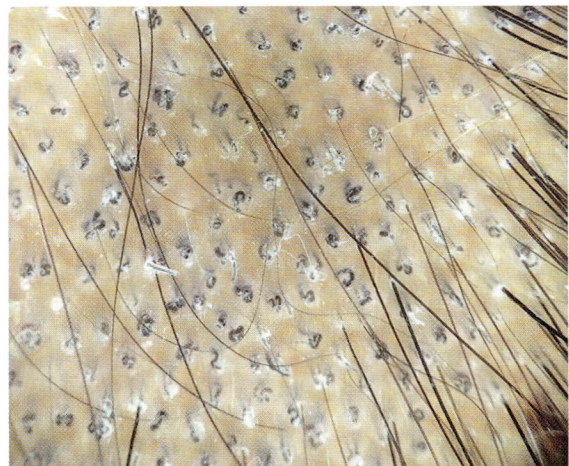

FIG. 30: Tinea capitis—multiple black dots and comma hair with few broken hairs.

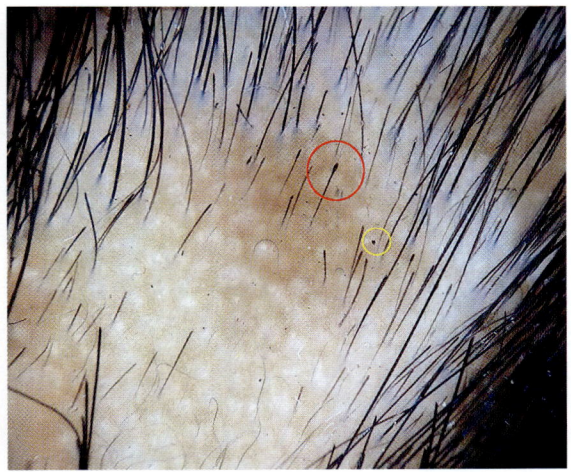

FIG. 31: Alopecia areata–multiple exclamation mark hairs (red circle) and few black dots (yellow circle).

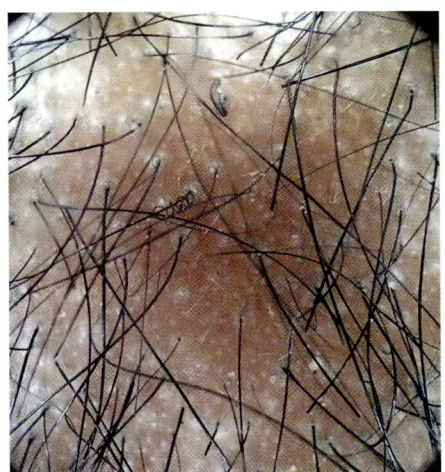

FIG. 32: Trichotillomania—hair shafts of variable lengths with many broken/fractures hairs.

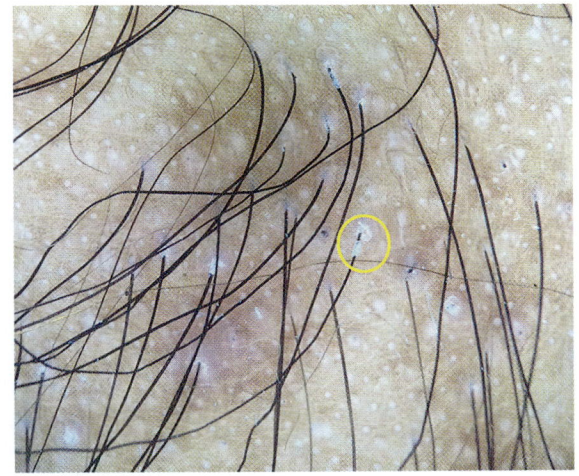

FIG. 33: Lichen planopilaris—peripilar tubular casts with normal interfollicular areas and white dots.

- Trichoscopy (hair and scalp dermoscopy) allows identification of hair and scalp diseases based on analysis of trichoscopy structures and patterns.
- Structures visualized by trichoscopy include hair shafts, hair follicle openings, the perifollicular epidermis, and cutaneous microvasculature.
- Trichoscopy allows distinguishing between normal terminal hairs and vellus (or vellus-like) hairs, which by definition are 0.03 mm or less in thickness and <3 mm in length.
- *Follicular patterns:*[8]
  - *Yellow dots:* Infundibulum of the follicle with sebum [in androgenetic alopecia (AGA)] and degenerating keratinocytes (in alopecia areata).

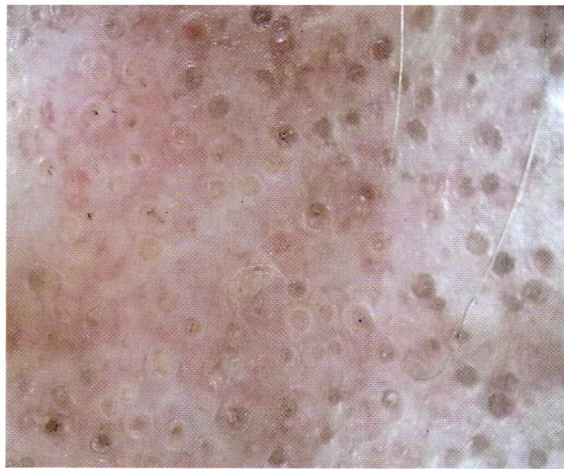

FIG. 34: Discoid lupus erythematosus–large yellow dots with radial, thin arborizing vessels arising from the dot.

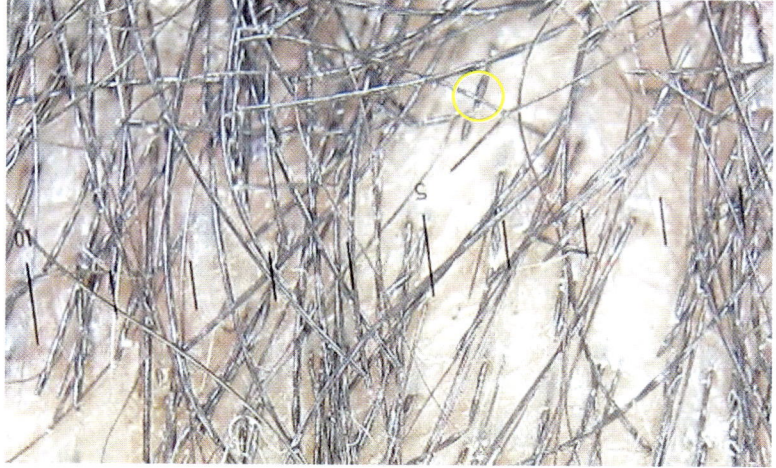

FIG. 35: Monilethrix–uniform elliptical nodes and intermittent constrictions and with variation in hair shaft diameter, yellow dots.

- - *White dots:* Seen in scarring alopecias that spare interfollicular epidermis [lichen planopilaris (LPP) or folliculitis decalvans].
  - *Black dots:* Denotes cadaverized hairs
  - *Red dots:* In discoid lupus erythematosus
- Vascular patterns:
  - *Interfollicular simple red loops:* Seen in normal scalp and most of the inflammatory conditions as multiple regularly spaced hairpin-like structures. Absent loops indicate epidermal atrophy.

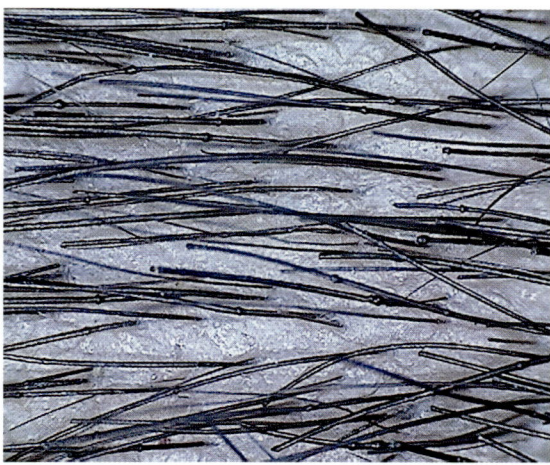

FIG. 36: Trichorrhexis invaginata (bamboo hair), hair shaft telescopes into itself (invaginates) at several points along the shaft.

-
  - *Interfollicular twisted loops:* Twisted coils and are best seen with the probe placed tangentially to the scalp surface.
    - Conditions characterized by acanthosis, such as psoriasis and folliculitis decalvans show this pattern.
  - *Arborizing red lines:* These are seen as lines that underlie the loops in normal and affected scalp. These represent the subpapillary plexus.
- *Pigment pattern:*
  - Normal scalp shows a diffuse pigmented brownish honeycomb pattern.
  - It comprises of a grid wherein the pigmented lines represent the rete ridges, and the amelanotic holes represent the suprapapillary epidermis.
- The method enables visualization of microexclamation hairs (in alopecia areata) or comma hairs (in tinea capitis) and hair shaft structure abnormalities, including genetic hair dystrophies, such as monilethrix, trichorrhexis invaginata, or trichorrhexis nodosa.
- Three to four hairs per unit are observed occasionally. A lower number of hairs is characteristic for hair loss (i.e., telogen effluvium and androgenetic alopecia); an abnormally high number is characteristic for tufted folliculitis.

NAILFOLD CAPILLAROSCOPY[9]

Nailfold capillaroscopy is shown in **Figures 37 to 42**.
- It is useful to recognize *peripheral microangiopathy* in autoimmune connective tissue diseases.
- It differentiates primary from secondary Raynaud's phenomenon.
- It differentiates the patients of scleroderma as having "early", "active", or "late" pattern.
    It is a significant test as it is a part of American College of Rheumatology (ACR)/European League Against Rheumatism (EULAR) criteria for classification of systemic Sclerosis (SSc). NFC has been given a score of 2.
- *Physiologically*: The capillaries have a hairpin-shape and are arranged in two parallel longitudinal rows.
- Uniformity of capillary width, length, and intercapillary distance

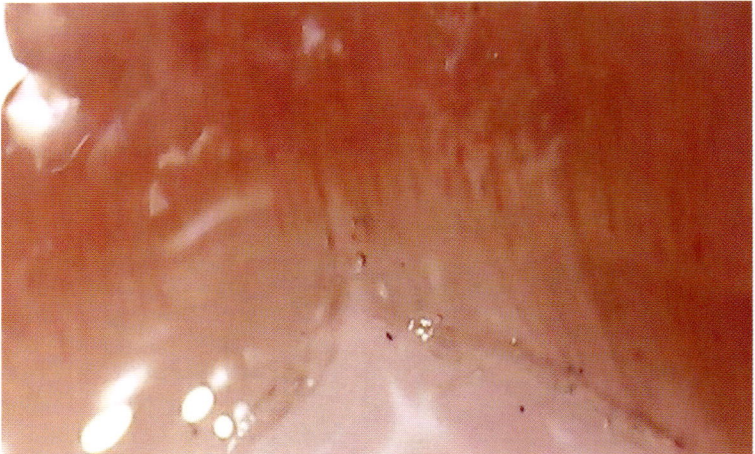

FIG. 37: Normal nailfold capillaroscopy (NFC) picture.

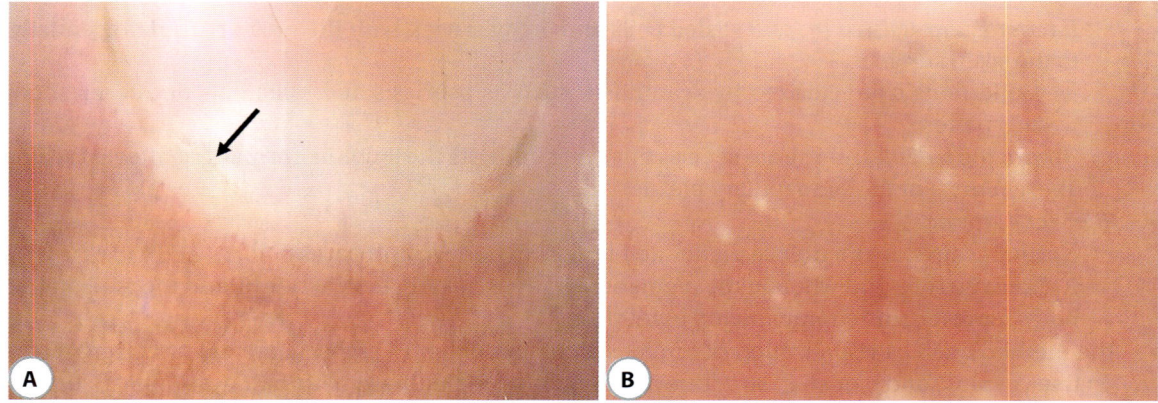

FIGS. 38A AND B: Early pattern. Well-preserved capillary architecture.

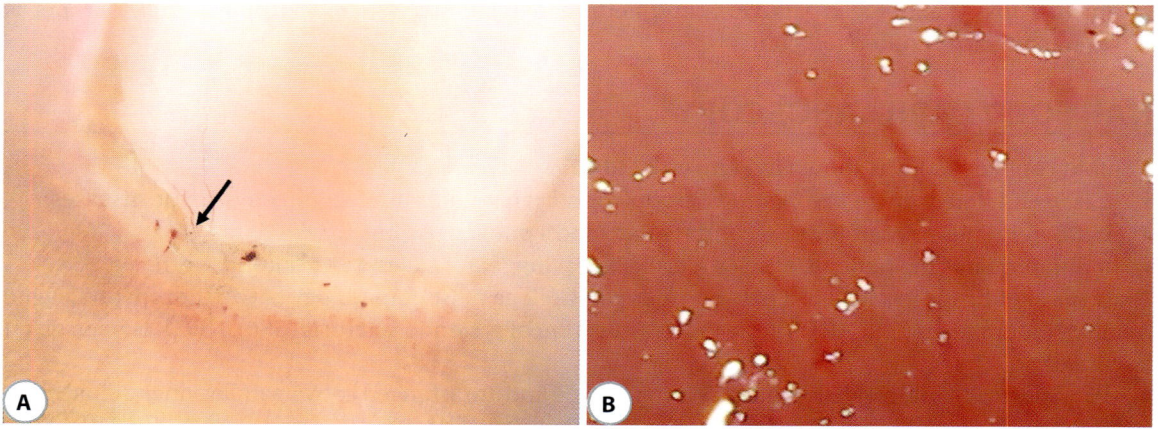

FIGS. 39A AND B: Active pattern. (A) Microhemorrhages; and (B) Giant capillaries.

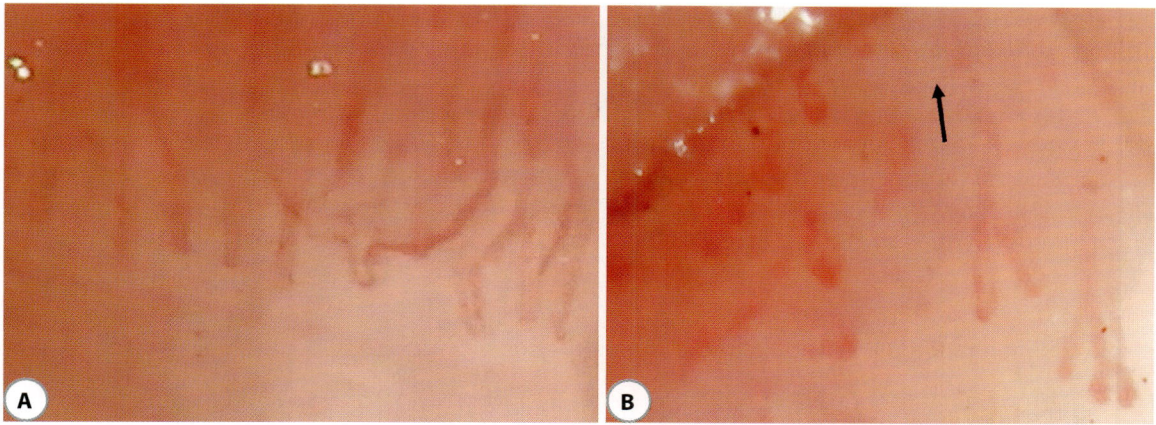

FIGS. 40A AND B: Late pattern. (A) Meandering capillaries; and (B) Capillary dropouts.

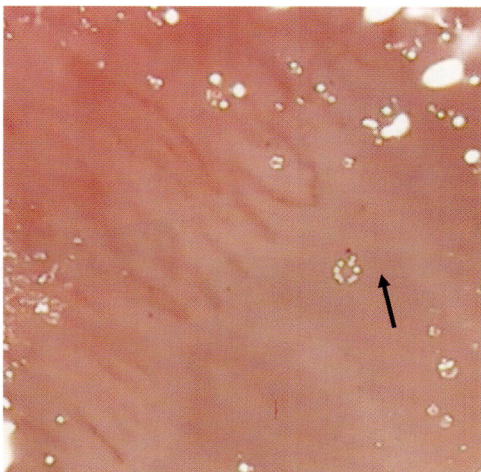

FIG. 41: Irregularly organized capillaries.

Systemic Lupus Erythematosus and Dermatomyositis

Nailfold capillaroscopy represents a tool for the prediction of microvascular heart involvement by considering the systemic microvascular derangement at the capillary nailfold.

WOOD'S LAMP

Wood's lamp apparatus is shown in **Figures 43A and B.**
- Invented by Robert W Wood in 1903
- Utilized in dermatology in 1925 by Margarot and Deveze

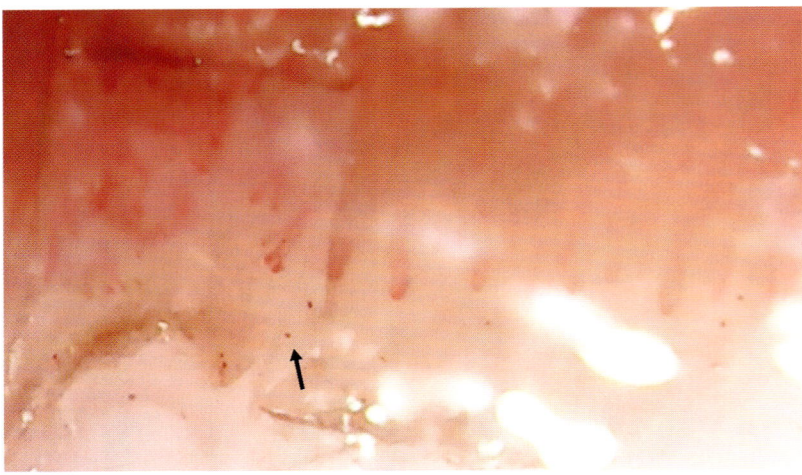

FIG. 42: Ragged cuticles, hemorrhagic spots, budding capillaries.

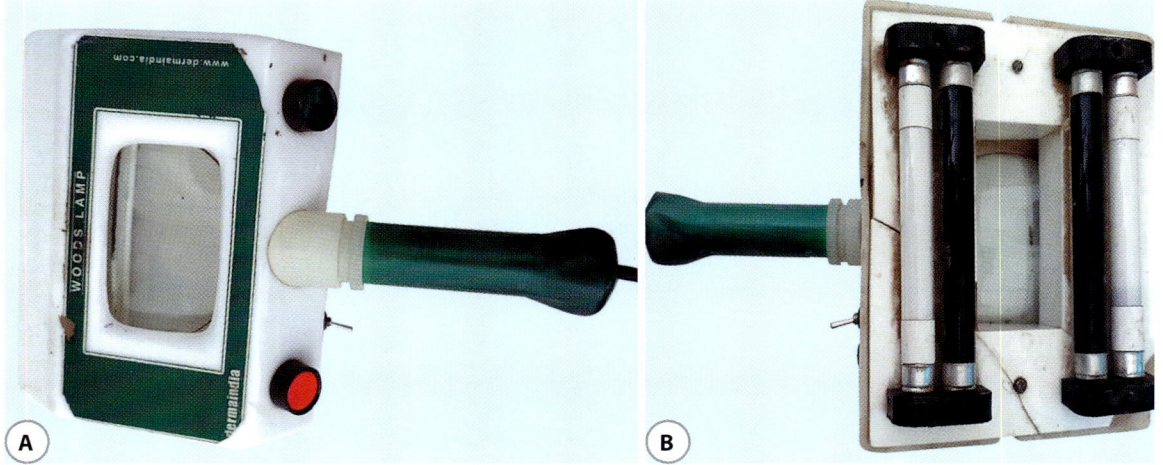

FIGS. 43A AND B: Wood's lamp apparatus.

Principle[10]

- Wood's lamp emits long wave UV rays—black light
- Generated by mercury arc
- *Filter:*
    - 1.9% barium silicate
    - 9% nickel oxide
- Filter is opaque to all lights except 320–400 nm, peak at 365 nm.
- Fluorescence of tissues occurs when Wood's (UV) light is absorbed and radiation of a longer wavelength is emitted.

Technique of Wood's Lamp Examination

- Prewarm for 1 minute before use.
- Hold the lamp 4–5 inches away from skin.
- Do not wash the area to be examined—results in dilution of pigment and gives false negative results.
- False positive fluorescence could be due to reflection from:
    - White apron—light blue
    - Salicylic ointment—green
    - Petrolatum—purple/bluish

Various dermatoses where Wood's lamp is useful aid in diagnosis **(Figs. 44 to 47)**.

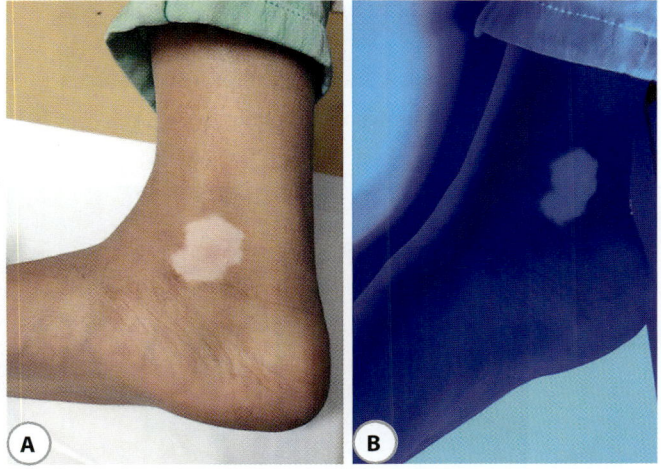

FIGS. 44A AND B: Autofluorescence as seen in vitiligo due to collagen.

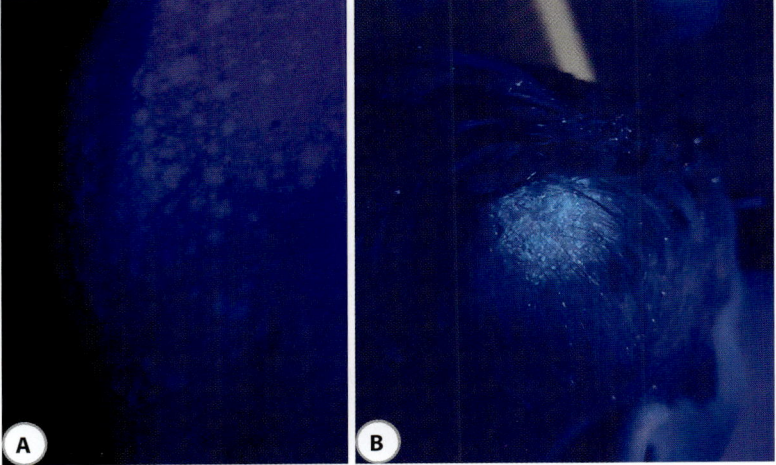

FIGS. 45A AND B: (A) Pityrialactone Causing fluorescence in *T. versicolor*; and (B) Pteridine causing fluorescence in *T. capitis* (*Microsporum canis, M. audouinii, M. distortum, M. ferruginum, M. gypseum,* and *Trichophyton schoenleinii*).

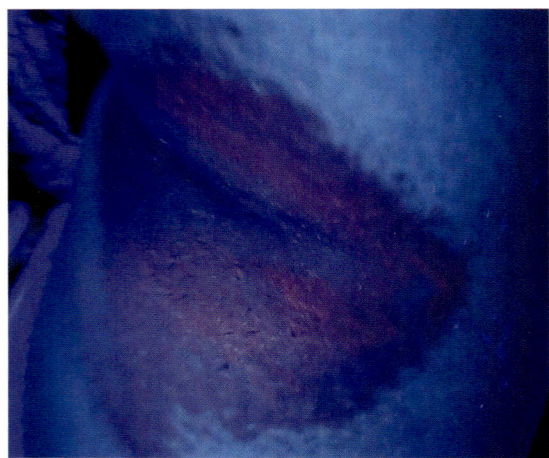

FIG. 46: Coral red fluroscence in erythrasma.

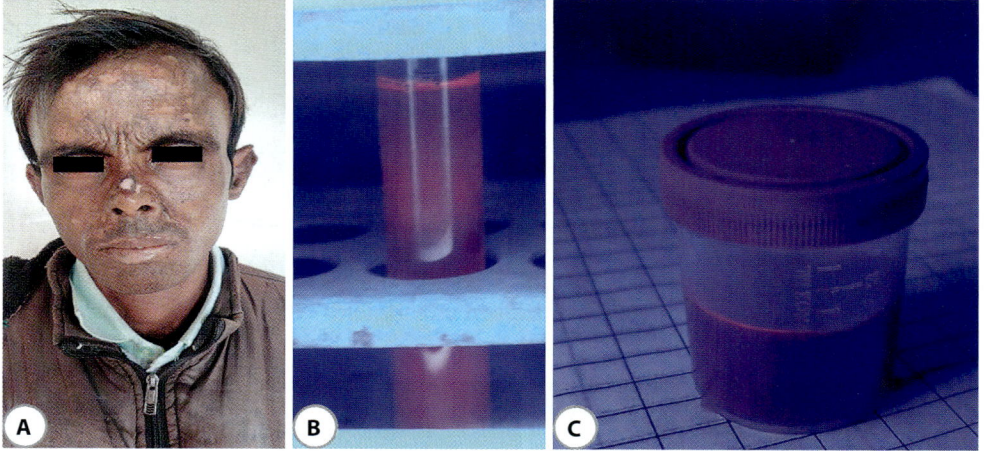

FIGS. 47A TO C: Coral red florescence in Günther's disease.

Interpretation
- *Vitiligo*: Porcelain-white florescence **(Figures 44A and B)**
- *Pityriasis versicolor and Tinea capitis*: **(Figures 45A and B)**

Steps of Mineral Oil Preparation
Steps of mineral oil preparation are given in **Figures 48A to E**

Lichen planus **(Figs. 49A and B):**
- Apply a drop of oil on surface of papule.
- See with dermatoscope.
- It is seen due to increased granular cell layer.

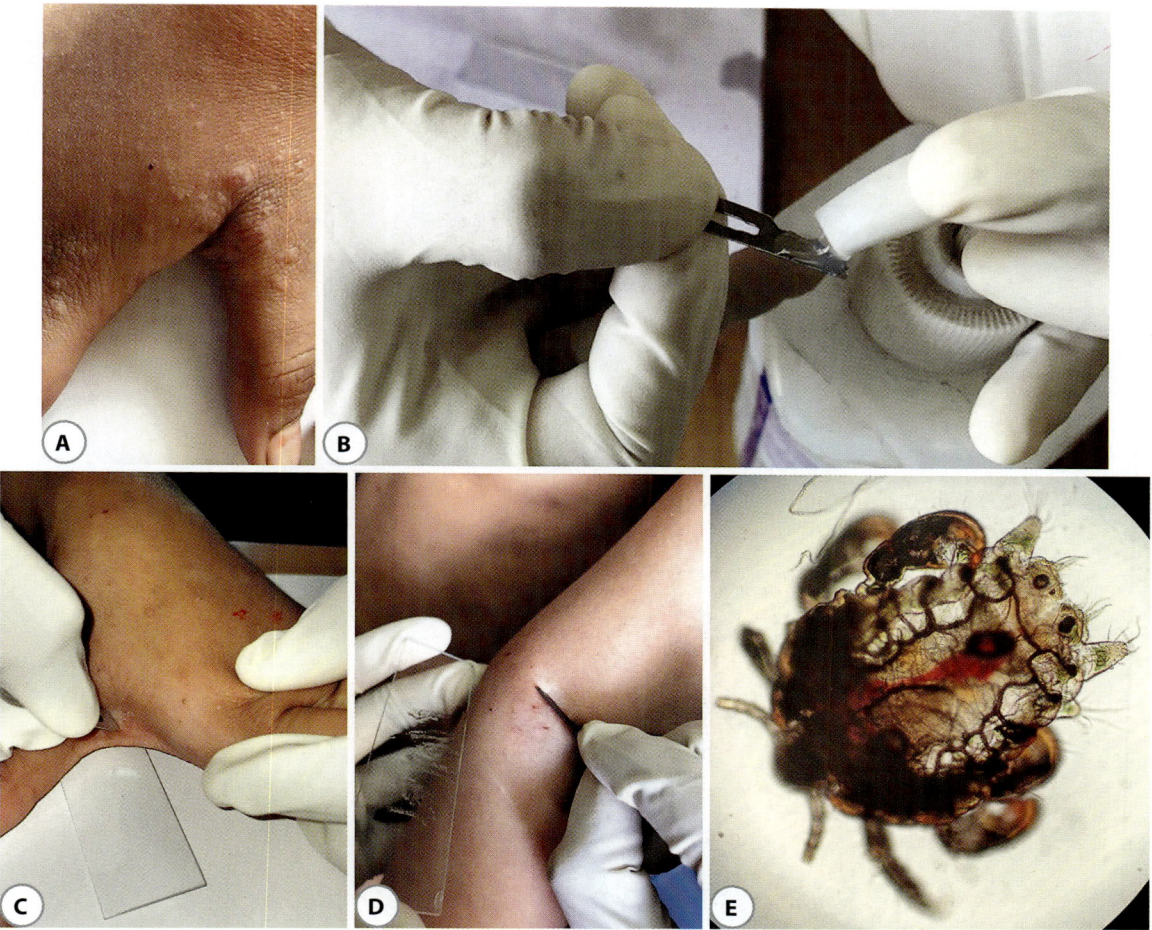

FIGS. 48A TO E: (A and B) 15 no. scalpel is dipped in mineral oil to provide viscous surface so that scales, mite, and debris can adhere easily; (C) Scabietic burrow is scraped with a 15 no. scalpel blade; (D) Transfer the scraping to glass slide; and (E) Mite seen under microscope.

HAIR PULL TEST[11]

Hair pull test is shown in **Figure 50**.

Prerequisites:
- No shampooing for 24 hours
- Grab approximately 60 hairs.
- Pull gently to slightly raise the scalp skin.
- Keeping a constant pull, fingers are moved toward the distal end of the hairs
- Proportion of hairs epilated are counted.
- *10% or more* epilated hairs indicates severe and active hair loss

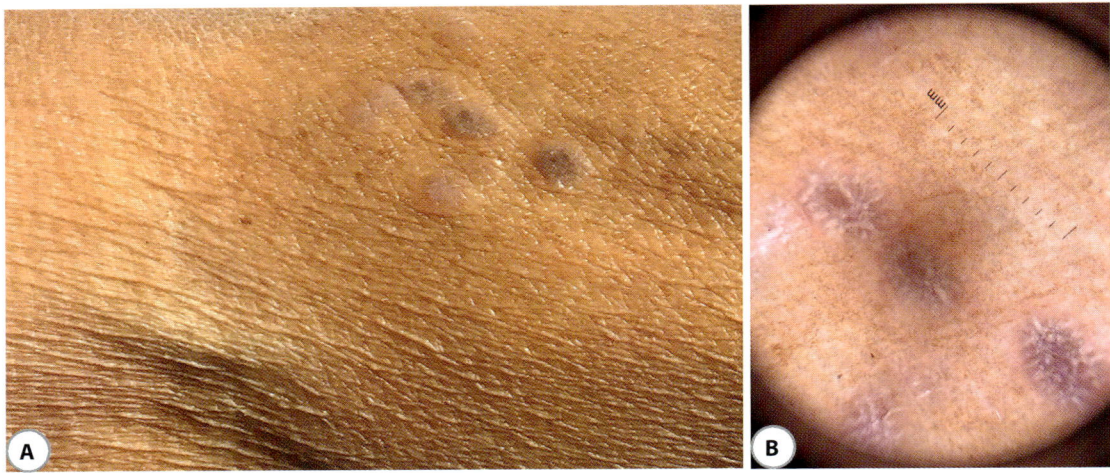

FIGS. 49A AND B: (A) Lichen planus; and (B) Wickham's striae.

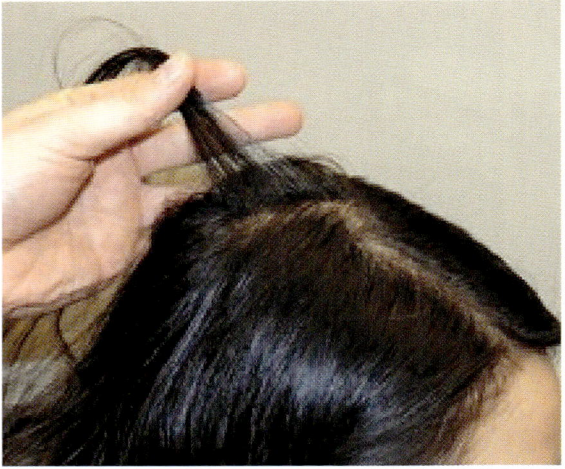

FIG. 50: Hair pull test.

- This test is based on the concept of "gentle" pulling of the hair to bring about shedding of telogen hairs.
- *The test is positive in cases of:*
    - Telogen effluvium
    - Anagen effluvium
    - Loose anagen syndrome
    - Early cases of patterned alopecia
    - Advancing edge of alopecia areata
- Negative tests do not exclude the diagnosis.

PATHERGY TEST

Pathergy test is defined as a state of *altered tissue reactivity* that occurs *in response to* minor *trauma*.

Pathogenesis[12]

Skin injury by needle prick triggers a cutaneous inflammatory response leading to *increased release of cytokines in the epidermis or dermis* resulting in a *perivascular infiltration* observed on skin biopsy.

Conditions with positive pathergy phenomenon:
- Behçet's disease **(Figs. 51A and B)**
- Pyoderma gangrenosum
- Sweets syndrome
- Eosinophilic pustular folliculitis
- Inflammatory bowel disease
- *Site:* A hairless area on the *flexor aspect of the forearms* is usually chosen as the test site.
- 20–22 gauge sterile *needle* is inserted *vertically or diagonally* at an angle of 45° to a *depth of 3–5 mm*. The needle should reach the *dermis* for a proper response.
- Readings are taken after *48 hours* of the needle prick.
- A *1–2 mm papule* that is usually felt by palpation and which is surrounded by an erythematous halo is formed on the skin.
- *Erythema without induration is interpreted as a negative result.*

Oral Pathergy

Oral pathergy is given in **Figures 51A and B**.
Pustule or ulcer of any size is considered positive.

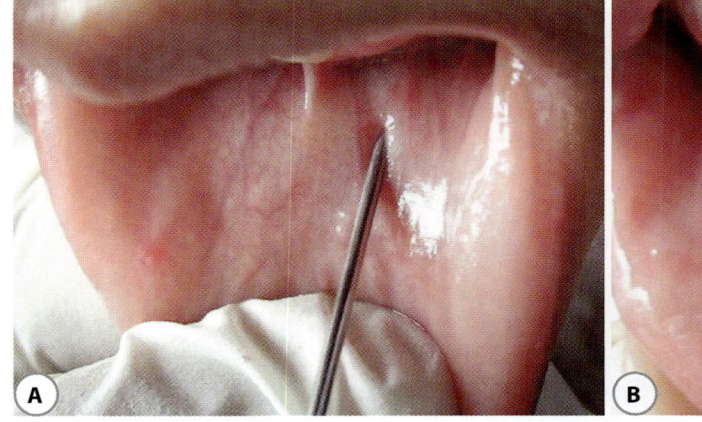
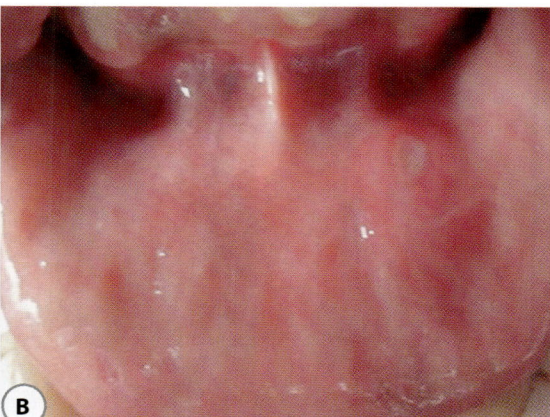

FIGS. 51A AND B: Oral pathergy.

TESTS FOR SEXUALLY TRANSMITTED INFECTIONS

Gram's Stain

Urethral Discharge

Urethral discharge is shown in **Figure 52**.
- *Neisseria gonorrhoeae*
- *Chlamydia trachomatis*
- *Trichomonas vaginalis*
- *Mycoplasma genitalium*
- Herpes simplex virus (HSV)
- *Adenovirus*

Sampling Technique
- *Site*: Men/women–urethral/rectal/oropharynx/endocervical canal and vagina
- *Rectal swab:* Proctoscope–swab stick 3 cm into anal canal and rotate for 10 seconds.
- *Pharyngeal swab:* Tonsillar crypts and bed of the pharynx

Results
- Gonorrhea
- More than 5 neutrophils per oil immersion field (1,000×) in urethral smear in the absence of gram-negative, intracellular diplococci is suggestive of nongonococcal urethritis **(Fig. 53)**.

Genital Ulcer Disease
- *Treponema pallidum* (syphilis) **(Fig. 54)**
- *Haemophilus ducreyi* (chancroid) **(Figs. 55A and B)**
- *Calymmatobacterium granulomatis* [Granuloma inguinale (GI)]
- *Chlamydia trachomatis* [lymphogranuloma venereum (LGV)]
- *Haemophilus ducreyi* **(Figs. 56A and B)**, school-of-fish appearance

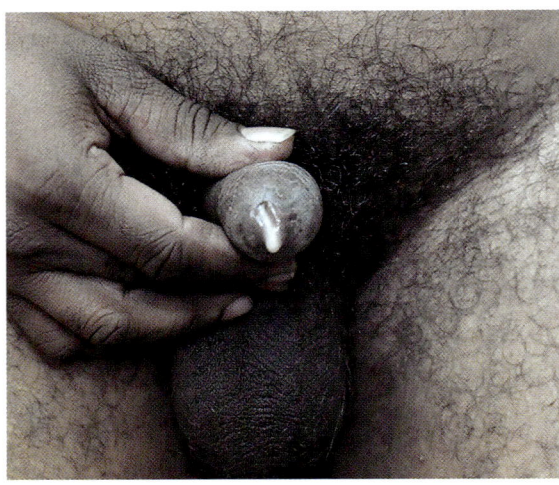

FIG. 52: Urethral discharge.

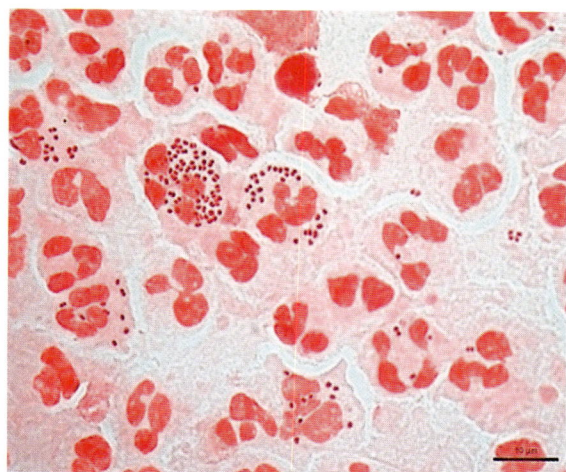

FIG. 53: Gram-negative intracellular diplococci.

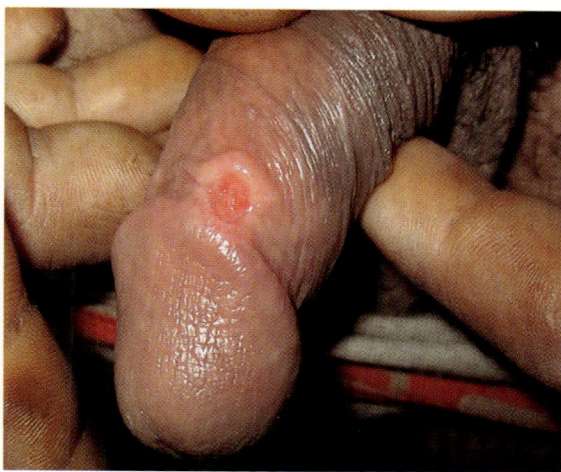

FIG. 54: Primary chancre.

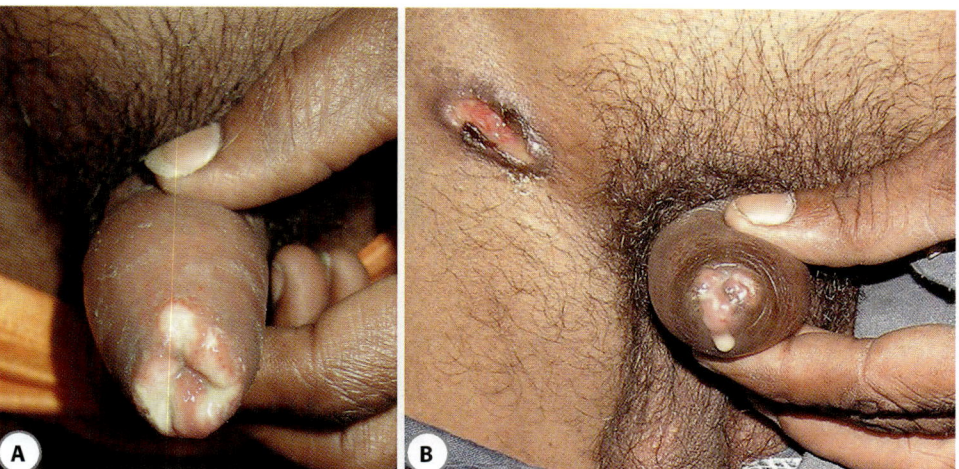

FIGS. 55A AND B: (A) Chancroid- multiple ulcers covered with slough; and (B) Chandroidal ulcer in groin, sub-preputial discharge.

- A small piece of tissue should be obtained from the ulcer edge using curettage, blade, or forceps.
- Place the specimen on one glass slide and crush it between two glass slides *(Rajam and Rangiah method)*.
- Stain with Leishman/Giemsa stain **(Figs. 57A and B)**.

Dark Ground Microscopy

Principle of dark ground microscopy is shown in **Figure 58**.

Condenser prevents the transmitted light from directly illuminating the specimen.

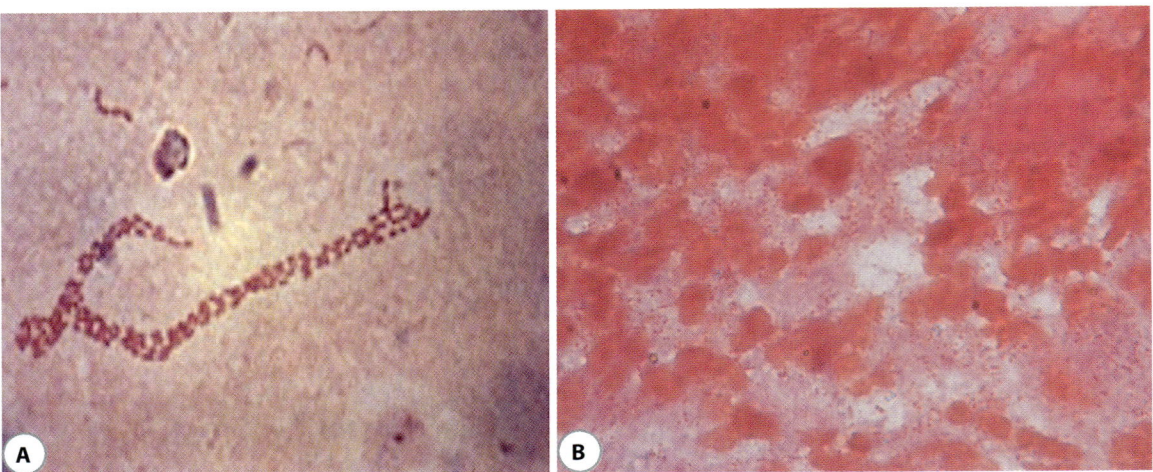

FIGS. 56A AND B: Crushed smear preparation—"School of fish" appearance.

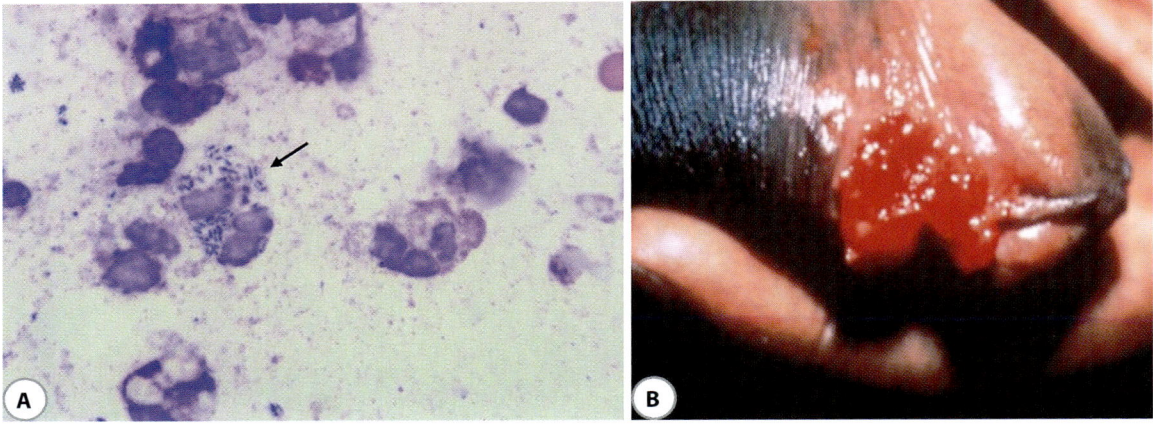

FIGS. 57A AND B: Granuloma inguinale: (A) Safety pin appearance in Giemsa stain; and (B) Beefy red ulcer.

Principle[13]

Only oblique scattered light reaches the specimen and passes onto the lens system causing the object to appear bright against a dark background.

Method

- Do not use antiseptics. Use saline or tap water.
- Compress the base of lesion to accumulate clear serum exudes.
- Collect the specimen by pressing the glass slide directly onto the lesion.
- Examine immediately to see *T. pallidum* **(Fig. 59)**

Chapter 13: Bedside Tests in Dermatology

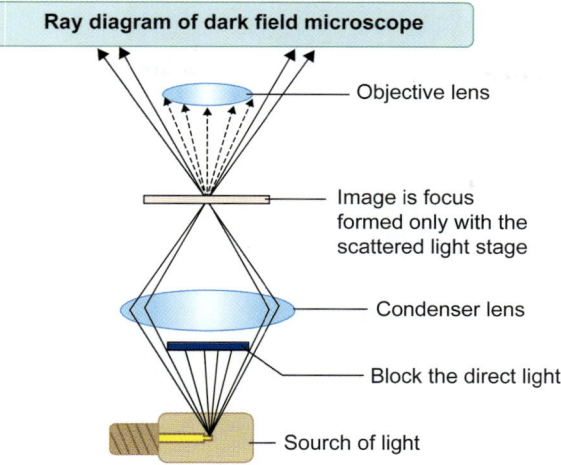

FIG. 58: Principles of dark ground microscopy.

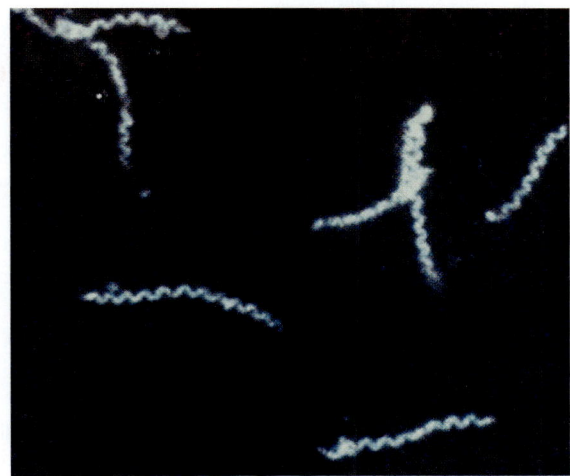

FIG. 59: *Treponema pallidum* as seen in disseminated gonococcal infection (DGI).

Wet Mount Preparation (Figs. 60 to 62)
Vaginitis
- *Trichomonas vaginalis*
- *Candida albicans*
- *Gardnerella vaginalis*
- *Mycoplasma, Ureaplasma,* and anaerobes

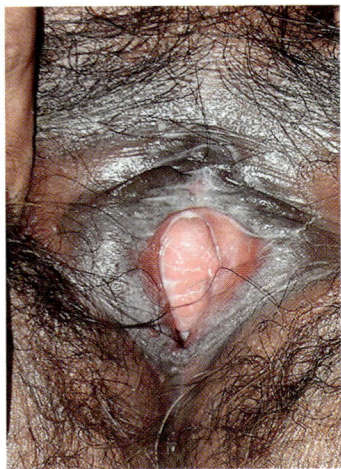

FIG. 60: Vaginal discharge.

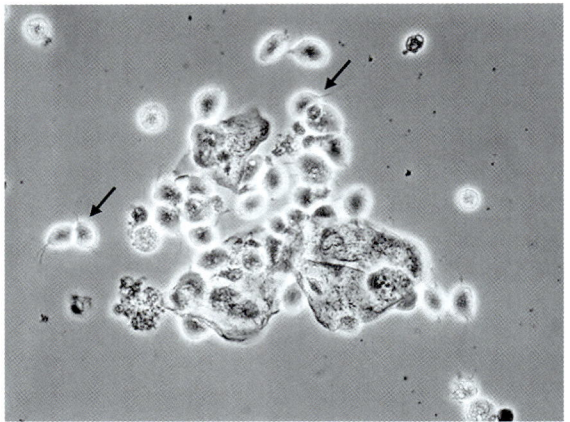

FIG. 61: Motile trichomonads in wet mount.

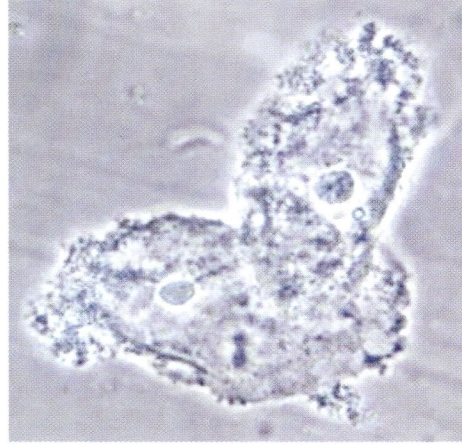

FIG. 62: Clue cells—vaginal epithelial cell studded with coccobacilli.

Cervicitis

- *Neisseria gonorrhoeae*
- *Chlamydia trachomatis*
- *Trichomonas vaginalis*
- HSV

Sampling Technique
- Speculum examination
- Vaginal swab is collected from posterior fornix using a sterile swab.
- The specimen is mixed with a drop of normal saline on a slide.
  Using warmed saline or warming the slide enhances the motility of the trichomonads.
- Trichomonas vaginalis

REFERENCES

1. Mittwer T, Bartholomew JW, Kallman BJ. The mechanism of the gram reaction. II. The function of iodine in the gram stain. Stain Technol. 1950;25(4):169-79.
2. Weinberg JM, Koestenblatt EK, Tutrone WD, Tishler HR, Najarian L. Comparison of diagnostic methods in the evaluation of onychomycosis. J Am Acad Dermatol. 2003;49(2):193-7.
3. Durdu M, Baba M, Seçkin D. The value of Tzanck smear test in diagnosis of erosive, vesicular, bullous, and pustular skin lesions. J Am Acad Dermatol. 2008;59(6):958-64.
4. Micheletti RG, Dominguez AR, Wanat KA. Bedside diagnostics in dermatology: Parasitic and noninfectious diseases. J Am Acad Dermatol. 2017;77(2):221-30.
5. Banerjee S, Biswas N, Kanti Das N, Sil A, Ghosh P, Hasanoor Raja AH, et al. Diagnosing leprosy: Revisiting the role of the slit-skin smear with critical analysis of the applicability of polymerase chain reaction in diagnosis. Int J Dermatol. 2011;50(12):1522-7.
6. Rudd M, Eversole R, Carpenter W. Diascopy: A clinical technique for the diagnosis of vascular lesions. Gen Dent. 2001;49(2):206-9.
7. Kaliyadan F. The scope of the dermoscope. Indian Dermatol Online J. 2016;7(5):359-63.
8. Rakowska A, Slowinska M, Kowalska-Oledzka E, Warszawik O, Czuwara J, Olszewska M, et al. Trichoscopy of cicatricial alopecia. J Drugs Dermatol. 2012;11(6):753-8.
9. Bolognia JL, Schaffer JV, Cerroni L. Dermatology, 4th edition. Amsterdam: Elsevier; 2017. p. 685
10. Mora ER, Martínez AF, Hernández-Núñez A, Martínez JB. Trichomycosis axillaris: Clinical, Wood lamp, and dermoscopic diagnostic images. Actas dermosifiliogr. 2017;108(3):264-6.
11. Jackson AJ, Price VH. How to diagnose hair loss. Dermatol Clin. 2013;31(1):21-8.
12. Ozluk E, Balta I, Akoguz O, Kalkan G, Astarci M, Akbay G, et al. Histopathologic study of pathergy test in Behçet's disease. Indian J Dermatol. 2014;59(6):630.
13. Sastry AS, Bhat SK. Essential of Medical Microbiology. 1st edition. New Delhi: Jaypee Brothers Medical Publishers (P) Ltd.; 2016. pp. 527-38.

CHAPTER 14

Signs in Dermatology

PSORIASIS

Auspitz Sign

Auspitz sign is named after Heinrich Auspitz, described originally in psoriasis, but also present in actinic keratosis and Darier's disease. It is described as the pinpoint bleeding seen on removal of Buckley's membrane due to increase in vasculature and suprapapillary thinning.

CONNECTIVE TISSUE DISEASES

Lupus Erythematosus

- *Carpet tack sign (Tin-tack sign and cat tongue sign)*: In cases of discoid lupus erythematosus, on removal of adherent scales, horny plugging is seen that has occupied patulous hair follicles. This sign is also seen in seborrheic dermatitis.
- *Shuster's sign*: Cribriform scarring of the concha after a plaque of discoid lupus erythematosus is called Shuster's sign.
- *Heugh–Gottron sign*: It is dystrophic and ragged cuticle seen in lupus erythematosus.
- *Raccoon sign*: In neonatal lupus erythematosus, an erythematous, slightly scaly eruption is present on the face, especially periorbitally resembling the eyes of a raccoon

Systemic Sclerosis

- *Ingram's sign*: It is the inability to retract the lower eyelid.
- Mizutani's *sign* (Round *finger pad sign*)**:** The name describes the sign itself. It refers to the round appearance of the finger pad rather than a peaked contour on finger pads. It is most obviously seen on the ring finger.
- *Stafne's sign*: It is the widening of the periodontal ligament space secondary to increase in the collagen synthesis and increase in the bulk of the ligament, accommodated at the expense of alveolar bone, thus causing an increase in the width of the periodontal ligament space.
- *Barnett's sign (scleroderma neck sign)*: It is ridging and tightening of the skin of the neck on extending the head with a visible and palpable tight band over platysma in the hyperextended neck.

Dermatomyositis

- *Samitz's sign*: Dystrophic and ragged cuticle seen in dermatomyositis
- *Holster sign of dermatomyositis*: Confluent macular violaceous erythema and edema present on the lateral side of hip and thighs (the holster area)
- *Gottron's sign*: Confluent macular violaceous erythema and edema seen on the dorsa of hands, metacarpophalangeal joints, and proximal interphalangeal joints collectively is called Gottron's sign.
- *Shawl sign*: Confluent macular violaceous erythema and edema on the posterior neck and shoulders
- *V-sign*: Confluent macular violaceous erythema and edema on the anterior neck and chest in patients of dermatomyositis is called "V" sign.

AUTOIMMUNE BULLOUS DISORDERS

Asboe-Hansen Sign (Blister Spread Sign)

Gustav Asboe Hansen first described this sign in 1960, when he demonstrated enlargement of bulla by applying finger pressure to small, intact, and tense bulla in patients with pemphigus and bullous pemphigoid. In the traditional bulla spread sign, pressure is applied to the blister from one side, whereas in eliciting Asboe-Hansen sign, pressure is applied at the center of the blister and perpendicular to the surface due to smaller size of the lesion.

Nikolsky's Sign

Nikolsky's sign is named after the Russian dermatologist Pyotr Vasilyevich Nikolsky who described it in 1894. It is a popular and respected sign in dermatology, which refers to easy peeling of skin on applying tangential pressure over a bony prominence and classically seen in pemphigus, toxic epidermal necrolysis (TEN), and staphylococcal-scalded skin syndrome. Nikolsky's sign can also be elicited in the oral cavity with the help of cotton-tipped applicator.

Hypopyon Sign

Hypopyon sign describes the presence of small, discrete, vesicles either flaccid or tense that become secondarily infected and pus accumulates in the lower half of the pustule. It is a clinical sign seen in pyodermas and secondarily infected vesiculobullous disorders [e.g., pemphigus, bullous pemphigoid, and linear immunoglobulin A (IgA) dermatosis], where there is a transverse fluid level comprising of purulent material at the bottom when the patient is in a standing position and is called hypopyon sign.

ERYTHRODERMA

Deck-chair Sign

Though classically described in papuloerythroderma of Ofuji, characterized by sparing of abdominal body folds, it can also be seen in case of erythroderma.

Pavithran Nose Sign

Pavithran nose sign is sparing of the nose and perinasal areas in case of erythroderma.

STEVENS–JOHNSON SYNDROME/TOXIC EPIDERMAL NECROLYSIS

Pseudo-Nikolsky Sign

Pseudo-Nikolsky sign is elicited by applying tangential pressure on erythematous/dusky skin in patients with Stevens–Johnson's syndrome (SJS). It is also known as epidermal peeling sign. Underlying pathology is necrosis of the cells in SJS/TEN.

LEPROSY

Tinel Sign

Tapping over the feeding nerve results in tingling sensation over the area supplied by the nerve.

Froment's Sign

The adductor pollicis muscle is supplied by the ulnar nerve. Book test is performed by asking the patient to hold a book between the thumb and side of the index finger. If the adductor muscle of the thumb is paralysed, flexion of the interphalangeal joint takes place. This is known as Froment's sign positive.

Wartenberg Sign

Wartenberg sign is used in the evaluation of ulnar nerve. The patient is asked to adduct all the fingers with the metacarpophalangeal, proximal interphalangeal, and distal phalangeal joints extended. If the little finger drifts away into abduction, Wartenberg sign is positive.

Frequently Asked Questions in Dermatology

Q.1. What is red dermographism?
Ans. *Red dermographism* refers to a skin reaction to superficial trauma that differs from typical dermographism. It is triggered more easily by rubbing and results in an erythematous band where a diffuse, palpable wheal appears. This reaction is most noticeable when the skin is stretched and is often associated with cholinergic dysfunction, especially in children with autism.
- *White dermographism* is a blanching response caused by capillary vasoconstriction following skin stroking. It is more commonly observed in individuals with atopic conditions.
- *Yellow dermographism* likely occurs due to the deposition of bile pigments in the skin.

Q.2. What is black dermographism?
Ans. *Black dermographism:* This is a black or greenish discoloration of the skin occurring after contact with certain metallic objects.

Q.3. State the importance of Dead Sea in dermatology.
Ans. The Dead Sea derives its name from the fact that its high salinity prevents the survival of most forms of life. Located about 400 meters below sea level, it holds the distinction of being the lowest point on Earth that is inhabited and is also the world's most hypersaline lake. Renowned for its balneologic properties and for providing climatotherapy, the Dead Sea is particularly beneficial for treating dermatological and rheumatological conditions. Its unique mineral composition, combined with the thick haze over the area and filtered sunlight, are key factors contributing to its balneologic properties.
- The salt concentration of the Dead Sea is around 320 g/L, predominantly consisting of potassium chloride, magnesium chloride, calcium chloride, and sodium chloride, along with their bromides. Overall, the salinity makes up 33% of the lake's content, far higher than the ocean's typical 3%. Studies have shown that regular bathing in the Dead Sea's mineral-rich waters can help treat certain skin conditions, with the minerals penetrating the skin and offering therapeutic benefits.
- Another notable feature of the Dead Sea is its "black mud", which is rich in organic compounds and known as "bituminous tar". This mud is prized for its high mineral content and its ability to retain heat, which aids in improving blood circulation and removing dead skin cells, contributing to skin rejuvenation.
- The mineral-rich haze that envelops the Dead Sea also plays a role in its therapeutic effects. Inhalation of bromides, which are natural sedatives, has been found to improve the condition of individuals with psoriasis, particularly those whose condition is exacerbated by stress.

- Additionally, the local drinking water contains a high concentration of bromine, which can enter the body through the skin. While less effective than inhalation, this exposure still provides calming and anti-inflammatory benefits. Bromine is also known for its antibiotic properties, making it helpful in treating inflammatory and dry skin disorders like psoriasis, eczema, and ichthyosis.

Q.4. What is black box warning?
Ans. A black box warning is the strictest warning put in the labeling of prescription drugs or drug products by the Food and Drug Administration (FDA) when serious adverse reactions or special problems occur, particularly those that may lead to death or serious injury.

Q.5. What is black triangle?
Ans. When a medicine is first licensed for use in clinical practice, the number of patients that have been exposed is generally relatively small compared to the number that will eventually receive it. Relatively uncommon reactions may, therefore, not have been detected. New medicines are marked with a black triangle (▼).

Therefore, all reactions (minor or serious) to any medicines with the black triangle symbol (▼) should be reported.

Q.6. Describe Coast of Maine versus Coast of California.
Ans. The irregular borders of the café-au-lait spots in McCune–Albright syndrome are often compared to a map of the Coast of Maine. By contrast, café-au-lait spots in other disorders such as neurofibromatosis (NF) have smooth borders, which are compared to the Coast of California.

Q.7. What are Lisch nodules?
Ans. These are iris melanocytic hamartomas, associated with NF type 1 (NF-1). When present in multiple numbers, these lesions are considered a key diagnostic feature of NF-1. They are found in over 90% of individuals with NF-1 by the time they reach their second decade of life.

Q.8. What is an "id reaction"?
Ans. Id reaction is an immunologically driven skin inflammation that occurs without the presence of a viable organism or other local triggers. It typically manifests as an acute, papulovesicular rash located away from the original area of dermatitis. The papules and vesicles often merge together. This condition is also referred to as autosensitization dermatitis.

Q.9. What is the significance of rapid plasma reagin (RPR) titers?
Ans. In the RPR test for syphilis, the sample is initially tested undiluted. If the result is positive, the sample is then diluted with an equal volume of diluent. If the diluted sample remains positive, it is reported as a 1:2 result. Further dilutions are made (1:4, 1:8, 1:16, 1:32, etc.), and if a dilution still produces a positive result, the corresponding titer is noted. If a sample with a 1:32 dilution turns negative after further dilution (e.g., 1:64), the highest positive dilution is recorded as 1:32. A decreasing titer after treatment indicates that the patient is responding to the therapy.

Q.10. What is Hoigné's syndrome?
Ans. Hoigné's syndrome refers to psychosis and seizures following the injection of procaine penicillin. It is an acute, toxic, nonallergic reaction to the intramuscular administration of aqueous penicillin G procaine. The reaction is to the procaine and not to the penicillin component. Treatment given is intravenous (IV)/intravascular (IM) diazepam.

Q.11. What is Brocq's phenomenon?
Ans. Brocq's phenomenon refers to the occurrence of subepidermal hemorrhage when a classical lichen planus lesion is gently scraped. This differs from psoriasis, where scratching the lesion surface typically leads to pinpoint bleeding.

Q.12. What is Job's syndrome?
Ans. It is one of the immunodeficiency syndrome characterized by recurrent episodes of eczema, increased susceptibility to sinopulmonary infections, and markedly raised levels of immunoglobulin E (IgE).

Q.13. What is normal chest expansion?
Ans. Normal chest expansion in healthy adults varies as per age. In 18–34 years age group, it is 3.74 cm for female and 3.72 cm for male; in 35–64 years age group, it is 3.57 cm for female and 3.66 cm for male; and in those of 65 years and more, it is 2.63 cm for female and 2.66 cm for male.

Q.14. What is repeated open application test (ROAT)?
Ans. Repeated open application test is a cruder and cheaper form of thin-layer rapid-use epicutaneous (TRUE) test. In repeated open application test, patients apply the suspected product to a quarter sized area on the forearm twice a day for 1 week. If patient is allergic, local reaction will occur confirming allergy. Patch testing is one-time occlusive test that does not always duplicate low level chronic daily exposure.

Q.15. What is Quinquaud's disease?
Ans. Folliculitis decalvans, also known as Quinquaud's disease, is a rare type of scarring hair loss characterized by the development of follicular pustules, which can form annular or circinate patterns. These pustules quickly develop into crusts, ultimately leading to permanent hair loss due to scarring.

Q.16. What is accelerated nodulosis?
Ans. Accelerated nodulosis refers to the swift appearance of rheumatoid nodules in a small number of patients undergoing methotrexate treatment. These nodules usually shrink or disappear once the medication is stopped and can return if methotrexate is reintroduced.

Q.17. Enumerate types of calcinosis cutis.
Ans.
- *Dystrophic calcinosis cutis:* It is the deposition of calcium salts in inflamed or damaged tissue. Metabolism of calcium and phosphorous is normal. It may be localized, such as within acne scars or epidermoid cyst, or widespread. It is seen in dermatomyositis or scleroderma.
- *Metastatic calcinosis cutis:* It is seen in chronic kidney disease (CKD) patients with aberrations in calcium or phosphorus metabolism. Serum calcium–phosphorus is elevated.
- *Idiopathic calcinosis cutis:* It occurs when no underlying cause is identified for tissue calcification.

Q.18. What is Meirowsky phenomenon?
Ans. It is also called immediate pigment darkening (IPD). Darkening of existing melanin, perhaps by oxidation, begins within seconds and completes within minutes to a few hours after exposure to ultraviolet (UV) radiation of longer wavelengths; it is particularly noticeable in light-skinned individuals. IPD is not photoprotective as it does not lead to a hardening effect as seen in delayed tanning.

Q.19. What is persistent light reactivity?

Ans. In cases of persistent light reactivity, photodermatitis is thought to be caused by topical or systemic medications that continue to affect the skin long after the suspected trigger has been stopped. Patients with this condition may experience heightened sensitivity to light, including visible light, and can become severely debilitated by the condition.

Q.20. What is the difference between hydroa aestivale and hydroa vacciniforme?

Ans. The difference between hydroa aestivale and hydroa vacciniforme is given in **Table 1**.

TABLE 1: Difference between hydroa aestivale and hydroa vacciniforme.		
Characteristics	**Hydroa aestivale (actinic prurigo)**	**Hydroa vacciniforme (Bazin's hydroa vacciniforme)**
Onset	Childhood onset, often resolution by adolescence or can persist indefinitely	• Childhood onset, remitting by adolescence • Occurs acutely within few hours of sun exposure
Sex	Girls are mostly affected	Both sexes affected
Distribution of lesions	Face, ears, and extremities, also in photo protected parts (buttocks, etc.)	Face and dorsa of hands
Morphology of lesions	Erythematous papulonodular lesion with hemorrhagic crusting	Papules and plaques develop umbilicated vesiculation followed by hemorrhagic crusting and varioliform scarring

Q.21. Describe features of Moynahan's syndrome.

Ans. Patients with Moynahan's syndrome have many lentigines on face, trunk, and extremities. Mnemonic LEOPARD has been applied to the clinical symptoms associated with this syndrome.
- *L*entigines
- *E*lectrocardiographic defects
- *O*cular hypertelorism
- *P*ulmonary stenosis
- *A*bnormal genitalia
- *R*etarded growth
- *D*eafness

Q.22. What is pyoderma faciale?

Ans. Pyoderma faciale is an acute disease of women aged 15–40 years with no previous history of acne. Pyoderma faciale is characterized by severe pustules, nodules, cysts, and draining sinus tracts. History of flushing is present in many patients and some authors consider it as severe variant of acne rosacea.

Q.23. What are satellite warts?

Ans. Satellite warts or fairy ring warts are annular warts that may develop after treatment that produces blisters [e.g., liquid nitrogen and topical 5-Fluorouracil (5-FU) bleomycin].

Q.24. What is blueberry muffin baby?

Ans. This term applies to babies exhibiting blue–red or indurated macules or papules on the face, trunk, or scalp present at birth or within first 2 days of life. They represent extramedullary dermal erythropoiesis and is seen in congenital rubella syndrome, toxoplasmosis, cytomegalovirus infection, neuroblastoma, leukemia, erythroblastosis fetalis, and twin transfusion syndrome.

Q.25. Describe pseudoporphyria.

Ans. Pseudoporphyria is a bullous photosensitivity that clinically and histologically mimics porphyria cutanea tarda (PCT).

No abnormalities are found in serum or urine porphyrin.
- *Pathophysiology:* It is not fully understood. Phototoxic injury to the dermal microvascular endothelium leads to a subepidermal split beneath the basal lamina.
- *Epidemiology:*
    - Race—fair skinned people are at risk
    - Age—2-81 years
- *Causes:* Chronic renal failure patients treated with hemodialysis:
    - Nonsteroidal anti-inflammatory drugs (NSAIDs)
    - Antibiotics—tetracycline, nalidixic acid, cefepime, and fluoroquinolones
    - Antifungals—voriconazole
    - Diuretics—furosemide, chlorthalidone, and bumetanide
    - Chemotherapy—5-FU
    - Sulfone—dapsone
    - Vitamin A derivatives—isotretinoin
    - Others—oral contraceptive pills, muscle relaxants, and narrowband ultraviolet B (Nb-UVB)
- *Clinical features:*
    - Increased skin fragility, erythema, appearance of tense bullae, and erosions on sun exposed skin
    - Classic features of hypertrichosis, hyperpigmentation, and sclerodermoid changes found with PCT are unusual with pseudoporphyria
    - Pseudoporphyria that mimics erythropoietic protoporphyria is seen in children taking naproxen for juvenile rheumatoid arthritis.
- *Differential diagnosis:*
    - Bullous pemphigoid
    - Epidermolysis bullosa
    - Epidermolysis bullosa acquisita
    - Bullous lupus erythematosus (LE)
    - PCT
    - Erythropoietic protoporphyria.
- *Treatment:*
    - Photoprotection—use of broad-spectrum sunscreens.
    - Avoidance of offending drugs.
- *Prognosis:* Good if offending agent is removed but patients are left with permanent scarring.

Q.26. What are the causes of acquired cutis laxa.

Causes of acquired cutis laxa are:
- Hypersensitivity reactions to penicillins or other drugs
- Systemic lupus erythematosus (SLE)
- Sarcoidosis
- Systemic amyloidosis
- Multiple myeloma
- Rheumatoid arthritis
- Nephrotic syndrome
- Celiac disease

- Syphilis
- Alpha-1 antitrypsin deficiency
- Following episodes of urticaria or angioedema
- Inflammatory skin diseases—eczema and erythema multiforme

Q.27. Name the syndromes associated with sarcoidosis.

Ans. Various syndromes associated with sarcoidosis are:
- Heerfordt's syndrome
- Lofgren's syndrome
- Sarcoidosis-lymphoma syndrome
- Melkersson–Rosenthal syndrome
- Blau syndrome
- Sjögren's syndrome
- Mikulicz's syndrome

Q.28. Enumerate causes of palmoplantar pits.

Ans. The causes of palmoplantar pits are:
- Cowden syndrome
- Nevoid basal cell carcinoma syndrome (Bazex syndrome)
- Keratosis follicularis
- Darier's disease
- Keratosis punctata of palmar creases
- Cole disease
- Buschke–Fischer–Brauer disease (punctate palmoplantar keratoderma type-1)
- Pitted keratolysis

Q.29. What are the various indications of UVA-1?

Ans. The various indications of UVA-1 are:
- Scleroderma
- Morphea
- Mycosis fungoides
- Lichen sclerosus et atrophicus
- Scleredema
- Granuloma annulare
- Pityriasis lichenoides chronica
- SLE
- Necrobiosis lipoidica
- Sarcoidosis
- Graft-versus-host disease
- Granulomatous slack skin
- Vitiligo

Q.30. What are the indications of UVB therapy?

Ans.
- Psoriasis
- Vitiligo
- Atopic dermatitis

Other non-FDA approved indications are lichen planus, pruritus in human immunodeficiency virus (HIV), actinic prurigo, mycosis fungoides, parapsoriasis, pityriasis rubra pilaris, scleroderma, seborrheic dermatitis, and polymorphic light eruptions.

Q.31. What are the differential diagnoses of sterile pustules.

Ans. Differential diagnoses of sterile pustules are:
- Eosinophilic folliculitis (Ofuji's disease)
- Subcorneal pustular dermatosis (Sneddon–Wilkinson's disease)
- Infantile acropustulosis
- Acrodermatitis continua of Hallopeau
- Pustular drug rash secondary to epidermal growth factor receptor (EGFR) inhibitors
- Acute generalized exanthematous pustulosis (AGEP)
- Generalized pustular psoriasis (von Zumbusch type)
- Transient neonatal pustular melanosis
- Pustulosis palmaris et plantaris (PPP).

Q.32. What is homeostatic model assessment of insulin resistance (HOMA-IR) and β-cell function (HOMA-β)?

Ans. "Homeostatic model assessment of insulin resistance (IR) and β-cell function (β)" is used to assess insulin resistance and β-cell function through fasting insulin and sugar levels or C-peptide levels.

$$\text{HOMA-IR} = \text{fasting insulin (mIU/L)} \times \text{fasting glucose (mg/dL)}/405.$$

Interpretation:
- Normal <3
- Moderate insulin resistance 3–5
- Severe insulin resistance >5.

Q.33. What is quantitative insulin sensitivity check index (QUICKI)?

Ans. "Quantitative insulin sensitivity check index" or QUICKI is used to monitor insulin sensitivity in type 2 diabetes mellitus patients through fasting blood samples.
It is calculated as follows:

$$\text{QUICKI} = 1/[\log(I0) + \log(G0)]$$

Where I0 = Fasting insulin level and G0 = fasting glucose levels.

Q.34. Explain the mode of action of LASERS.

Ans. *LASER is an acronym:* Light amplification by stimulated emission of radiation.

Lasers are sources of high intensity light with the following properties:
- Monochromatic, i.e., the light is of a single wavelength
- Coherent, i.e., the light beam waves are in phase
- Collimated, i.e., the light beams travel in parallel.

Mechanism of action of lasers:
- *Selective photothermolysis:* Different wavelengths of lasers are varyingly absorbed by various chromophore producing localized and selective tissue destruction.

- *Photothermal effect:* Heat produced by laser produces destruction of tissues.
- *Thermomechanical effect:* Attainment of very high temperatures rapidly causes disruption of cells due to pressure, cavitation, and differential expansion.
- *Photoacoustic effect:* High energy pulses cause fragmentation and shattering of pigments.

Q.35. What is R20 protocol?
Ans. This protocol is used for pigment removal as in nevus of Ota or tattoo removal.
- 4 LASER treatments spaced 20 minutes apart in 1 day, repeated after 4–6 weeks.
- When using R20 protocol, it is advised to use fluence level 50–70% lower than standard.
- The 20 minutes wait period time allows laser frosting or whitening that occurs in response to Q-switched laser to subside, thus, preventing next pulses of energy from being blocked.
- Advantage of this protocol are low cost of treatment and faster removal of tattoo.

Q.36. What is trichoscopy?
Ans. The term "trichoscopy" was introduced in 2006 by Lidia Rudnicka and Malgorzata Olszewska. It refers to the use of dermoscopy to examine the scalp and hair. This innovative, noninvasive technique provides a simple yet effective bedside method for diagnosing various common hair and scalp conditions.

Trichoscopic findings can generally be categorized into hair signs, vascular patterns, pigment patterns, and interfollicular patterns. In addition to aiding in the diagnosis of alopecia, trichoscopy can help avoid unnecessary biopsies. When a biopsy is necessary, it assists in selecting the most appropriate site. Furthermore, trichoscopy serves as a valuable tool for tracking treatment progress through photographic evaluation during follow-up visits.

Q.37. State the use of statins in dermatology.
Ans. Statins are competitive inhibitors of 3-hydroxy-3-methylglutaryl coenzyme A (HMG-CoA) reductase.
- Include atorvastatin, cerivastatin, fluvastatin, pravastatin, lovastatin, and simvastatin.
- Reduce lipoprotein C level. Its main indication is in atherosclerosis.
- In dermatology, it is used to combat hyperlipidemia caused by retinoids and cyclosporine A.

Off-label uses—alopecia areata, vitiligo, lichen planus, subacute cutaneous LE, erythema multiforme, psoriasis, bullous pemphigoid, systemic sclerosis (SSc), mycosis fungoides, toxic epidermal necrolysis, and Behçet's disease due to its immunomodulatory effects.

Q.38. What are the uses of tranexamic acid in dermatology.
Ans. Tranexamic acid is a plasminogen inhibitor with antifibrinolytic activity.

Its various uses in dermatology are:
- It is used mainly to control bleeding in congenital hemangiomas and telangiectasia.
- Oral-250 mg twice daily/topical/intralesional use in melasma and also used in nonhereditary, antihistamine unresponsive angioedema, or hereditary angioedema.

Q.39. What are retinoic acid metabolism blocking agents (RAMBAs)?
Ans. These are the compounds that block the catabolism of endogenous vitamin A, called RAMBAs. These drugs have less side effects. Also, there is a reduction of the post-treatment teratogenicity period due to their favorable pharmacokinetic profile; few examples are rambazole and liarozole.

Q.40. Define ointment, gel, lotion, and cream.
Ans.
- *Ointment:* It is oil based, homogeneous, semisolid preparation with high viscosity, which is applied over skin.
- *Gel:* It is semisolid emulsion in alcohol base and is thicker than solution.
- *Lotion:* It is similar to solution but thicker and tend to be more emollient in nature than solution and is usually oil mixed with water.
- *Cream*: It is emulsion of oil and water in approximately equal proportions.

Q.41. Define Phadiatop test.
Ans. Phadiatop test is a commercially available qualitative serological test employed for screening of allergic sensitization in patients with suspected allergic diseases.
- It is used to differentiate between atopic and nonatopic patients.
- It uses an immunoCAP with mixture of representative allergens including grasses, weeds, cat, dog, mites, and molds.

Q.42. What is diaper dermatitis?
Ans. The term napkin dermatitis implies an inflammatory eruption of the napkin area. Such an eruption may have many causes.
- Maceration by water
- Friction
- Urine
- Antibiotics
- Diarrhea
- Developmental anomalies of the urinary tract

Clinical features: Primary irritant diaper dermatitis typically occurs between the 3 and 12 weeks of life. It is characterized by widespread redness on the convex surfaces of the buttocks, genitalia, lower abdomen, pubic area, and upper thighs, while the deeper groin folds are usually unaffected.

In some infants, the rash is limited, more or less confined to the margins of the napkin area (tidemark dermatitis) and often due to friction from the diaper's edges or prolonged contact with the impermeable material of napkin. In acute cases, the redness may appear shiny, and the skin may peel in large sheets. In long standing cases, fine scaling is more commonly present. Postinflammatory hypopigmentation may be a striking feature in racially pigmented infants.

Q.43. What is Jacquet's dermatitis?
Ans. Jacquet's dermatitis is a rare, severe form of irritant contact diaper dermatitis. It is characterized by punched-out erosions or ulcerations with crater-like borders and is typically associated with frequent liquid stools, poor hygiene, infrequent diaper changes, or occlusive plastic diapers. It is more common in children with chronic diarrhea or incontinence, such as those with spina bifida or Hirschsprung disease.

Q.44. What are acne vaccines?
Ans.
- A component vaccine targets *Propionibacterium acnes* surface sialidase
- Heat inactivated whole bacteria vaccine—reduce *P. acnes*-induced inflammation in vivo.

Q.45. What are the indications of nailfold capillaroscopy (NFC)?

Ans. Nailfold capillaroscopy is an affordable, noninvasive technique used to examine the microcirculation at the nailfold.

Key indications for capillaroscopy include:
- Assessing patients with Raynaud's phenomenon
- Monitoring the progression from primary to secondary Raynaud's phenomenon
- Early detection of SSc
- Differentiating between SSc-related conditions, such as localized SSc and eosinophilic fasciitis, which typically show normal capillaroscopic patterns
- Identifying severe microangiopathy and assessing prognosis in SSc
- Monitoring treatment response and disease activity in dermatomyositis
- Evaluating SLE

Method to perform NFC:
- The patient must remain in an acclimatized room for 15–20 minutes with its temperature around 20–22°C.
- A drop of immersion oil is placed on the cuticle of the fingers for better visualization of the capillaries.
- The distal row of capillary loops extends into the dermal papillae, offering a longitudinal view of its three segments (afferent, efferent, and transition), arranged parallel to the skin surface.

The following parameters are typically assessed during capillaroscopy:
- The number of capillary loops per millimeter
- The presence of dilated capillaries, including those with ectasia or megacapillaries
- Signs of devascularization, along with microhemorrhages and capillaries that are tortuous, meandering, or branched
- Devascularization can be evaluated either by counting the loops per millimeter or by using a devascularization score ranging from 0 to 3, where 0 indicates no devascularization and 3 represents extensive areas of avascularity.

Q.46. Name histopathologic types of seborrheic keratosis.

Ans. Histopathologic types of seborrheic keratosis are as follows:
- *Acanthotic:* One of the most common type, in this type, epidermis is broad and composed of basaloid cells. The base of the lesion demonstrates a "flat bottom".
- *Hyperkeratotic (papillomatous):* Epidermis shows a papillomatous, "church spire" proliferation.
- *Adenoidal (reticulated):* The epithelium is elongated and reticulated with moderate-to-prominent pigment deposition.
- *Clonal:* It shows nesting pattern. Within the epidermis are "clones" of basaloid epidermal cells surrounded by normal keratinocytes termed as Borst–Jadassohn phenomenon.
- *Irritated (inflamed):* Earlier-mentioned variants with squamous eddies, i.e., exocytosis, apoptosis, acantholysis, scale-crust formation, spongiosis, and trichilemmal keratinization
- *Miscellaneous:* Desmoplastic and psoriasiform

Q.47. Explain iPLEDGE.

Ans. The iPLEDGE program is a computer-based drug safety program designed to further public health goal to eliminate fetal exposure to isotretinoin through a special restricted distribution approved by the FDA. The program strives to ensure that:
- No female patient starts isotretinoin therapy if pregnant.
- No female patient on isotretinoin therapy becomes pregnant.

The iPLEDGE program requires registration of all wholesalers distributing isotretinoin, all healthcare professionals prescribing isotretinoin, all pharmacies dispensing isotretinoin, and all male and female patients who have been prescribed isotretinoin.

Q.48. Desmoglein (Dsg) and hair—what do you know?

Ans. In stratified squamous epithelia like the epidermis, desmogleins are typically expressed in a manner that is specific to the differentiation stage of the cells. Similarly, the hair follicle is organized into a hierarchy of cell types based on their degree of differentiation. Undifferentiated stem cells in the bulge region are capable of producing epidermal cells, sebaceous gland cells, and hair bulb matrix cells. These matrix cells then differentiate into at least six distinct cell types, which undergo keratinization as they move upward through the hair shaft and inner root sheath **(Table 2)**.

TABLE 2: Location of different types of desmogleins (Dsg) in various parts of hair follicle.

	Dsg1	Dsg2	Dsg3
Bulge	–	+++	+
Basal cells of outer root sheath (ORS), below bulge	–	++ to +++	+/–
Matrix	–	++	+/–
Suprabasal cells of ORS, from suprabulbar to bulge region	– to ++	++ to –	+++ to ++
Basal cells of interfollicular epidermis and infundibulum		+	++
Trichocytes (precortical cells)		+	+
Suprabasal cells of ORS at isthmus, from lower to upper isthmus	++++	+ to –	+++ to –
Medulla	+	–	+++
Suprabasal cells of epidermis	+++	–	+/–
Inner root sheath (IRS)	+++	–	–

Q.49. Name the syndromes associated with lentigines.

Ans. Syndromes associated with lentigines are as follows:
- Xeroderma pigmentosum
- LEOPARD [Lentigines (dark-brown skin spots similar to freckles), ECG conduction abnormalities, ocular hypertelorism (widely spaced eyes), pulmonary stenosis (a narrowing of the pulmonary wave), abnormal genitalia, retardation of growth leading to short stature, and deafness of hearing loss owing to inner ear defects]
- Peutz–Jeghers
- Laugier–Hunziker
- Carney complex—nevi, atrial myxoma, myxoid neurofibroma, ephelides (NAME) + lentigines, atrial myxoma, mucocutaneous myxoma, blue nevi (LAMB)

Index

Page numbers followed by *b* refer to box, *f* refer to figure, *fc* refer to flowchart and *t* refer to table.

A

Acantholytic cells 6*f*, 226*f*
Accelerated nodulosis 259
Acne vaccines 265
Acquired cutis laxa, causes of 261
Actinic prurigo 260
Actinomycetomas, modified two-step treatment for 216*t*
Activated partial thromboplastin time 44
Adalimumab 193
Adenosine monophosphate 163
Aicardi Groutières syndrome 50
Alefacept 167
Alopecia areata 237*f*
Aminoimidazole-4-carboxamide-1-beta-D-ribofuranoside 163
Aminolevulinic acid 129, 129*t*
Angiotensin-converting enzyme 54
Antibiotics drugs, order of 212*t*
Antibody 72
Anti-CD20 antibodies, newer 20
Antigen-presenting cells 25, 26
Antihistamines 205
 classification of 206*t*
 first-generation 208*f*
 second-generation 207, 208*t*, 208
Anti-inflammatory 157
 properties 164
Antinuclear antibody 58*t*, 72, 72*f*, 75, 148, 192
 negative lupus 56
 relevance of 57
 titers
  clinical significance 57*t*
  correlation of 57*t*
  relevance of 57
Antiphospholipid antibody 44
Antiproliferative 157
Anti-Scl-70 antibody 74
Antistreptolysin O 148
Antisynthetase syndrome 95
Apoptosis 14
Asboe-Hansen sign 255
Atopic dermatitis 158, 168, 203
 newer neurokinin-1 inhibitors for 204
 pathway inhibitors for 203, 204
 small molecules inhibitors for 203*t*, 203
 topical phosphodiesterase-4 inhibitors for 203
Auditory canal, external 139
Auspitz sign 254
Autoantibody 99
Autofluorescence 243*f*
Autoimmune blistering disease 11
 sites of predilection in different 7
Autoimmune bullous disorders 158, 255
Autoimmune connective tissue disease 57, 57*t*, 58*t*, 72, 72*f*, 75, 176
Autoimmune disorders 63*fc*
 evaluate pregnant women with 63
Autoimmune vesiculobullous diseases 9*t*, 12, 12*t*
 based on clinical features 9
 treatment of 15, 15*t*, 19*t*
 target antigens 14, 14*t*
Autoimmune vesiculobullous disorders 3, 8
 significance of age 6
Azathioprine 157, 159
 off-label indications for 158

B

Bacillus Calmette-Guérin 91
Bacterial isolates 211*t*
Bamboo hair 239*f*
Basal metabolic rate 27
Bazin's hydroa vacciniforme 260
Bees, swarm of 228*f*
Beta-cell function 263
Biological agents 166
Biologics 192
 adverse effects 195
 for atopic dermatitis 203*t*
 for dose escalation 194
 in psoriasis 191-194, 196
  dosing schedule 193*t*
 kind of 197
 minimal response criteria with psoriasis 193
 monitoring guidelines 192
 newer 193
 side effects of 196*t*
Black box warning 258
Blister, management of 16
Blister spread sign 255
Blood pressure 144
Blood test 124
Blueberry muffin baby 260
Bohan and Peter classification 90*t*
Branched septate hyphae 224*f*
Brocq's phenomenon 259
Buccal mucosa, bilateral 6*f*
Bull's eye lesion 31
Bullous fixed drug eruption 29
Bullous pemphigoid 8, 9, 12, 12*f*, 168, 227*f*
 tense blisters on erythematous skin 9*f*
 variants of 11

Bullous pyoderma gangrenosum 135, 146, 151
   histopathology of 150*f*
Burning 7
   micturition 7

C

Calcinosis 72
Calcinosis cutis 78, 93*f*
   types of 259
Capillary
   architecture, well-preserved 240*f*
      budding 242*f*
      dropouts 241*f*
      meandering 241*f*
Carbamazepine 25
Carbol fuchsi 231*f*
Carcinogenesis 161, 177
Cardiovascular system 67
Cat tongue sign 49
Central nervous system 72, 196
   lupus flare 63, 63*t*
   significance of
Cervicitis 252
Cetirizine 207
Chancre, primary 249*f*
Chancroid 249*f*
Chandroidal ulcer 249*f*
Chest expansion, normal 259
Chest X-ray 55, 142
Chicago sky-blue stain 225*f*
Chlamydia 28
Cicatricial pemphigoid 175
Circles, pattern of 235
Clods, pattern of 235
Clue cells 252*f*
Coast of California 258
Coast of Maine 258
Coccobacilli 252*f*
Complete blood count 19, 99
Computed tomography 142
   high-resolution 99
Concealed pyrexia 110
Connective tissue diseases 65, 254
Coral red florescence 244*f*
Coronavirus disease 2019 88
Corticosteroids, role of 145
Cranial radiation therapy 34
C-reactive protein 55

Cream 265
Crest syndrome, clinical features in 78
Cribriform scarring 149*f*
Crushed smear 250*f*
Culture and sensitivity pattern 211
Cyclophosphamide 174
   levels 178
      raise 178
   pulse in pemphigus 19
Cyclosporine 166, 178
Cytoplasmic antineutrophil cytoplasmic antibody 148
Cytotoxic 157
   agents 178
Cytotoxic T lymphocytes 26

D

Dapsone hypersensitivity syndrome 36
Dark ground microscopy 249
   principles of 251*f*
Dead sea in dermatology 257
Deck-chair sign 255
Deformities, risk factors for development of 119
Denileukin diftitox 132
Dense dermal infiltrate 123*f*
Deoxyribonucleic acid 19, 54, 60
Dermal papillae, tips of 13*f*
Dermatitis herpetiformis 9, 12, 13*f*
Dermatology
   antibiotics in 210
   bedside tests in 221
   immunosuppressants in 157
   life quality index 192
   nosocomial infections in 214
   signs in 254
   systemic drugs in 157*t*
   use of
      statins in 264
      tranexamic acid in 264
Dermatomyositis 58, 65, 77, 88, 90, 90*t*, 96*t*, 97, 98, 158, 167, 241, 255
   adult 96, 96*t*
   autoantibodies 99, 99*t*
   Bohan and Peter classification for 90
   childhood 167

cutaneous
   classical signs of 92
   diagnostic criteria for 91
   lesions of 100
   major criteria for 91*b*
   manifestations of 92*t*
   minor criteria for 92*b*
   uncommon presentations of 93
diagnosis of 98, 98*t*
etiopathogenesis of 91, 91*t*
evaluation of 98*t*
first-line systemic therapy for 100
investigate 98
juvenile 96, 96*t*, 97*f*
management of 100, 101
principles of management of 100
rash of 97*t*
role of rituximab in treatment of 101
sine myositis 91
systemic 96
with malignancies 96
Dermatoscopy, principle of 233*f*
Dermatosis, benign 107*b*
Dermographism
   black 257
   red 257
Dermoscopy 231
   patterns of 234
Desloratadine 207
Desmogleins 267
   types of 267*t*
Dexamethasone-cyclophosphamide pulse therapy 18
Diabetics 18
Diaper dermatitis 265
Diascopy 230
   test 232*f*
Direct Coombs test 55
Direct immunofluorescence
   false-positive 13
   histopathology 12*t*
Discoid lupus erythematosus 49*f*, 52*f*, 59, 60, 238*f*
   lesion of 48, 49
   predictors of systemic disease 62
   risk of progression 49

Disseminated gonococcal infection 251*f*
Dots, pattern of
Drug hypersensitivity syndrome 34
Drug rash with eosinophilia and systemic symptoms
  common drugs implicated in 36
  criteria for 28*t*
  pathogenesis of 36
Drug reactions 22
  severe cutaneous 24
Dupilumab 201, 202
  adverse effects of 202
  contraindications 202
  indications of 202
  mechanism of action of 201

E

Edema 109
Efgartigimod 20
Electrocardiogram 55
Electroporation 174
Emergency room, severe cutaneous adverse reactions in 37
Endocrinopathy 77
Eosinophilia 28
Eosinophils, abundant 227*f*
Epidermal necrolysis, drug causality for 34
Epidermal ulceration 150*f*
Epidermotropism 123*f*
Erosions, multiple 6*f*
Erythema
  degree of 123*f*
  diffuse 9*f*
  heliotrope rash 89*f*
Erythema multiforme 30*t*, 32, 32*t*
  major 29
Erythema nodosum leprosum 116*f*, 117
  classify 118
  necroticans 116*f*
Erythematous 39*f*, 51*f*
  base, multiple erosions with 5*f*
  papules, multiple discrete 45*f*
  plaques, multiple 122*f*
  scaly annular polycyclic plaques 47*f*
  scaly plaque 48*f*

Erythrasma, coral red fluroscence in 244*f*
Erythrocyte sedimentation rate 55
Erythroderma 102, 107, 111, 212, 255
  complications of 110
  developing 103
  drug-induced 108*t*
  frequency, adult-onset 103*b*
  in children 105
  proteins and scales lost in 109
  treat 108
Esophageal dysfunction 72
Etanercept 166, 193
European Alliance of Associations for Rheumatology 60
European League Against Rheumatism criteria 73
European Organization for Research and Treatment of Cancer classification 127*t*
Extracorporeal photochemotherapy 130, 131
  indications of 130
  mechanism of action of 130
  side effects of 131
Extracorporeal photopheresis 125
Eye, right 140*f*

F

Face
  and neck, diffuse pigmentation on 69*f*
  heliotrope rash 89*f*
Fatigue, significance of 51
Female pattern hair loss 236*f*
Fexofenadine 207
Finger tips, stellate scars on 70*f*
Flagellate dermatitis 94*f*
Focal proliferative lupus nephritis 56
Folate supplementation 172
Folylpolyglutamate synthase 163
Froment's sign 256
Fungal microscopy, diagnostic steps in 223*b*

G

Gastric antral vascular ectasia 87
Gastrointestinal system 67

Gel 265
Generalized exanthematous pustulosis, acute 29, 29*f*
  clinical features of 36
  common drugs causing 37
  differential diagnoses of 37
Generalized tonic-clonic seizure 44
Genital ulcer disease 248
Giant capillaries 240*f*
Giemsa stain 226*f*, 228*f*, 250*f*
Gilliam and Sontheimer classification 45, 46*fc*
Glucose transporter-1 137
Gottron papules
Gottron sign 93*f*
Gottron's papules 90*f*
Graft of normal skin 87
Gram's stain 248
Gram-negative intracellular diplococci 249*f*
Gram-positive cocci 223*f*
  chains 222*f*
  clusters 222*f*
Gram-stain 221, 223*f*
  chemicals for 222*f*
  staining materials 222*f*
Granulocyte-colony stimulating factor 151
Granuloma inguinale 250*f*
Günther's disease 244*f*
Guselkumab 193

H

H1 antihistamines 205
H2 antihistamines 208
Hailey-Hailey disease 227*f*
Hair follicle, parts of 267*t*
Hair pull test 245, 246*f*
Hair shaft
  diameter diversity 236*f*
  telescopes 239*f*
Heart failure, congestive 196
Heart rate 144
Hemangiomas 140*f*
  multiple 141, 142*f*
  novel treatment modalities 145
Hematological adverse drug reactions 162*t*
Hematopoietic 169

Hemorrhagic
  crusting 136f
  cystitis and bladder cancer 176
  spots 242f
Hepatic toxicity 170
Hepatitis A 28
Hepatitis B 28
  surface antigen 148
Hepatitis C 28
Hepatotoxicity 161
Herpes iris of Bateman 31
Hidradenitis suppurativa,
  treatment of 196
Histone deacetylase inhibitors 125
Hoigné's syndrome 258
Holster sign 93f
Homeostatic model assessment 263
Human immunodeficiency 148
  virus 22, 192
Human leukocyte antigen 22, 25, 26
Hyalinized cytoplasm 226f
Hydroa aestivale 260, 260t
Hydroa vacciniforme 260, 260t
Hyperlipidemia 182
Hypersensitivity 160
Hypertension 181
Hypopyon sign 255

I

Id reaction 258
Imatinib-induced drug reaction 28f
Immunoglobulin A 9, 12
Immunoglobulin G 9, 12, 13f
  granular deposits of 13f
Immunological domain 60
Immunosuppressant action 164
Immunosuppressive agents 178
Impetigo, clinical of 223f
Indirect Coombs test 55
Indirect immunofluorescence
  false-positive 13
  histopathology 12t
Indolent clinical behavior 127
Infantile hemangiomas 135-137, 137t, 138fc
  approach 138
  clinical guidelines for
    propranolol use in 144t

complications associated with 139, 139t
deforming face 140f
features of 139t
first-line therapy for 143
natural course of resolution of 139
risk factors for 137
role of laser therapy 146
syndromes associated with 140
theories of origin for 137
treatment modalities 143b
upper lip and right Ala nasi 140f
Infected cells, fusion of enlarged 227f
Infection, susceptibility to 161
Inflammatory skin diseases 158
Infliximab 167, 193
Inosine monophosphate 163
Insulin resistance 263
Interferon alpha 125
Interleukin 191
Interleukin-23 inhibitors, dosage 193t
Interstitial lung disease 67
  approved drug for 87
Intravenous immunoglobulin 101
iPLEDGE 266
Iris lesion 31
Isolated epithelial cells 226f
Itching 7
Itolizumab 193

J

Jacquet's dermatitis 265
Janus kinase 203, 204
Jet with contrail sign 235f
Job's syndrome 259

K

Keratinizing, dermoscopy colors of 234t
Keratinocyte 26, 91
Kikuchi–Fujimoto disease 51

L

LASERS, mode of action of 263
Lebrikizumab 202
  adverse effects of 202

Lentigines, syndromes associated with 267
Lepra reaction
  management of 118
  types of 117
Lepra reactions 112
Leprosy 256
  current situation in India 119
  disabilities, disability grading for 119
  national strategic plan for 120
  reaction 117
    classification of type-1 118t
    types of 117t, 118
  reconstructive surgeries for deformity 120
Lesions
  arcuate-shaped 122f
  close-up of 122f
  cutaneous 46
Leukocytes, ring of 226f
Levocetirizine 207
Licensed indications 158
Lichen
  planopilaris 237f
  planus 236f
Lip and tongue 39f
Lisch nodules 258
Liver 28
Liver function test 19, 55, 192
Loratadine 207
Lotion 265
LUMBAR syndrome 141f
Lung involvement, patterns of 67t
Lupoderma 86
Lupus band test 59, 59t
Lupus erythematosus 46, 47f, 158, 254
  acute cutaneous 46, 51f, 60
  cells 59
  cutaneous 45, 46fc
  drug-induced 54, 54t
  subacute cutaneous 47, 47f, 59, 60
    drug-induced 54t
  tumid 49
Lupus foot 63
Lupus hair 52
Lupus nephritis
  class of 55, 56
  clinicopathological correlations in 55t
  stages of 55

Lupus panniculitis 50*f*
  suspect 49
Lupus pernio 50
Lupus profundus 50
Lupus, subtypes of 59*t*
Lymph node biopsy 124
Lymphadenopathy 28
Lymphocytes, atypical 123*f*

M

Magnetic resonance imaging 142
Major histocompatibility complex
  class 210
Malar area, bilateral 47*f*
Malignancy 52
  highly radioactive 131
  risk of 96
  screening for 100
  secondary 172
  underlying 7
Malondialdehyde modified
  epitopes 72
Mast-cell stabilizers 209
Mechanic's hands 95
  and feet 95*f*
Meirowsky phenomenon 259
Melanocytic, dermoscopy colors
  of 234*t*
Membranous 55, 56
Metabolism and excretion 178
Methicillin-resistant
  Staphylococcus aureus 212
Methotrexate 162, 165, 166, 166*fc*,
  167, 169, 174
  efficacy 167
  in human immunodeficiency
    virus infected 169
  induced hepatic fibrosis, risk
    factors for 170
  induced pancytopenia, risk
    factors for 169
  mechanism of action of 163*fc*
  osteopathy 171
  potential drug interactions with
    172
  therapy, contraindications 173
  toxicity 39, 40
Methyl aminolevulinate 129, 129*t*
Microhemorrhages 240*f*
Microsporum canis 243*f*

Mineral oil preparation, steps of
  244
Mixed connective tissue disease
  57, 58
Mizolastine 208
Molecular structure 191
Monilethrix, uniform elliptical
  nodes 238*f*
Monoclonal plasma cell disorder
  77
Morphea 168
Motile trichomonads 252*f*
Motor examination 114
Moynahan's syndrome, features
  of 260
Mucosal examination 5
Mucous membrane pemphigoid
  175
Multinucleated giant cell 227*f*
Musculoskeletal 183
Musculoskeletal system 68
Mycobacterium leprae 230*f*
Mycoplasma 28
Mycosis fungoides 175
  histopathological of 128
  nodular stage of 128
  poor prognostic factors for 128
  role of radiotherapy in 131
  TNMB staging of 127, 127*t*
  types of 132
Myelodysplastic syndromes 151
Myeloid leukemia, acute 151
Myelosuppression, monitoring for
  162
Myelotoxicity 161
Myoclonic 44

N

Nailfold capillaroscopy 239
  indications of 266
  normal 240*f*
Nausea 160
Neodymium-doped Yttrium
  Aluminum Garnet 143
Neonatal lupus erythematosus,
  evaluate 48
Nerve 114
  examination 114, 114*t*
Neurokinin-1 203
Neurologic 182

Neutrophilic dermatoses 176
Neutrophils, numerous 228*f*
Nevus depigmentosus 232*f*
Nikolsky's sign 15, 255
  types of 9
Noninvasive tests 171
Nonlesional sun exposed 59
Nose 140*f*
Nuclear antigens, extractable 56

O

Ointment 265
Olopatadine 208
Omalizumab 197
  administered 197
  dosage of 197, 198
  injection of 198
  mechanism of action of 197
Oral cavity 140*f*
Oral lesions, diagnoses for 7
Oral pathergy 247*f*
Organism, type of 212
Organized capillaries, irregularly
  241*f*
Organomegaly 77
Ovoid palatal patch 94*f*

P

Pain in throat 7
Palmoplantar pits, causes of 262
Palms hemorrhagic cheilitis 51*f*
Paraneoplastic pemphigus 9, 12
  malignancies in 8
  respiratory system examination
    8
Parker's ink preparation 224*f*
Pathergy 247
Pathergy test 247
Pautrier's microabscess 128
Pavithran nose sign 256
Peak plasma concentration 206
Pemphigoid, variants of 11
Pemphigus 8, 175, 212
  classify 10
  end points of therapy 15
  foliaceus 9, 9*f*, 12
  in pregnancy, management of
    20
  in ward 21

prognostic factors in 21
role of intravenous
   immunoglobulin 20
treatment of 15
type of 7
Pemphigus vulgaris 3, 9, 12, 12f,
   13f, 15
causes of death in 21
corticosteroids 16
pathogenesis of 14
role of rituximab in 20
severity grading of 15t
Periorbital edema 97f
Peripheral extension of blister 15
Peripilar tubular casts 237f
Persistent light reactivity 260
Petechiae 232f
PHACES syndrome 141f
Phadiatop test 265
Phenytoin 34
Phosphodiesterase-4 203
Photochemotherapy
   indications of 131
   mechanism of action of 131
Photodynamic therapy 129
   indications of 129
   mechanism of action of 130
   side effects of 130
   topical agents used in 129
Photosensitivity 7, 51
Phototherapy 166, 166fc
Pityrialactone causing fluorescence
   243f
Pityriasis rubra pilaris 94f
Pityriasis versicolor 224f, 225
Plaques
   multiple 122f, 123f
   single 113f
Poikiloderma, extensor
   distribution 93f
Poikilodermatous rash over face
   97f
Polymyositis 58, 72, 90, 158
Polyneuropathy 77
Port-wine stain 232f
Postinflammatory
   hyperpigmentation 136f
Potassium hydroxide 224f
   mount 223b, 223
Pregnant women, evaluation of
   63fc
Premethotrexate, evaluation 173

Prescleroderma 86
Proliferative disorders 167
Proliferative lupus nephritis,
   diffuse 56
Prostate-specific antigen 99
Proteins via skin, loss of 8
Pseudohyphae 224f
Pseudo-Nikolsky sign 256
Pseudopods, pattern of 235f
Pseudoporphyria 261
Pseudoscleroderma 79
Psoralen 125
Psoriasis 159, 179, 254
   area and severity index 192
   combination therapy in 165
   for biologic therapy 191, 191t
   indications of methotrexate
      therapy 164
   phosphodiesterase 4 inhibitor
      approved for 196
   red dots and scaling 235f
   small-molecule inhibitors for
      196
   treatment, biologics used for 191
   tyrosine kinase 2 inhibitor for
      196
Psoriatic erythroderma 102
Psychiatric reaction,
   corticosteroid-induced 63, 63t
Pteridine causing fluorescence
   243f
Pterygium inversum unguis 76
Pulmonary artery hypertension
   67
Pulmonary function test 99
Pulmonary hypertension, classify
   84
Pulmonary toxicity 171
Pulse therapy 16
Purpura 232f
Pus 211
Pustular psoriasis 111
Pyoderma faciale 260
Pyoderma gangrenosum
   associated with 152
   classic ulcerative 150
   classical and bullous 151, 151t
   clinical variants 149
   investigate 151
   manage 153
   suspected of 152
   syndromes associated with 153

Q

Quantitative insulin sensitivity
   check index 263
Quinquaud's disease 259

R

R20 protocol 264
Radial arrangement
Radiological test 124
Ragged cuticles 95f, 242f
Rapid plasma reagin titers,
   significance of 258
Raynaud 76
Raynaud's phenomenon 72, 75
   causes of secondary 76, 77fc
   diagnosis of primary 75
   evaluation 75fc
   myocardial 85
Reaction
   mild and severe type 1 118
   relapse and late reversal 118
   type-1 117
Red blood cell 148
Reflecting salt-pepper
   hypopigmentation 123f
Refractile 224f
Renal function test 19, 55, 192
Repeated open application test
   259
Reproductive 177
Residence 6
Residual skin disease, bexarotene
   for 125
Respiratory system 67
Reticular pattern 235f
Reticulohistiocytosis, multicentric
   98
Retinoic acid metabolism blocking
   agents 264
Retinoids 166
Rheumatoid arthritis 191
Rheumatoid factor 72, 148
Rheumatoid nodules 259
Ribonucleic acid 72
Ribonucleic acid polymerase 72
Ribonucleoprotein 72
Risankizumab 193
Rising creatinine 181fc
Rituximab 187
   adverse effects 190

contraindications of 189
infusion
    injection of 190
    protocols for 188
    rate chart for 189t
injection of 188, 191
maintenance dose, infusion rate chart for 190t
mechanism of action of 187
use of 188
Rowell syndrome 50

S

S-adenosyl methionine 163
S-adenosylhomocysteine 163
Samitz's sign 95
Sampling technique 248, 253
Sarcoidosis
    cutaneous 168
    syndromes associated with 262
Satellite warts 260
Scabies 235f
Scabietic burrow 245f
Scales, types of 109
Scalpel 245f
Scalpel blade 245f
Scaly plaques 48f
Scarring alopecia 52f
Sclerodactyly 70f, 72
Scleroderma
    classify 76
    renal crisis, association with autoantibodies 87
    sine scleroderma 86
Sclerodermatous skin 87
Sclerosing 55, 56
Sclerosis, multiple 196
Seborrheic keratosis, types of 266
Secukinumab 193
Sensory examination 113
Sertoli rosettes 10
Sexually transmitted infections, tests for 248
Sézary cells 110, 129
    circulating 107b
    in blood, causes of 129
    stains used identify 129
    types of 110
Sézary syndrome, triad of 110
Shawl sign 90f
Shulman's disease 80
Shuster sign 49, 49f
Sjögren's syndrome 58
Skin 77
    directed therapy 125
    failure, acute 27fc, 109
        causes of 35
        consequences of 35
        long-term complications of 35, 35t
    layer in 234
    lesions, type of 30
Slit skin smear 230
Sneddon syndrome 51
Staphlyococcus species 222f
Stem cell transplantation 81
    allogeneic hematopoietic 126
Sterile pustules, differential diagnoses of 263
Steroid-sparing drugs
    dose 19t
    mechanism of action
    monitoring guidelines 19t
    side effects 19t
    used in autoimmune vesiculobullous diseases 19
Stevens–Johnson syndrome 25, 26f, 30t, 34b, 256
    development of 25b
    lesional skin in 36
    pathogenesis of 26f
        drug-induced 25f
Streptocytes 10
Subepidermal
    cleft 12f
    edema 150f
Super antigen 210f
Suprabasal cleft 12f
Swallowing, difficulty 7
Synovial sarcoma 72
Systemic chemotherapy 126
Systemic lupus erythematosus 42, 46, 46b, 51-53, 54t, 57-59, 72, 97, 167, 241
    alopecia in 52
    causes of death in 62
    clinical domains in 59t
    diagnosis of 59, 60t
    evaluation of 54
    mucosal lesions in 52, 53f
    nonspecific markers of 46
    pediatric and adult 62
    rash of 97t
    risk factors for 45
    risk of progression 49
    significance of fever 52
    systemic examination of 44t
    vascular manifestations of 54t
Systemic Lupus International Collaborating Clinics classification system 60
Systemic scleroderma, central nervous system changes 85
Systemic sclerosis 58, 65, 79, 87, 168, 254
    antibodies in 72t
    causes of death 86, 87
    cutaneous 72
    diagnosis of 79
    diffuse cutaneous 72
    diseases associated 85
    eye changes 78
    futuristic therapies 88
    in pregnancy, course of 85
    limited cutaneous 74t
    manage 81
    nervous system affected 78
    overlap 72
    peak age of onset of disease 87
    prognosis of 85
    progressive 57
    scoring system of 86
    systemic involvement in 67
    very early diagnosis of 87

T

Target antigen 14, 72
Target lesion, typical and atypical 31t
Targetoid 31
T-cell lymphoma, cutaneous 35, 74, 74t, 98, 103, 121, 130, 131
    classify 126
    monitor disease activity in 131
    photochemotherapy in 131
    role of chemotherapy in 132
    systemic therapies for 132
    treatment of 125t
T-cell receptor 25, 210
Telangiectasis 72
Teratogenicity 172

Thibierge–Weissenbach syndrome 76
Tildrakizumab 193
Tinea capitis 237f
Tinel sign 256
Tin-tack sign 49
Tofacitinib 199-201
   biologics for treatment of 199
   formulations 200
   method of administration 200
Total skin electron beam therapy 125
Toxic epidermal necrolysis 23f, 25b, 25f, 26f, 47f, 256
   lesional skin in 36
   severity-of-illness score 34
Toxicity 196
   acute 170
   long-term 161
   medium-term 161
   monitoring 162
   short-term 160
   treatment of 40
Toy Soldier sign 128
Tralokinumab 202
   adverse effects of 202
Treponema pallidum 251f
Trichophyton schoenleinii 243f
Trichorrhexis, invaginate 239f
Trichoscopy 236, 264
   normal scalp on 236f
Trichotillomania, hair shafts of 237f
Tuberculoid leprosy
   lesion, histology of borderline 115f
   with type-1 reaction 112
Tuberculosis 196
Tumor necrosis factor 54, 191
   alpha inhibitor agents 91, 192

Tzanck
   preparation 227f
   smear 10, 225, 228f
      modified 229

U

Ulcer
   and vesicles right leg and dorsum of foot 148f
   beefy red 250f
   healed 115f
   multiple 249f
   oral over hard palate 45f
   with slough 148f
Ulceration
   cutaneous 94f
   hemangioma
      management of 146, 146t
   pyoderma gangrenosum, classic 151b
   with hemorrhagic crusting 39f
Ultraviolet
   indications of 262
   radiation and skin cancer 161
Upper arm, heliotrope rash on 89f
Upper respiratory tract infection 196
Urethral discharge 248, 248f
Urine 211
Urticaria 32, 32t
   biologics for treatment of 199

V

V sign 90f
Vaginal
   discharge 252f
   epithelial cells 252
Vaginitis 251

Vancomycin-resistant *Staphylococcus aureus* 214
Vascular
   malformations 137, 137t
   swelling 136f
   tumors, dermoscopy colors of 234t
Vasculitis 53, 175
Vellus hair, proportion of 236f
Vessel vasculitis, medium 53f
Vision, difficulty 7
Vital sign monitoring guidelines 144t
Vitiligo collagen 243f

W

Wartenberg sign 256
Weight 59, 60
   loss, significance of 7, 52
Welsh regimen and modifications 214
Wet mount 252f
   preparation 251
Whiff test 225
Wickham's striae 236f, 246f
Windmill maneuver 79
WONG variant 94f
Wood's lamp 241
   apparatus 242f
   examination, technique of 243

Y

Yeast, budding 224f

Z

Ziehl–Neelsen stain 230f